AF654454

Tribal Health and Malnutrition

About the Author

Prof. R.K. Mutatkar, a student of Prof. S.C. Dube and Leela Dube at Saugar University, joined Pune University in 1960, at Deccan College Post-graduate and Research Institute, at the Department of Sociology and Anthropology, under Prof. Irawati Karve. He became the first Head of the University Department of Anthropology and subsequently, the first Director of the Inter-disciplinary School of Health Sciences.

He pioneered teaching of Medical Anthropology in India, and initiated social science research on Leprosy at WHO in 1981. He chaired the Curriculum Development Committee for Anthropology at the UGC to prepare a model syllabus in 2001. He was Chairman of the first working group of "AYUSH in Public Health" for the Eleventh Five Year Plan. He established "The Maharashtra Association of Anthropological Sciences, (MAAS)," in 1976 at Pune and was Chairman of the Indian National Confederation and Academy of Anthropologists (INCAA).

Society for Indian Medical Anthropology (SIMA) organised a conference in his honour at Mysore in 2007 and dedicated the book, "Explorations in Indian Medical Anthropology" (2 Vols.) published by Concept Publishing Company (P) Ltd., to him. His book, "AYUSH in Public Health" (2 Vols.), brought out by Concept Publishing Company (P) Ltd., was released by Hon. Governor of Maharashtra on 13 August, 2016. His research study, "Society and Leprosy" (1978), was published by Gandhi Memorial Leprosy Foundation, Wardha, of which he has been a Member-Secretary. His field study of a Gwalior village in 1958, "Caste Dimensions in a Village" has been restudied by the Anthropological Survey of India.

Prof. Mutatkar has been the recipient of "Adiwasi Sevak" award of the Government of Maharashtra. He is also Hon. Governor's expert nominee on the Tribes Advisory Council, Maharashtra. He was honoured with International Gandhi Award for Leprosy, on 30th January, 2016, World Leprosy Day, by Hon. Vice President of India, Shri Hamid Ansari, at New Delhi.

TRIBAL HEALTH AND MALNUTRITION

R.K. Mutatkar

Jointly Published for
Maharashtra Association of Anthropological Sciences (MAAS)
by
CONCEPT PUBLISHING COMPANY PVT. LTD.
NEW DELHI-110059

© Maharashtra Association of Anthropological Sciences (MAAS)

All rights reserved. No part of this work may be reproduced, stored, adapted, or transmitted in any form or by any means, electronic, mechanical, photocopying, micro-filming recording or otherwise, or translated in any language, without the prior written permission of the copyright owner and the publisher. The book is sold subject to the condition that it shall not, by way of trade or otherwise, be lent, resold, hired out, or otherwise circulated without the prior publisher's written consent in any form of binding or cover other than that in which it is published.

The views and opinions expressed in this book are author(s) own and the facts reported by him/her have been verified to the extent possible, and the publishers are not in anyway liable for the same.

ISBN-13: 978-93-86682-42-0

First Published 2018

Published and Printed by

Concept
Since 1974

Concept Publishing Company Pvt. Ltd.
A/15-16, Commercial Block, Mohan Garden,
New Delhi-110059 (INDIA)
T: 91 11 25351460, 91 11 25351794
E: publishing@conceptpub.com; *W*: www.conceptpub.com

Cataloging in Publication Data--Courtesy: D.K. Agencies (P) Ltd. <docinfo@dkagencies.com>

Mutatkar, R. K. (Ramchandra Keshav), 1936- author.
Tribal health and malnutrition / R.K. Mutatkar.
pages cm
Includes bibliographical references and index.
ISBN 9789386682420

1. Tribes--Health and hygiene--India--Maharashtra. 2. Tribes--Nutrition--India--Maharashtra. 3. Tribes--Medical care--Government policy--India--Maharashtra. 4. Malnutrition--India--Maharashtra. I. Maharashtra Association of Anthropological Sciences. II. Title.

LCC GN635.I4M88 2018 DDC 362.10890095479 23

Dedication

The book is dedicated to the memory of three eminent personalities who initiated and made significant contributions to health policy planning in India. Affectionate close interaction with them helped to sharpen my medical anthropological perspectives about health issues of the marginalized people of India.

1. Dr. C.G. Pandit, Padma Bhushan, First Director, ICMR

The evening sessions at his Pune residence during his post-retirement period, in the company of heads of health institutions across India were an academic feast to discuss national policy issues. Dr. Pandit gave inaugural address at the International Symposium on Medical Anthropology at University of Pune on 19 December, 1978.

2. Prof. P.V. Sukhatme, Padma Bhushan, Director, Statistics, FAO (Rome)

As a pioneer agricultural statistician, he initiated international debates on hunger, poverty and nutrition. During post-retirement period at Pune, he initiated a community kitchen with the hypothesis of poor helping the poor, i.e. poor women making cheap and nutritious food affordable to poor people. He promoted the establishment of Interdisciplinary School of Health Sciences at Pune University with me as the first Director. He was President of our academic NGO "Maharashtra Association of Anthropological Sciences" at the time of his demise on 28 January, 1997.

3. Dr. Rajanikant Arole, Padma Bhushan

Creator of Jamkhed model of community health, whereby marginalized village women provided primary health care to the people. The initiation of para-medic cadre such as CHV, Health guide, ASHA has been the direct contribution of Jamkhed model.

Dr. Arole has been the Co-Project Director with me of an intervention programme "Comprehensive and Sustainable Human Development of the Tribal People of Maharashtra" (Adivasi Utthan Karyakram) until his sad demise on 25 May, 2011. The project model to address issues of tribal malnutrition has been accepted by the Government of Maharashtra, branded as Bharat Ratna A.P.J. Abdul Kalam Amrit Ahar Yojana.

Preface

"The efforts of applied anthropologists to assist development projects have met with varying success. When anthropologists themselves play a central role in planning and carrying out projects, they can take socio-cultural factors into account at each step. But all too often, development workers proceed to introduce rapid change without cautiously evaluating possible repercussions, ignoring or misunderstanding anthropological principles.... Over the course of time, anthropologists have seen many communities and ecosystems disrupted by the impact of development, and so they remain skeptical of the notion of "progress". They recognize the inevitability of modernization but usually take the position that people should have a choice of modernizing or remaining traditional, fully informed of the relative costs, risks, and benefits of either course" (Ann McElroy and Patricia K. Townsend, 1985: 409).

I

This book discusses the perspectives about policy issues regarding distinctiveness of tribal health, development and malnutrition. Every year, there are media reports followed by PILs since 1993 (writ petition) in various High Courts about malnutrition deaths in tribal regions. The issue of tribal malnutrition is responded by the Government as a seasonal epidemic of a malady to be addressed by health care facilities to prevent deaths of children suffering from acute malnutrition. The Government in response, undertakes urgent actions, usually by way of feeding programmes and intensive care in the respective primary health centres, rural hospitals and upward referrals. In short, the relief measures are taken to tide over the immediate crisis of child mortality visible in the public domain. There is apparently no programme to design and implement a sustainable model to prevent tribal children develop acute malnutrition, threatening mortality.

This book addresses the issues of tribal health and malnutrition from the Emic and Etic perspective. As a student of anthropology, I have tried to study the indigenous knowledge, practices and institutions, as part of tribal culture to understand the ground reality. There are tribal healers who have good knowledge of medicinal plants in the vicinity and the *Dais* who have been providing obstetric care during pregnancy and child birth. In the Government Health Care Programme, no consideration is given to the existing indigenous knowledge and practices of the people about health and nutrition. Probably, the solution lies in upscaling the indigenous knowledge of the tribal people and complementing it with modern scientific knowledge. If the services of local healers with knowledge of medicinal herbs and services of trained *dais* are co-opted in health care, scenario could be more positive.

The book has provided several quotes, liberally, not by way of literature survey mandatory of Ph.D. style research, but to put together the similar ideas pronounced by peer academics from diverse disciplines. The quotes are meant to support the discussion about academic and field issues, based on the reflection and experiences of respective scholars. The observations and opinions expressed by national and international scholars is validated by field situation presented in the book.

In this book, an intervention programme about tribal malnutrition jointly planned and administered by two NGOs with peoples' involvement, and funded by the Government of Maharashtra has been presented in Chapter 5.

Neonatal and infant mortality have not been exclusively tribal problems, since these are also problems in urban slums whose residents have largely been migrants from rural areas. During British Rule in India, these were also issues among the upper middle classes and poor people in urban centres, as most of the deliveries were managed at homes. Gender discrimination and early marriage also contributed to neonatal mortality. As reported, up to 1931 Census, there has been no wide diversion between fertility and mortality. Currently tribal malnutrition is a major issue, pronounced as a "National Shame", by leaders of the country, despite special constitutional provisions and administrative arrangements about tribal development.

There is always a debate as to whether academics should themselves design, implement and monitor intervention programmes. Due to constant interaction with doctors, more often from the field of leprosy, there was a challenge to respond to their remarks as to why we social scientists were only evaluating their programmes and finding faults or advised them, but not get involved into the programme with them as partners. The challenging offer from Tribal Development Department, Government of Maharashtra jointly to Dr. R.S. Arole and me, to develop a model as "partners in development" to address issues of tribal child malnutrition had to be accepted as a national duty. The offer first made to 13 NGOs in Maharashtra working among the tribal communities zeroed down to two of us.

Dr. Arole who had initiated community health work in a rural area around Jamkhed with a hospital as the base for referral services, first expressed reticence about working in tribal areas across the State of Maharashtra. I had personal experience of field knowledge of all tribal areas in Maharashtra as an anthropologist, and also by virtue of serving on several government expert committees about pseudo-tribal issues. I had no experience of grassroots level tribal development work. When Dr. Arole asked me, "shall we take this big bite?" I said, "with your experience of community health and my knowledge of tribal communities, we should take this bite." So, we decided to get involved in intervention programme based on holistic and integrative, inter-sectoral approach of anthropology and also primary health care, as reflected in the title, "Comprehensive and Sustainable Human Development of the Tribal People of Maharashtra". I was looking forward to learn from this experience of direct intervention among the tribal communities, which I had studied all these years from classical anthropological perspectives. The intervention programmes evolved in response to demands of the people, suggestions and consultations of our colleagues in the field, and from the discussions in the joint monitoring committee meetings with the government.

The book is essentially intended to document the design,

process and outcome of joint intervention by two voluntary organisations, both wedded to the concept of comprehensive and sustainable paradigm of development. Attempts have been made to make it a peoples' programme, "by them, for them and of them" which could address their concerns effectively. In a way, Chapter 5 could also serve the purpose as a handbook for others to further innovate and evolve into a useful tool to be used by community based organizations, constructive programmeme organizations and academics interested in interventions or intervention research.

II

Christopher Columbus and such other sea voyagers from European countries, many of them heading towards India for its black spices such as black pepper and clove, navigated to the shores of North American Continent, identifying the land as that of India and the people they confronted as Indians. Indigenous people got branded as "Indians or Red Indians". Some of the voyagers, who became ill, were treated successfully by the 'Indian' medicine men with herbs. These examples are well documented, by the voyagers.

"During the bitter cold winter of 1535–36, the three ships of Jacques Cartier were frozen fast in the fathom – deep ice of the St. Lawrence River near the site of Montreal. .... Soon Scurvy was so rampant among them that by mid-March twenty five men had died and the others ..... were so ill that hope for their recovery was abandoned. .... Cartier had the good fortune to encounter once again the local Indian Chief, Domagaia, who had cured himself of the same disease with "the juice and sappe of a certain tree". The Indian women gathered branches of the magical tree "boiling the bark and leaves for a decoction, and placing the dregs upon the legs". All those so treated rapidly recovered their health, and the Frenchmen marvelled at the curative skill of the natives."

"These Indians had never heard of vitamin C, and there was no value in the external application of their remedy. .... More than 200 years, after Cartier's experience, James Lind a British Naval Surgeon having read of these incident, launched the experiments which proved the dietary basis of Scurvy."

"Logan Clendenin reports that the Cartier account was noticed by James Lind of Edinburgh (1716-94), a British Naval Surgeon whose experiments with Scurvy patients led to the conclusions that lemon juice was the best preventive" (Virgil J. Vogel, 1970: 3-4, 86).

In Anthropology, the knowledge and practices of medicine of tribal communities is referred to as Ethno-medicine, commonly referred as folk medicine. Ethno-botany has developed as a sub-discipline of Botany. The book "AYUSH in Public Health" in two volumes compiled as a result of field research in Himachal Pradesh, Madhya Pradesh, Chhattisgarh and Maharashtra, published by Concept Publishing Co. (P) Ltd., in 2016 documents such knowledge in the rural areas of these States. For Maharashtra, the examples are from tribal areas across the State.

The current book deals with health issues of tribal people in India, with field examples from Maharashtra. The basic philosophy and principles of life, which evolves culture through historical process would be similar, for all communities including the Indian tribal communities and "American Indians". The universals of Man-Environment, Man-Man, and Man-Supernatural relationships create distinctive cultures of respective communities. This has also been referred as Psychic Unity of Mankind by some anthropologists. The tribal communities living in isolation in the forest, hill tops in difficult terrain, on islands, not too much disturbed by the invaders in historical times, lived autonomous lives establishing symbiotic relationship with nature. Now, they are citizens of respective Nation-States. In India, the tribal communities are governed by the Constitution of India like all citizens of India. Even the Jarawas, Onges and Sentinilies in the Andaman Islands who continue to live food gathering and hunting life style are Indian citizens. The Constitution of India using the principle of Equity has bestowed some special rights to the tribal people through affirmative action. However, they are not in a position to enjoy these rights with self-confidence and in the spirit of self-help. That is the index of their backwardness. The aim is therefore to empower them to develop themselves as full-fledged citizens of India according to "their own genius" without losing social identity, self-confidence and self esteem and contribute to clean the polluted mainstream with their gender friendly ethical life styles and human values.

There are multiple stakeholders in addressing the issues of tribal health and development. Following the principle of single window administration, Tribal Development Departments were created with a budgetary outlay equivalent to the S.T. population in the State. However, the Department functions like a post office doling out grants to Line Departments without having any authority to monitor the expenditure towards Tribal Development. The schemes of tribal development are more in the nature of relief operations for the survival of the tribal people rather than towards their capacity building for sustainable development. In Maharashtra, Hon. Governor has bestowed 5 per cent of TSP funds to PESA villages as untied funds to be managed by the respective *Gram Sabha*. Its management has yet to be assessed. Implementation of Forest Rights Act meets with hurdles created by regulatory Forest Department who supposedly continue the functional legacy of British Raj in their *Khaki* uniforms.

The Rights approach referring to Right to Work, Right to Food, emanating from Right to Life as per Article 21 of the Constitution of India, Right to Information etc. leads the tribal issues at the door step of judiciary. It appears that we continue to govern either in the "revenue spirit" or welfare spirit of provider and beneficiary, rather than the application of the Rights Approach or Human Development Approach. We continue to address the Revenue Collectors who have been collecting land revenue (*Lagan*) since Akbar's time, about planning and implementation of development vision, in preference to Chief Executive Officers of *Zila Parishads*, which were created to devote wholly to the issues of rural development and transformation, through massive community development movement initiated on Gandhi Jayanti on October 2, 1952.

III

In the first Chapter on Introduction, there is discussion about the reasons for distinct treatment to tribal issues, not clubbing it with rural issues. Anthropology as a discipline happens to have specialized on tribal studies for unravelling the process of social and cultural evolution. As a result, Anthropologists are considered as subject experts on tribal issues. In the universities, fieldwork training in remote tribal pockets for anthropology students is mandatory. Students and teachers have to stay with the people, in their villages and observe their day-to-day lives, participating in the activities, as much as possible, to understand the emic perspectives, i.e. their mind and behaviour through their eyes. Since health issues are an aspect of integrated culture, there is discussion about the anthropological meaning of health and disease. Nutrition and diet are traditionally the response of the people to the environment in the walking distance, in the neighbourhood of the village. People have learnt to adapt to the environment. With plural medical systems there are diverse explanations about disease, health and nutrition, some of which have been standardized as Ayurved, Unani, Siddha and Naturopathy in the respective classical texts.

The first two Chapters in the book are discussing conceptual base about health, poverty and nutrition. Chapter 2 discusses the wider debates about Poverty and Malnourishment among the experts which forms the national policy for categorizing the people of India as poor and not-so-poor. Government has committed itself to subsidize food and other such amenities to the poor by reducing the prices at public facilities and offering special schemes of development. Below Poverty Line (BPL) and Above Poverty Line (APL) are the two categories in which all families have been classified. "*Antyodaya*" is another category for Particularly Vulnerable Tribal Groups (PVTG).

Third Chapter on Emic Perspectives narrates my field experiences in the tribal areas since 1963, which provided me with insights about tribal culture. The fieldwork was done in classical anthropological style by living with the people, what is referred to as "going native". These experiences have framed the mental make up to look at issues from people's perspectives. This offers leads in framing conceptual framework for planning and implementing interventions.

Fourth Chapter presents two case studies of health research in two tribe dominant districts in Maharashtra. Bharatiya Agro-Industries Foundation (BAIF), a large NGO established by a disciple of Mahatma Gandhi, Sri Manibhai Desai was scheduled to extend its livelihood, horticulture development programme called "Wadi project" to tribal areas in Maharashtra; after its success in Gujarat. A baseline survey was undertaken by Maharashtra Association of Anthropological Sciences with the help of Pune University students from Department of Anthropology and newly established Interdisciplinary School of Health Sciences to help the BAIF organization to plan its strategies and later use it for post-intervention evaluation. Another experience based study was commissioned by the Planning Board of the State Government to understand the insights about a tribe dominant newly created district Nandurbar, since it was ranked the lowest in Human Development Index in the State in the year 2002 and sustained the position in 2012.

The Fifth Chapter presents a challenge, as an opportunity, not limiting itself to help plan and evaluate government schemes about health, development and addressing malnourishment among tribal children, but to undertake intervention programme in the tribal areas across the State of Maharashtra, jointly by two NGOs. A combination of my anthropological approach, and experience of committed Doctor-couple, Dr. Rajanikant and Dr. Mabel Arole in community health work in rural areas, helped to evolve a model to reduce malnutrition amongst tribal children. Since, the project was financially supported by the Government of Maharashtra, as a joint programme of two NGOs, with a Marathi title, mentioned in the G.R. as "Adiwasi Utthan Karyakram" (AUK), and not funded by foreign agencies, the work has been open to public scrutiny on all counts. The model has to be largely replicable in the public sector and not remain as a stand-alone successful case study of best practices. The State Government has accepted some programmes developed by the twin NGOs for implementation, in all tribal regions of Maharashtra, as government schemes.

Based on these intervention experiences, recommendations have been made which could be followed by governments, Panchayati Raj Institutions (PRIs), community based organizations, voluntary organizations usually referred to as NGOs, and social science academic departments and inter-disciplinary schools. It is being advocated to undertake interventions or intervention research projects to do further fine tuning in consultation with the community, ideally making it a people-centric activity of micro-planning and implementation. The indigenous knowledge of the tribal communities and the traditional health workers such as *vaidus* and *dais* who have been serving the people for hundreds of years need to be incorporated in the health care programmes in the public sector. Their skills could be further enhanced for community management. Their capacities have been proved in developing Jamkhed model as also in the AUK model presented in Chapter 5.

Epilogue summarises the issues about special treatment to

tribal communities which are required due to historical and geographical factors. Their problems of health and nutrition are the result of blocking their access to traditional resources of livelihood. The administrative mechanism which is the legacy of regulatory British Raj pattern has to be logistically minimized to restore back the functional implementation of their traditional pattern of self-governance, bestowed by 73rd Amendment of the Constitution, symbolized by PESA and Forest Rights Act (FRA). The benefits of science and technology have to be made accessible to them through affirmative action. Towards this, capacity building of tribal youth and CBOs are to be given priority, which was tried under AUK. Constitutional provisions for promotion of their development do not get translated in action due to delay in making rules and regulations, virtually denying them their rights. They are not empowered enough to challenge such forces by organizing themselves, for want of leadership.

The academic community through educational institutions, from Ashram Schools to Universities, can contribute by way of training, orientation and research to help micro-planning. Anthropologists as knowledgeable scholars about tribal culture and society, need to identify tribal strengths to further empower them. The model developed by two NGOs who have experience of community health and looking at people's concerns through their perspectives, could be further evolved for addressing region and ethnic group specific issues.

We are confident that this book of Practicing Anthropology and Socio-cultural Epidemiology on Tribal Public Health trying to present experience of interventions in tribal health and malnutrition, will provide motivation and insights to those who want to undertake policy research about Tribal Poverty and Human Development. It is time to shed off the ghost of value neutrality as a legacy of colonial anthropology and intervene with people-centric programmes of development and capacity building, following the universal human values and fundamental rights of the people. Anthropologists as citizens of the nation have to perform their fundamental constitutional duty, as so-called experts on tribal issues, to help the stakeholders towards tribal development. Mahatma Gandhi's talisman about remembering the last man will always provide direction to plan the intervention programmes and intervention research.

This book is expected to give a message to academics in anthropological and epidemiological sciences including those dealing with nutrition and diet in plural systems of medicine (AYUSH). Those researchers who are engaged in micro-level field exercises to understand the emic perspectives, would enrich their knowledge further and provide insights to present new hypotheses and theories if they designed and implemented interventions themselves. The least they could do is to get linked with field NGOs engaged in advocacy and development of tribal people. We do not compromise our scientific objectivity by undertaking interventions in line with the Human Rights and Universal Values of Humanity.

It would be useful to redesign our academic curricula to inculcate this knowledge and approach to the students. The UGC model curriculum in Anthropology (2001) need to be revised to incorporate issues of Action Anthropology and intervention research. Ethnography of processes of change or focused ethnography is more significant than ethnography of Culture as if it was a static entity in time freeze. This is the way to develop anthropology as a professional discipline, with our strengths to understand the quality of life as perceived by the people and helping them to widen their choices.

Pune **R.K. Mutatkar**
15th September, 2017

Acknowledgements

The book discusses the tribal issues about health and development in the context of child malnutrition, presenting the field reality from tribal Maharashtra. Chapter 5 forms the bulk of the book documenting the process of interventions in all tribe dominant regions of Maharashtra. Chapter 4 presents the studies undertaken in the tribal districts in western and northern Maharashtra. The opportunities of such work has given experience to reflect on the work which could be undertaken by anthropologists and other social sciences like Sociology, Social Work, Political Science and Public Administration. It would be desirable and productive if the economists combine quantitative, secondary data, with some qualitative data collected by them from the field.

I had close association with BAIF and with Manibhai Desai personally. He asked me to do qualitative assessment of their first interventions of horticulture based *Wadi* project starting with five families at Vansda in Gujarat. Before launching a major development programme in the tribal areas of Thane (now Palghar) and Nashik, BAIF asked us to undertake baseline survey, the results of which are presented in Chapter 4. We fondly remember Dr. Manibhai Desai and express our gratitude to BAIF for providing us opportunities to understand the process of intervention work which proved useful while designing AUK.

Human Development Report prepared by the State Government of Maharashtra, 2002, ranked the tribal district of Nandurbar created in 1998, as the lowest, 35th district. Indira Gandhi Institute of Development Research (IGIDR), Reserve Bank of India, commissioned quick strategy studies about livelihood, health and education of the three lowest ranked districts according to HDI. I was asked to study health and education issues in Nandurbar district which are presented in Chapter 4. I am thankful to IGIDR to provide an opportunity to analyse the district as a unit while usually we anthropologists study single village.

The book primarily documenting the process and impact of interventions to reduce malnutrition of tribal children in Maharashtra is not an academic research document. Chapter 5 provides the evolution of the process of involving the community in intervention activities as an example of practicing anthropology and community health, as a model of tribal public health. The primary data was collected by the local youth and tribal citizens (volunteers) of respective villages and hamlets, trained to function as human resources to operationalise AUK. A demographer Dr. Anjali Radkar from Gokhale Institute of Politics and Economics (GIPE) took pains to cull out the cohorts from this data for impact analysis about reduction of malnutrition. The evaluation report is presented as an annexure of Chapter 5. We are grateful to her for undertaking this task. Dr. A. P. Kulkarni, formerly at the GIPE and his team, took up the analysis of baseline survey done by the local tribal youth. The salient findings have been presented as annexure. We express our gratitude to them. Dr. Kalpana Mutatkar, an obstetrician and gynaecologist by training, formally served as an honorary consultant for couple of years, but provided her inputs during the entire project period, by visiting all the field sites several times.

I had the good fortune of having worked with Dr. Arole as a Co-Programme Director, who initiated the community health and development approach in rural India. He gave me full freedom to implement AUK programme and offered guidance by participating in all meetings and workshops of coordinators and at government meetings. Unfortunately, he passed away on 25 May, 2011.

Prof. P.V. Sukhatme, a pioneer agriculture statistician had all his energy for helping the poor and a vision for making villages livable, to dissuade urban migration by the rural folk. Constant contact with him provided insights about identification of poor, which need to be a priority research agenda of the field anthropologists. He undertook interventions in sanitation and water in rural areas, to test his hypothesis about the relative roles of infections and nutrition in childhood morbidity. Chapter 2 on poverty and malnourishment is based on interaction with him. The book is dedicated to the memory of Prof. Sukhatme and Dr. Arole.

Another senior mentor, Shri Janardan Maharaj Valvi, a pioneer tribal educationist in Nandurbar from the hilly region of Dhadgaon-Akkalkua (our field centres), was respected by all politicians and the people. He was a great help for our work in the difficult area of Dhadgaon and Akkalkua. Our association since 1962 was cut short due to his sad demise on 16 August, 2012. We pay our respects to them.

We are happy to put on record our gratitude and appreciation of the government system which reposed its confidence in us by giving us a free hand to pilot-test and undertake mid-term corrections. The Tribal Development Department headed by a Cabinet Minister and a Minister of State; the bureaucracy headed by Principal Secretary, Tribal Commissioner and Additional Tribal Commissioners, down the line with Project Officers of Integrated Tribal Development Projects (ITDP) in the Scheduled Area, provided all help and advice in the field, as also in the joint monitoring committee meetings.

The community represented by the male and female tribal volunteers, tribal peer supervisors and local tribal coordinators responded to our transparent attempts in a learning mode in addressing their concerns. They experienced and enjoyed freedom of action at their level. We have learnt from this partnership with the government and the people, and have experienced a wider holistic perspective which is the soul of Anthropology.

Department of Tribal Development, Government of Maharashtra

We are grateful to the Hon'able Ministers of Tribal Develoment, Shri Madhukar Pichad, Shri Babanrao Pachpute, Shri Vijaykumar Gavit and Ministers of State, Shri Padmakar Valvi and Shri Rajendra Gavit for their personal interest in the Adiwasi Utthan Karyakram and occasional interaction during a period of nine years.

The initiatives and sympathetic monitoring by Principal Secretaries, Commissioners, Additional Commissioners, Joint Commissioners and Project Officers of Tribal Development made it possible for the Government-NGO partnership to develop a replicable model involving the tribal communities.

We are grateful to

Shri Ramesh Kumar, Shri B. Nagrale, Dr. P.S. Meena, Shri Suneel Porwal, Shri Uttam Khobragade, Dr. Rameshchandra Sagar, Shri Mukesh Khullar, Principal Secretary; Shri Rajesh Kumar, Shri Bhaskar Mundhe, Shri Thakur, Shri Parag Jain, Shri T.K. Bagul, Shri D.S. Rajurkar, Shri Sambhajirao Sarkunde, Tribal Commissioners; Shri S.B. Hingonekar, Shri Chandrakant Khade, Shri Suneel Limaye, Shri Shivaji Dudhwadkar, Shri Karvande, Shri K.T. Singh, Addl. Tribal Commissioners; Shri V.S. Patil, Shri Dashrath Panmand, Jt. Tribal Commissioners.

Maharashtra Association of Anthropological Sciences : AUK

We express our sincere gratitude to the AUK workers for their sincere contribution to people friendly interventions for sustainable results. It is not possible to thank all the field level volunteers who took the brunt of implementing the five year project for eight years. They exhibited their capacity building competence at Nashik confluence on 22 Novembers, 2012. The project coordinators at Pune and in the respective field stations, and the supporting administrative infrastructure functioned with great sincerety and commitment. We never had to face adverse remarks from government auditors since our administration and accounting was transparent. Credit also goes to Accounts personnel at the Tribal Commissioner's office who were very sympathetic and understanding, offering us advice in case of difficulties. All the accounts of supplementary food and meals to pregnant women were maintained by the tribal lady volunteers. We owe our rgards to them and their management acumen.

AUK Central Office: Pune

State Project Coordinators

Dr. Purshottam Agashe (2004-07), Dr. Laxmikant Nagapure (2004-05), Dr. Mukund Pande (2004-05), Shri Ganpat Pandit (2005-13), Dr. Shailesh Dalvi (2006-13).

Consultant

Dr. Kalpana Mutatkar (2007-09).

Asst. Project Coordinator

Shri Pravin Kasote (2006), Shri Balasaheb Bheke (2007-09), Dr. Sanjay Dakhore (2007-08).

Project Assistant

Ms. Suvarna Kareliya (2005-06), Shri Sushil Kahat (2007-11).

Admistration

Shri Prabhakar Tumkar, Accounts Assistant (2004-06), Shri Nandu Dighe, Office Assistant (2006-13), Ms. Aarti Pardeshi, Typist (2006-08), Shri J.J. Dange, Accountant (2007-13), Ms. Swati Dandare, Typist (2008-2013).

Driver

Shri Vilas Jadhav (2004-12), Shri Akil Saiyad (2004-09), Shri Sujit Ghule (2012-13).

Field Area Coordinators and Assistants (AUK)

Jawhar, District Thane: Shri Mushtaq Kotwal; Shri Umesh Sapkale, Shri Vishnu Bhore, Shri Ravindra Dhum.

Mokhada, District Thane: Shri Mushtaq Kotwal (Hon.), Shri Vilas Patil; Shri Suresh Jadhav, Vilas Pahu, Devram Dive, Sudhakar Zinjurde.

Karjat, District Rajgad: Shri Madhav Mathpati (Hon.); Murlidhar Patil; Somnath Waghmare, Rajendra Bhagat, Bhagwan Bhagat.

Akole, District Ahmadnagar: Ms. Ratna Kamble (Hon.); Vilas Patil (Hon.); Shri Sudhir Telore, Ganpat Khade.

Dhadgaon, Dist. Nandurbar: Shri Vitthal Kadam; Shri Rohidas Pawara; Mansingh Rahse.

Akkalkua, District Nandurbar: Shri Ganpat Vasave; Karansingh Padvi.

Dharni, District Amravati: Shri Naresh Panzade; Shri Omprakash Waghmare, Santosh Wyavahare.

Zarizamni, District Yavatmal: Shri Bharat Khandare; Ayya Aatram, Vasudeo Todsam, Ravindra Sidam.

Etapali, District Gadchiroli: Late Shri Khapne (Hon.); Shri Rakesh Durge; Shri Mahesh Donarkar, Somaji Pallo, Nandu Narote

Special gratitude : This book would not have been word processed for printing without the commitment of Shri Santosh Sidhankar. Smt. Sharvari Nisal, with an experience of computer processing of the two volumes of the book, "AYUSH in Public Health", published in 2016, by Concept Publishing Co. Pvt. Ltd., New Delhi, prepared this book for final printing. I am grateful to them for making their services available to me.

Contents

List of Abbreviations and Acronyms

ANM	Auxiliary Nurse Midwife
ASHA	Accredited Social Health Activist
AYUSH	Ayurved, Yoga & Naturopathy, Unani, Siddha, Homoeopathy
AUK	Adivasi Utthan Karyakram
ATSP	Additional Tribal Sub-Plan
AWW	Anganwadi Worker
APL	Above Poverty Line
BAIF	Bhartiya Agro-Industries Foundation
BPL	Below Poverty Line
BCC	Behavioural Change Communication
BAMS	Bachelor of Ayurvedic Medicine & Surgery
BDO	Block Development Officer
CRHP	Comprehensive Rural Health Project
CBO	Community-based Organization
CHV	Community Health Volunteer
CEO	Chief Executive Officer
EGS	Employment Guarantee Scheme
FAO	Food & Agricultural Organization
FRA	Forest Rights Act
GIPE	Gokhale Institute of Politics & Economics
GOM	Government of Maharashtra
GOI	Government of India
HC	Health Centres
ICMR	Indian Council of Medical Research

IEC	Information, Education, Communication
ISM	Indian Systems of Medicine
IIPS	International Institute of Population Sciences
IMR	Infant Mortality Rate
ILO	International Labour Organization
IGIDR	Indira Gandhi Institute of Development Research
ITI	Industrial Training Institute
ICDS	Integrated Child Development Services
IDSP	Integrated Disease Surveillance Programme
ITDP	Integrated Tribal Development Project
JSY	Janani Suraksha Yojana
KVIC	Khadi Village Industries Commission
LBW	Low Birth Weight
MBBS	Bachelor of Medicine & Bachelor of Surgery
MADA	Modified Area Development Approach
MNREGA	Mahatma Gandhi National Rural Employment Guarantee Act
MAAS	Maharashtra Association of Anthropological Sciences
MPW	Multi-purpose Worker
MMR	Maternal Mortality Rate
MDG	Millenium Development Goals
NABARD	National Bank for Agriculture & Rural Development
NRHM	National Rural Health Mission
NHM	National Health Mission
NGO	Non-Governmental Organization
NT	Nomadic Tribe
OBC	Other Backward Class
PIL	Public Interest Litigation
PHC	Primary Health Centre
PESA	Panchayat Raj Extension to Scheduled Areas
PDS	Public Distribution System
PER	Protein Efficiency Ratio
PVTG	Particularly Vulnerable Tribal Group
PRI	Panchayati Raj Institution
RCH	Reproductive & Child Health
RUTF	Ready to Use Therapeutic Food
SHG	Self-Help Group
SEZ	Special Economic Zone
SC	Scheduled Caste
ST	Scheduled Tribe

TBA	Traditional Birth Attendant
TSP	Tribal Sub Plan
TDD	Tribal Development Department
TRTI	Tribal Research & Training Institute
UGC	University Grants Commission
VJ	Vimukta Jati
WHO	World Health Organization

List of Photographs

MAHARASHTRA ASSOCIATION OF ANTHROPOLOGICAL SCIENCES (MAAS)

MAAS as an academic voluntary organization was established at the University of Pune in 1976, with the active support of the Vice-Chancellor, Prin. Devdutta Dabholkar, as a platform to bring together academics, litterateurs, activists, administrators and political workers, to discuss issues around tribal development, health, environment, gender, culture and education in the anthropological holistic perspective. MAAS was Asian Partner of London School of Hygiene and Tropical Medicine for ten years to undertake operational research on TB and HIV Government of Maharashtra offered an intervention project on tribal malnutrition, covering all tribe dominant areas in the State to develop a doable model. Government of India bestowed a Centre : AYUSH in Public Health, to assess AYUSH under NRHM and undertake epidemiological research and training in Himachal Pradesh, Madhya Pradesh, Chhattisgarh and Maharashtra. MAAS is an accredited Research Centre under Savitribai Phule Pune University, and recognized as SIRO by DST, GOI.

Established by Prof. R.K. Mutatkar, MAAS had illustrious Presidents, such as, Prof. G.B. Sardar, prominent thinker, and President Marathi Sahitya Sammelan, Janardan Walvi, a Bhil educationist, Prof. P.V. Sukhatme, Padmabhushan, Director, FAO-Statistics, Prof. A.R. Kulkarni, Chairman, ICHR, Prof. R.K. Mutatkar, anthropologist, Prof. P.B. Vidyasagar, Vice-Chancellor, Swami Ramanand Tirth Marathwada University, Nanded. Current President is Prof. S. Parasuraman, Director, Tata Institute of Social Sciences (TISS), Mumbai.

Chapter 1
Introduction

Anthropology as a Science of Man in totality deals with biological and cultural evolution of "Man and His Works". To a common man, anthropology deals with the past and with the tribal people, their queer customs and dance forms. Anthropology was a compulsory subject at the Indian Civil Services examination, probably to understand peoples' traditions and customs, which could help good governance without hurting the people. British rulers were careful not to step on the hard aspects of culture and have another experience of the armed rebellion of 1857.

Since the discipline of anthropology with the basic concepts like Culture and Structural-Functional theory emerged out of the studies of "primitive people in isolated islands" or "American Indians", tribal communities continue to be the prime subject matter in the curricula of anthropology. Anthropologists are invited as experts about the issues concerning tribal identity in relation to constitutional provisions about Scheduled Tribes.

Although applied and action anthropology or practicing anthropology are not rated academically high, anthropologists in the West were hired during Second World War to advise the winning powers about relationship with the losing nations and their people. The author of the classic book "Mirror for Man", Clyde Kluckhohn, became a principal adviser to General Douglas MacArthur, "upon the problem of pacifying and democratizing the Japanese after Second World War". He was one of those who advised against "forced abdication of Emperor Hirohito, on the grounds" that this would be "unacceptable to the Japanese, who regarded the Emperor as a deity."

"It is just this sort of thing that makes anthropology relevant to the problems of modern life on a national and international scale in the important task of reconciling domestic conflict, as well as conflict between cultures. We are shown how knowledge of the past and of non-literate cultures can help us with the solutions to contemporary world problems, that indeed, anthropology has predictive power in the realm of politics, social attitudes, and above all in human relations of every sort" [Ashley Montagu in Foreword to *Mirror for Man by Kluckhohn*, pp. xvii-xviii, 1985 (first ed. 1949)]

In India, foreign anthropologists were invited as consultants while Community Development Programme for rural reconstruction was launched on October 2, 1952. Among the Indian anthropologists were Prof. S.C. Dube and Prof. D.N. Majumdar.

The tribal communities and tribal belts became a functioning part of the democratic set up in Indian Republic. Elected representatives of tribal people occupied formal positions in elected bodies from village to national level. Following the constitutional provisions, to facilitate tribal development, that is, full participation in the governance at all levels, Tribal Development Departments to implement Tribal Sub-Plan were constituted as Single Window for comprehensive development. Several tribal states have been formed, districts and talukas have been reformulated to facilitate autonomous self-governance. What is the scenario after 70 years of Independence?

On the one hand, the tribal areas have become accessible with transport and communication. In the social sector, there is tremendous growth and investment in primary and secondary education exclusively for tribals. The health care facilities available to caste villages, have reached tribal areas on a reduced population ratio per facility, although not functioning satisfactorily. PESA and Forest Rights Act have been legislated, although not implemented; lacking transparency, commitment and sincerity, on the part of continuing British pattern of bureaucracy, which has a revenue and forest regularity authority mind-set.

What we receive from the Media plate are the stories and statistics of malnutrition and mortality of tribal children, problems of food security and large scale seasonal migration for livelihood. Judiciary is on the side of the tribal people, entertaining PIL's on these issues and by way of *Suo Motu* injunctions asking the governments to report action.

The two NGOs, "Comprehensive Rural Health Project, Jamkhed (CRHP)" and "Maharashtra Association of Anthropological Sciences (MAAS), Pune" were jointly offered an intervention programme addressing these issues as reported in Chapter 5 of this book. Hon. High Court of Mumbai was duly informed about this AUK programme by the Government of Maharashtra and the NGOs were instructed to file the reports about activities to the government, for informing the Hon. High Court.

The issues about tribal situation in India regarding their increasing deprivation after Independence, despite the affirmative provisions in the Constitution of India, have been discussed in the successive committees appointed by the government, as also in academic journals, although not presented in scientific research journals.

The monthly journal "Seminar" has devoted its 661st issue of September 2014 to the symposium on "The Malnourished Tribal". Mr. Harsh Mander in his paper on "Unequal Destinies" has discussed the implications of colonial policy about forest rights.

"The greatest blow to their survival, and communal dignity, was the colonial policy of introducing state control over forests, thereby depriving them of traditional sources of nutrition and livelihood. As Amita Baviskar described in an essay in the World Bank report mentioned earlier, from "communal owners of the forest, they became encroachers, tenants and poachers." This policy remained unchanged even after independence: of all the government departments in independent India, the forest department mostly retains its colonial culture. No wonder Verrier Elwin famously recounted that paradise for a tribal person is miles and miles of forests with no forest guard. The forests became a major source of state revenues, and tribal people found themselves increasingly debarred from hunting and gathering in the forests, and from their traditional systems of shifting cultivation. Soon forests themselves dwindled. As they could no longer gather, hunt, or grow food from the past abundance of forests, hunger and penury were natural outcomes. (*Journal "Seminar"–"The Malnourished Tribal"* Journal No. 661, September 2014, pages 49 & 50, "Unequal destinies" by Harsh Mander).

Development and Poverty among the Tribals

"The critical determinant of tribal poverty is the expansion of state or state sponsored capitalism on the primitive social base during the colonial rule and intensification of the same in the post-Independence period. It appears that during the later period of colonial rule, the expansionist policy in outlying tribal areas had to be curbed because of compulsions of the political situation inside the country. .... Independent India, however, has different strategic, political and economic imperatives. It can more relentlessly pursue the unfinished task of creating a unified national market" (B.K. Roy Burman, p. 381).

"In the early nineteenth century the colonial rulers adopted a policy of massive exploitation of forest resources in the interest of state sponsored capitalist enterprises like railways, shipping and others. This reduced the areas on which the forest dwellers could depend on for their livelihood. At the same time, hardly any investment was made to augment production of housing materials, fuel wood, fodder and so on."

"This process was compounded by the policy adopted by the state in the matter of the preparation of record of rights. All lands which were not under current economic use by the individual tribal households were generally considered as state owned. .... In States such as West Bengal, Maharashtra and in parts of Gujarat, a good number have turned into landless labourers" [B.K. Roy Burman, in Tarlok Singh (ed.), 1990:382].

The First Review Committee of the Indian Council of Social Science Research in 1973 under the Chairmanship of Dr. Malcolm Adiseshiah with Prof. S.C. Dube, anthropologist as its member, had constituted a standing committee on Social and Cultural Anthropology under the Chairmanship of Prof. L.P. Vidyarthi. One of the recommendations about research priorities has been :

"In the field of applied anthropology, emphasis should be placed on the problems of the poorer sections of the community. In this context, the study of poverty—the concept of poverty, its socio-cultural determinants, levels of poverty, its manifestations and ways of banishing it—in the context of tribal culture and social structure should be given top priority" (*ICSSR*, 1973, vol. 2-38).

However, poverty and its health implications have never been taken as a research agenda by anthropologists. As tribal studies have been given up as a preserve of anthropology, poverty has been abandoned by other disciplines, to be addressed only in economics. What about tribal poverty and health?

Dr. N.P. Bhanage as Director, Tribal Research and Training Institute, Government of Maharashtra, Pune had published, in 1993, a book reviewing in an abridged version, the 25 reports of committees and commissions about tribal issues during 1947 and 1992. It is a matter of reflection that despite so many reports making useful recommendations, the tribal situation in India is projected as about hunger, malnutrition and child mortality.

Recently the report of the "High Level Committee on Socio-Economic, Health and Educational Status of Tribal Communities of India" (2014), under the Chairmanship of Prof. Virginius Xaxa available. The Committee has discussed among other issues, legal and administrative framework for Scheduled Tribes and Scheduled Areas, about disease patterns, traditional healers and *dais*; human resources for health and public health research.

The gender friendly sex-ratio among the tribal communities has been pointed out by the committee which has never been studied by the mainstream society which asks tribal people to join them.

"The tribal population has shown favourable sex-ratio as compared to other social groups in the country, with 990 females per 1000 males (Table 7.2). The sex-ratio of tribal population reflects nearly equal share of males and females as seen in Himachal Pradesh and West Bengal (each with 999/1000 males) or favourable to females as in Goa (1046 females), followed by Kerala (1035 females), Arunachal Pradesh (1032 females), Odisha (1029 females), Chhattisgarh (1020 females) Meghalaya (1013 females) and Maharashtra (977 females)". (Government of India, 2014: 193).

(*Ref*: Report of The High Level Committee on Socio-Economic, Health and Educational Status of Tribal Communities of India, Ministry of Tribal Affairs, Government of India May, 2014.)

In Maharashtra, a High Level Committee under the Chairmanship of Sri Vijay Kelkar was constituted to address the issues of regional imbalances among the geographical regions, which constituted Maharashtra. Apart from geographical regions, the Committee considered all tribal areas as one region, and has analysed the issues such as cultural deprivation, health care, land alienation, education, deprivation of forest and water rights. The administrative and governance issues such as the Tribal Sub-Plan and PESA have also been addressed. A separate Tribal Health Plan has been recommended. It has been observed that according to

YASHADA, a Government Institution for Development Administration based at Pune, among the 356 Talukas in Maharashtra, the bottom 15 are all tribal majority talukas. Nandurbar and Gadchiroli districts continue to be at the lowest order in HDI among the 35 districts (Kelkar Committee : October 2013).

Adivasi and Scheduled Tribe (ST)

ST is a constitutional term. The President and subsequently the Parliament was to notify the tribal groups or parts thereof, as Scheduled Tribe for the purpose of the Constitution. Many caste groups or non-tribals claim ST Status. Tribal people are believed to be living in geographical isolation for a long time, have been basically the collectors of food, using simple technology and not yet drawn into the market economy. Traditionally, they have been self-governing people, not having interaction with the outside world. They have their own deities and dialects which have no script. However, there is no agreed definition of the term Tribe, nor a national tribal policy approved by the Parliament. The generic term *Adivasi*, probably coined by Thakkar Bapa, was accepted by Mahatma Gandhi as one of his constructive programme.

Caste and Schedule Caste (SC)

Indian society is organized as per *varna* and caste hierarchy. Traditionally, castes are endogamous groups having a traditional occupation. Agriculture is the main and open occupation. SC refers to the fifth *varna*, out of four-fold *varna* hierarchy and hence called *pancham* (fifth), who suffered from the stigma of untouchability. Caste-peasantry village is a part society linked through social organisation and market economy with other parts of the country. The *Adivasi* have a very limited geographical spread and range of marital ties usually not going beyond 20 km. radius. As a result, there is vast difference between the vision of SC and ST.

Although, SC and ST are put together as constitutional categories, their concerns and issues are totally different. Academically, while anthropologists have been studying tribal communities, sociologists have been studying Caste and Scheduled Castes. Persons or groups who want to get the benefit of constitutional benefits of reservation, claim ST status but not SC status. The most sought after and relatively easy status to claim is that of nomadic community or OBC.

Role of Voluntary Organization (VO) in Tribal Development

The workers of VO have to function as facilitators between Government Agencies and the Community by building bridges with the elected representatives of the people and CBOs. CBOs have to be created, if necessary. The volunteers/social workers from the community have to be oriented to play the role of change agents and development functionaries who are accountable to the people and also to the VOs.

In the tribal areas, the most common activity of VO has been to run a school or an *Ashram* School, for which major funding has been available from the Tribal Development Department. In Maharashtra, of about 1000 *ashram* schools, half are run by the voluntary organizations, with government funding.

It is probably for the first time that the Government of Maharashtra offered partnership relationship with the government, jointly to two voluntary organizations, CRHP and MAAS, to address primarily the issues of malnutrition amongst tribal children across the state and gave freedom to devise the plans for implementation. What has evolved is a replicable model implementable in the government system, by involving the community in management.

A. ANTHROPOLOGY AND TRIBAL COMMUNITIES

It is common knowledge that Anthropology as a discipline developed out of the documentation of other people's culture, usually by voyagers and navigators. With the hypothesis about the biological evolution of *Homo Sapien,* there was curiosity to unravel the processes of cultural-social evolution and the existence of plural cultures or cultural diversity. The studies of isolated communities which were thought to be in time freeze could possibly provide insights about the process of cultural evaluation. There has been a debate about unilinear or multi-linear evolution, about diffusion, culture contact and acculturation. Some classics like studies of Trobriand Islands, Tikopia, studies of American

Indian ethnic groups, helped to develop and discuss hypothesis about evolution, diffusion, psychic unity of mankind, culture and personality etc. Marx and Engels analysed history from 'primitive' cooperative ownership of using natural resources equitably, to satisfy the needs, as analysed by Lewis Morgan in "Ancient Society". It was claimed that the Russian edition of "Ancient Society" was cheaper than the American edition due to tacit support to Marxist argument about economic and socio-cultural evolution.

In India, the Western and Indian scholars like Verrier Elwin, J.P. Mills, Grigson, S.C. Roy, Haimendorf and many others wrote monographs of ethnic tribal communities by following the standardised method of "going native". The same conceptual model was later followed for writing village monographs (*ICSSR: A Survey of Research in Sociology and Social Anthropology*, Vol. III, 1972).

"Early tracts by anthropologists and colonial administrators describe these isolated communities, mostly living in remote hills and forested regions, as distinct, relatively homogenous and self-contained social and cultural entities. These studies were mostly preoccupied with their culture and social arrangements, and dwelt less on their material conditions – of poverty, illness and hunger. However, as tribal expert Virginius Xaxa observes, although their housing and clothing were very elementary and their survival basically at subsistence levels, desperate poverty in the form of hunger deaths was generally absent, except for periodic episodes of famines and epidemics" (*Harsh Mander*, 2014: No. 661 p. 49).

Field trip to remote tribal area has been mandatory for a university degree in Anthropology in India, with a view to develop objective faculties of studying people and their culture, by interacting with alien people, not in regular contact. Examples of some of my field trips have been given in Chapter 3 about documenting Emic Perspectives.

Tribal Development Issues: Committee Reports

Along with the struggle for Independence to free India from the British Rule, discussions were continuously held to improve the social, economic and educational standards of marginalised communities in India, who were referred as depressed classes and aboriginal tribes. With the formation of provincial governments in directly ruled British Presidencies such as Bombay Presidency, legislative councils with elected representatives, through the process of indirect elections, were also constituted. One of the first committees, known as Starte Committee was constituted in Bombay to inquire and recommend measures for the upliftment of depressed classes and aboriginal tribes (1930). Dr. B.R. Ambedkar as a MLC was a member among other MLCs and Sri A.V. Thakkar. Provincial Government of Bombay under the leadership of Sri B.G. Kher appointed a committee under the Chairmanship of D. Symington to study and recommend measures for improvement of conditions of Bhils and others in West Khandesh (1938).The backward areas identified by this Committee were put together to form a tribal district of Nandurbar in 1998, which continues to be the most backward district in Maharashtra, according to Human Development Reports of the State Government of 2002 and 2012.

The leaders like Mahatma Gandhi and Jawaharlal Nehru took great interest in tribal development. Tribal development was one of the constructive programmes of Mahatma Gandhi, which was promoted by his disciple A.V. Thakkar, popularly known as Thakkar Bappa. The Thakkar Committee report on excluded and partially excluded area in 1947 has used the term "Scheduled Area", which was adopted in the Constitution. The Committee has promoted the value of education and contact foı their development, as also the need to protect them from land alienation and serfdom under the moneylender. The Committee had made the distinction between poor people among the rural folk and the aboriginal community found predominantly in certain areas. The Committee has strongly recommended that the officials posted in aboriginal areas obtain working knowledge of the language and dialect of the local people.

Dr. Verrier Elwin in his report (1960) on special multi-purpose tribal blocks acknowledged Nehru's five fundamental principles: "*Panchsheel*" as providing the basis of the Government's policy approach to tribal development:

1. People should develop along the lines of their own genius and we should avoid imposing anything on them. We should try to encourage in every way their own traditional arts and culture.

2. Tribal rights in land and forest should be respected.
3. We should try to train and build up a team of their own people to do the work of administration and development. Some technical personnel from outside will, no doubt, be needed, especially in the beginning. But, we should avoid introducing too many outsiders into tribal territory.
4. We should not over administer these areas or overwhelm them with a multiplicity of schemes. We should rather work through, and not in rivalry to their own social and cultural institutions.
5. We should judge results, not by statistics or the amount of money spent, but by the quality of human character that is evolved.

There have been numerous committees in Independent India, which have suggested the strategies for tribal development. The expert committee under the chairmanship of Prof. S.C. Dube in 1972 recommended 'hamlet' instead of a "revenue village" as a unit of development effort, since in many tribal areas a village does not represent anything except a conglomeration of hamlets for revenue purposes. Almost all the committees have recommended involvement of voluntary organizations to undertake specific projects for which the budget should be provided from the normal development funds of the Government.

(N.P. Bhanage, Director, TRTI, Pune, *"Tribal Commissions and Committees in India"*, Himalaya Publishing House, 1993).

Constitutional Provisions

The Constitution of India in the Directive Principles of State Policy has mentioned the duty of the State to promote educational and economic interests of SC, ST and other weaker sections of the people and to protect them from social injustice and all forms of exploitation. The State has also to perform the duty of organizing Village Panchayats and endow them with powers and authority to enable them to function as units of self-government. Part X and Part XVI of the Constitution provides for provisions in regard to administration of the Scheduled and Tribal Areas and special provisions relating to certain classes including SC and ST with regard to reservation and National Commission. Fifth Schedule to the Constitution is regarding provisions as to the Administration and Control of Scheduled Areas and Scheduled Tribes.

In pursuance of Article 339 of the Constitution, the President appointed Dhebar Commission to report on the administration of Scheduled Areas and Welfare of the Scheduled Tribes, the report of which was submitted in October 1961. The Commission has criticized the British policy of isolationism, which led to exploitation of tribals by *zamindars*, landlords, moneylenders and contractors.

The 73rd Amendment to the Constitution has now bestowed special powers to the *Gram Sabha* in tribal villages in decision-making and implementation of development projects.

Planning Commission was formed to frame Five Year Plans for comprehensive development of India. Poverty elimination has been a political agenda of all political parties which becomes an election agenda.

"Since the early seventies, alleviation of poverty has been at the centre of the political dialogue. .... Disparities between regions, between rural and urban areas, and between different sections of the population were increasingly coming to the fore. It was clear that regions like hill areas, drought prone and desert areas, tribal areas, flood affected areas and others which had remained backward required special attention in development" [Tarlok Singh, (ed.) 1990: vii].

Development process required construction of dams as hydro-electricity projects, natural resource management, transport and communication.

"Post-independence, the requirements of planned development brought with them the spectre of dams, mines, industries and roads on tribal lands. With this came the concomitant processes of displacement, both literal and metaphorical—as tribal institutions and practices were forced into an uneasy existence with or gave way to market or formal state institutions (most significantly, in the legal sphere), tribal peoples' found themselves at a profound disadvantage with respect to the influx of better equipped outsiders into their areas. The repercussions for the already fragile socio-economic livelihood base of the *adivasis* were devastating—ranging from loss of livelihoods, land alienation on a vast scale, to hereditary bondage."

"What has been the impact of government policies on tribal

livelihoods? Where should Central and State Governments focus to improve the situation? To answer these questions we quote in detail from a Planning Commission (2000) document:

"As tribal people in India perilously, sometimes hopelessly, grapple with these tragic consequences, the small clutch of bureaucratic programmes have done little to assist the precipitous pauperization, exploitation and disintegration of tribal communities. Tribal people respond occasionally with anger and assertion, but often also in anomie and despair, because the following persistent problems have by and large remained unattended to: land alienation; indebtedness, relation with forests, and government monopoly over MFPs, and non-implementation of the Forest Rights Act, 2006; ineffective implementation of Panchayats (Extension to the Scheduled Areas) Act of 1996 (PESA, 1996) for Schedule V areas; involuntary displacement due to development projects and lack of proper rehabilitation; shifting cultivation, such as podu; poor utilization of government funds; and poor delivery of government programmes." (*Journal "Seminar" – "The Malnourished Tribal"* Journal No. 661, September 2014, pp. 16 & 17, "Children of a Lesser God" by N.C. Saxena).

India as a land of plurality and diversity is a role model of tolerance and co-existence. But as a land of disparities, India ranks very low on different indices measuring quality of life. In one Nation-state with the unifying democratic instrument of one person one vote, it looks up to equality of opportunity to all citizens. History has however, created disparities within geographical regions and within communities. The tribal communities, internationally referred to as indigenous communities are most deprived, having been forced to live in geographical isolation, after they lost their kingdoms or sovereignty to powerful armies of the outsiders. This has been a global phenomena as amongst the American Indians or Australian aborigines. Indian situation is not comparable since the tribal communities are referred in Hindu mythology. Lord Rama was helped by the forest dwellers in war with Ravana. In historical times, the local Hindu or Muslim kings did not disturb the ownership of food resources of the tribal people.

Tribals in India are not the same as "indigenous people" labelled by ILO. They are also not the same as American Indians or Australian Aborigines who were militarily overpowered by the outsiders. References of tribals are found in the *Ramayana* and *Mahabharata*. In the *Ramayana*, Lord Rama representing the irrigated agricultural communities tried to develop a symbiotic relationship with the forest dwellers symbolized by the Monkey-God Hanuman and his tribe. It is reasonable to believe, with knowledge of Anthropology that the animals and birds who fought for Rama on issue of attempted adultery by Ravana, were the totemic clan names of the forest dwelling tribal communities. In *Mahabharata*, the Bhils were exploited, symbolized by Eklavya being forced to sacrifice his thumb to continue the archery combat superiority of ruling kings. Chhatrapati Shivaji Maharaj had befriended the tribals and incorporated them in his struggle for freedom. There have been several instances of tribal warriors in different parts of the country who fought the British.

The British Raj, however, claimed ownership of the forests to use the resources for their opulent life style and for creating infrastructure such as rail-roads. Forest department is visibly a regulatory department donning the uniform of para-military forces.

Constitution of India invoking the principle of Equity has tried to create a governing system whereby autonomy of the tribal regions and communities is continuing simultaneously making provisions for their development in line with the mainstream Indian society. Tribal States, Districts and Blocks have been created or restored, and identified as Scheduled Areas. A separate administrative mechanism by way of Tribal Sub-Plan has been established. Head of each State, the Governor, has been bestowed with special constitutional powers to guide and correct the respective governments in order to protect and promote tribal interests.

Despite all these measures, tribal communities continue to be deprived of their natural resources, their geographical and cultural habitat, to the extent of getting malnourished/undernourished and remain hungry.

The tribal economy has traditionally been a subsistence economy in which food security is sought through collection of forest products, fishery and seasonal cereal production using primitive technology. Historically, the tribals have never been the producers of food as they could get enough from nature through collection of food. The inseparable relationship of tribals and forest has been proved historically when during famines in the past, tribals did not suffer as much as caste peasantry, since the tribals continued to get food from the forests.

Land has never been an issue of ownership or property in tribal economy. Tribal economic organization has always been labelled as primitive communism in anthropological literature. Natural resources including land have been used but have never been owned by individual families. At best, there has been community ownership of natural resources. Till a few years ago, in 1970, my personal experience has been that the tribals in Mokhada taluka of Thane district could not definitely pronounce the ownership of a particular piece of land which was being tilled by them. This also resulted in their exploitation. Even among the caste-peasantry, the revenue clerk, *Patwari,* who maintained land records and collected land revenue could embezzle land, since the peasants were totally illiterate. Having seen a large estate in the tribal area on west coast of Bombay, owned by a Brahmin family of Pune, I asked, how did he settle down in this area. I was told by the owner that his grandfather used to be a *Patwari* in that area. Further query was not necessary.

In a field observation in 1995, among the Dongria Kondhs of Orissa, it was seen that the land acquired by the local community through *Podu* (shifting cultivation) was found to be distributed equally among the tribal families in a village, on which about 18 varieties of crops necessary for consumption were cultivated. In Bastar, a riverboat in 1997 was found to be owned by the community for crossing the river from one bank to another, without any fee being charged, and without any assigned boatman. The tribal society does not have the division of labour as in the hierarchical caste society. As a result, all the tribal people perform all tasks necessary for their living in a spirit of cooperation.

Over the ages, tribal people got into "time freeze" due to geographical isolation and adjustment with the nature for meeting their essential needs, developing a symbiotic relationship with the plant and animal life in the local environment. Every contact with the outside world was a harrowing experience of economic and other forms of exploitation for the tribal communities. As a result, the tribal psyche and life style developed into what is commonly referred as backwardness. Backwardness operationally signifies lack of capacity to develop and utilize the infrastructural facilities to improve quality of life. On the other hand, development efforts imposed from outside have always been misunderstood as attempts for exploitation and attack on the autonomy and freedom. The bigger the schemes of development projects, the larger has been the exploitation.

The Raja of Aheri in Gadchiroli district in personal communication in December 1963 expressed displeasure about infrastructure development like roads and bridges. According to him, the outsiders used the infrastructure facilities to enter the tribal area and deprived the tribals of their natural resources. It is common knowledge, as to how large irrigation projects dehabilitated the tribals, since the tribals lacked the capacity to benefit from the potential benefits of irrigation and power generation. The Industrial Training Institutes (ITIs) in tribal areas have been failures since not many tribal boys and girls possessed the requisite minimum qualification for recruitment to the ITIs.

The tribal psyche, which is stability and equilibrium conscious, in a way, opposed to change, is the result of limited geographical and cultural worldview. The tribals managed their own affairs through centuries. They developed their capacities to develop symbiotic relationship with the environment and met all their needs from the immediate vicinity of around twenty km. Every contact with the outside world gave them experience of exploitation. The tribals, therefore, neither had the knowledge nor the capacity to develop themselves to improve their quality of life beyond subsistence levels. Backwardness in the tribal context, to repeat again, therefore, refers to their incapacity to use the opportunities and infrastructure of development. The tribals have been variously referred as noble savage, wild flower or those living the culture of poverty. Some caste Hindu leaders refer them as part of the mainstream, who got secluded due to geographical isolation and offered them opportunities for assimilation in the mainstream. This offer is spurned by many tribal leaders, who believe that the big brotherly attitude is an attack on their cultural identities. The Government of India has pursued the policies of Integration in preference to that of Assimilation.

Anthropology and Tribal Development

In this book, we are focusing on the tribal issues of malnutrition in Maharashtra which is similar all over the country, except probably in the North-East.

Although anthropology is not an exclusive study of Tribal Culture and Society, the popular image of the discipline of anthropology is an expert discipline of tribal issues. Since researchers from other discipline do not venture to go to relatively inaccessible tribal areas and interact with the people, anthropologists continue to own the study of tribal communities. Classical anthropological studies are about studying other people, from the perspectives of study population, through their eyes and spectacles. "Going Native" summarizes the classical anthropological methods of study which were followed by those who shifted their attention to village and peasantry.

After decolonization, the national development agenda has been under pressure of globalization leading to economic neo-colonialism. It impacts the life of people who remained isolated from the mainstream market economies. The national priorities are about the development and empowerment of the marginalized, as citizens of a democratic Nation-State. Anthropologists cannot and should not disown these national responsibilities as fundamental duties, to safeguard the fundamental rights of people. The development paradigm has now shifted from welfare and provider-beneficiary relationship to rights approach and human development. The folk tale about a benevolent monkey on a riverside tree trying to save a tiny fish struggling in flooded river by sticking to the trunk of a tree, takes the fish out of water on his palm, with disastrous result of death of the fish. It is believed that "benevolent development policies, and schemes" designed at macro-level and their centralized implementation sometimes lead to unproductive and fruitless results, since these do not address the emic perspectives of the people and their concerns.

Anthropologists are expected to understand and analyse these processes and make people-centric recommendations. The Ministers of Tribal Development during informal interaction, accept that their schemes were survival schemes and not development schemes.

Why should the tribe dominant districts and blocks get ranked lowest on the Human Development scale, despite very large budgetary outlay to the tribal development departments? Why should there be more deaths and malnourishment amongst tribal children as compared to rural and urban poor? Anthropology as a discipline, historically inalienable from the tribal world, has to find ways of coming out of this starvation and death trap, by developing a model of comprehensive and sustainable development, through community management. As anthropologists, we know that it is far easier to work amongst the tribals, who are honest, than to work amongst the hierarchical caste-peasantry who are a part of exploitative market economy.

B. ANTHROPOLOGY OF HEALTH AND NUTRITION

In common man's paradigm, health refers to one's capacity to undertake work with optimum efficiency, commensurate with age, gender, occupation, class etc. The work is usually measured in terms of productive activity, measurable in wage labour, whether in a factory, farmland or at home. Prof. P.V. Sukhatme eminent agricultural statistician of India who led statistics division at FAO, a UN organization at Rome, is credited with having discussed nutrition with a view to determine a viable policy on poverty and malnutrition (Prof. P.V. Sukhatme, 1982: 12-13).

In common parlance, the terms 'malnourished' and 'undernourished' are used as synonyms, possibly due to its vernacular expression as *'kuposhan'*, in preference to starvation, which is linked with famine. When malnourishment of tribal children is discussed at all levels including at the High Courts and Supreme Court of India, it is in the context of under-nourishment and is linked with poverty and food security. The discussion encompasses the policies about employment, migration, owning land or being landless, facility or denial to use the forest land and forest food products. The children are deprived of schooling since they have to engage in collecting or working for food etc. Affirmative action besides linkage with historically created deprivation due to membership of such branded groups as Scheduled Castes, Scheduled Tribes etc. is also administered in terms of measurement of poverty linked to availability of food calories, commonly known as Below Poverty Line (BPL) or Above Poverty Line (APL). The prices of available food grains in Public Distribution System or Ration Shop varies as per BPL and APL category. The Particularly Vulnerable Tribal Groups (PVTGs) classified in each State of India are eligible for "Antyodaya" ration card which provides food products in PDS shops at further reduced rates.

With reference to requirement of food at the individual level, there could be intra-individual variations which are classified in Ayurveda as per concept of *Prakriti*: *Vata, Pitta, Kapha,* and their combinations.

The most controversial concept discussed in relation to food and poverty relates to understanding of what is hunger. The FAO definition has been, "if a person eats below the level of average requirement he becomes thin and wastes away and if he eats above the average he becomes fat and is exposed to the hazard of obesity."

There are no agreed definitions of the criteria of "proper nutrition" and "malnutrition". Whether malnutrition is reflected in abnormally low size and/or consumption, or in terms of certain clinical signs of nutritional inadequacy and or functional impairment, such as the inability, and/or functional impairment, to work productively, are debated issues.

Beside productivity, there could be issues about lower levels of immunity due to under-nutrition or hunger, resulting into catching infections faster. With infections like diarrhoea, so common, wherever potable water supply is not available; or respiratory infections due to paucity of protective clothes, especially to neonates and infants, would result in mortality or chronic morbidity. In tribal area, lack of health care facilities in the public or private sector (due to low purchasing capacity) coupled with lack of affordable transportation and communication, and difficult terrain, are compounding factors for mortality and morbidity. The institutions or the infrastructure facilities are set up with bureaucratic, statistical budgetary formula of ratio of population per facility. In tribal area, facilities are created for lesser population of beneficiaries as compared to caste-peasant rural areas. However, this does not conform to the ground level criteria as to how much time is required to access the facility and at what cost?

It is now commonly accepted that while the issues of under-nutrition are grave until the age of 2 years, Anganwadi is usually attended by +3 children who may get access to supplementary food. Similarly in mixed villages of caste-peasantry and tribal communities residing in the hamlets, tribal children do not access to the Anganwadi located in the mainstream village occupied by caste groups. Besides there are other issues like mid-day meal or food supplies in Ashram Schools which continue to be organized through contract system, who are professional businessmen and work for profits, unmindful of the food habits and requirements of different age groups.

Former Prime Minister Dr. Manmohan Singh had expressed concern about malnutrition as a "National Shame". The judiciary has been addressing issues of tribal malnutrition in a *Suo Motu* injunction or being liberal in adjudicating the Public Interest Litigation (PIL) and directing the governments to take time bound remedial action. Supreme Court had gone to the extent of directing the government to ensure food security by giving food grains free of charge from the stocks of food which had the potential danger of rotting.

"Man is more than an animal and does not live by bread alone; and for this reason the purely biochemical and physiological points of view are not sufficient to formulate dietary regimens adequate for his welfare. The relation of food to human existence involves factors that go above and beyond the relation of biochemical nutrition to physical life. .....In some societies, no new relationship can be initiated or no transaction carried on without gifts of food. This gift has no function other than to be a medium of relatedness" (Rene Dubos, 1965: 86-87).

Human food has medical, spiritual, ritual, economic and social value. Foods to be offered to deities on various ritual occasions, foods to be offered to guests, on social occasions such as marriage and festivals, to different caste groups are standardized in various cultural groups. M.N. Srinivas has written about hierarchy of caste and hierarchy of food going collaterally. The philosophical treatise, '*Gita*' has discussed the moral value of food categories influencing human behaviour, named as '*Sattva*', '*Rajas*' and '*Tamas*'. Same is discussed in classical Ayurvedic texts, as also in other medical systems, such as Unani. Food taboos as per climatic seasons, age, gender, caste, different kinds of afflictions, during pregnancy and lactation, are some of the commonest and universal culture specific norms. Heads of States start their diplomatic parleys with formal banquets. In so-called drugless therapies like Naturopathy, medicinal value of food is very important. Diet recipes may be classified as soft aspects of culture, but they are hard aspects when it comes to offerings to deities on ritual occasions. Lady doctors from all systems of medicine follow the traditionally prescribed food regimen and food taboos, during their own pregnancy and lactation.

"It is in fact food which is responsible for the development of an individual and for the appearance of disease. The only difference is that food is wholesome in the case of the individual and unwholesome in the emergence of the disease. .... A straightforward definition of wholesome food is that which maintains the balance of *Dhatus* and retrieves the balance after it has been disturbed. .... Eatables of many different kinds share common properties since they are all articles of food. .... From the stand point of effects, food may be wholesome or unwholesome. There will be countless variations in food when the diverse properties joins and disjoins. What is necessary from the practical point of view is to know which specific items of food are wholesome and which are unwholesome. .... However, the use of the entities must take into account the role of '*pathya*' which ensures that what is prescribed is favourable to the flow of substances through the body channels and that it is agreeable to the patient." (M.S. Valiathan, 2003 : 96-98).

The biological evolution of man is closely linked to evolution of items of food consumed by apes and ape-man, from the stage of quadruped to biped, descending from the trees. The evolution of jaw, linked to type of raw or cooked food consumed, thereby limiting the tight or loose hold on the bones of the head, encasing the brain, and affecting its size, are researchable issues in the evolution of Man.

"Man is a cooking animal. The beasts have memory, judgement, and all the facilities and passions of our mind in a certain degree; but no beast is a cook" (Boswell, 1970) as quoted by Kanchan Mukhopadhyay (2011).

"The entire history of the human-being has been divided into two parts, time when they used to gather and hunt their food that was grown naturally and time when they started cultivating and rearing their food. Gaining command over the sources of food through domestication has been called a revolution; undoubtedly that revolution has remained the most significant one in human history. Processing food for preserving or consuming the same, cooking is a part of that effort, marks another extremely significant dividing line between the humans and the non-humans" (Kanchan

Mukhopadhyay: *Anthropology of Food in India: The Scope and the Prospect*, pp. 157-158, *Journal of the Indian Anthropological Society*, Volume 46: 2 & 3, July/Nov. 2011).

The discovery of making fire by man, or domestication of fire, has made a major difference in human living. With or without pots, food can be cooked on fire, leaves being used for wrapping a product to be cooked on open fire by baking or roasting.

Domestication of cattle and plants led to surplus production which necessitated protection by a special force, and markets. Protection led to kingship, extortion or taxes, for taking responsibility of law and order. Surplus production also led to storage in baked earthen pots or bamboo baskets, and processing for increasing the storage life. We have seen, in the tribal areas, food being cooked exclusively in earthenware.

It is believed that current problems of hunger and undernutrition among the tribal people is due to denial of free access to their natural food resources in forests. Besides food shortages, there is shortage of medicinal herbs which also affects commercial production of Ayurvedic and Unani drugs.

Another area of inquiry is about the efficacy of parameters of health and nutrition according to modern bio-medical concepts. The parameters in different systems of medicine are different. What is required by the body for maintenance of health and for its promotion, for prevention of illness, are not exclusively bio-chemical phenomena.

Health, Nutrition and Culture

Health is an aspect of culture. In classical anthropology, there is no specific ethnography about health issues. There is description about foods offered to Gods, guests at rituals etc. There is also documentation about the Shamans, *Bhagats* and their magico-religious practices, not as much about their knowledge and practices about treatment of diseases and about the medicinal herbs. Medicinal herbs were later discussed in Ethno-botany. Although, the magico-religious practices of shamans or *bhagats* may have psychological effect about cure of ailment, better than the placebo effect, these practices are shunned in modern health care practices dominated by Allopathic Medical System. They are branded as exploitative and superstition. On the other hand,

Mother Teresa's faith cure miracles are formally recognized. The basic issues of mind-body interaction in causing and healing the ailments are grey areas in scientific research, although the role of mind is increasingly being recognized in modern science. Spiritual, healing miracles of Mother Teresa are formally recognised.

Health refers to the total fitness of an individual, which would ensure performance of social roles to his optimum efficiency (Mutatkar, 1981). Health is an aspect of culture like economic, political, social and religious aspects of life. Culture being an integrated whole, all aspects are interrelated. In any traditional society, the integration is close knit, the static or equilibrium spirit overriding the dynamic nature of culture. Health aspects could be classified into softer or visible aspects such as ill health or disease, which needs treatment. Ideas about prevention and promotion of health and causation of illness are part of hard core of culture, which would fall in the area of belief. Cause effect relationship about health and illness, therefore, fall in the areas of belief system. The plural treatment therapies, which may be herbal or of synthetic drugs in modern medicine, are guided by results, which could be classified as material culture as soft aspects of culture. Magico-religious procedures are also followed in health, more so in tribal society, but not totally absent in the developed societies. There is no vacuum of knowledge or practices, in matters of health and medicine in any society. There are professionals in tribal society, generally referred to as *bhagat* or *vaidu*, who have good knowledge of herbal medicine. Tribal people have faith in them since they are a part of the community, their kin, and are always available.

There are references to people in Caucasia whose longevity is a matter of international curiosity and a subject of research.

"Among the other peoples of the Caucasus, a rugged mountain area in the southern part of the Soviet Union, there is an exceptional concentration of the people who claim to be over 100 years old. Even more impressive than their sheer survival to an advanced age is their health and vigour."

"What is probably happening is not a prolongation of old age but rather a slowing down of the whole ageing process. Menopause seems to be delayed, the birth of children to women said to be over fifty is not unusual, and men claiming to be over ninety have fathered children."

"Despite the emphasis on feasting and hospitality, overeating is frowned on and obesity is regarded as illness. Caloric intake is low from an American or European perspective. The everyday diet emphasizes milk products, cereals, an abundance of fresh vegetables, fruits and nuts" (Ann McElroy and Patricia K. Townsend, 1985: 244-246).

"In many areas of the world, people whose nutritional pattern appears, according to Western standards, to be inadequate, actually present a picture of health. In sections of Africa where mixed cultivation is still practised and cash crops have not been taken up, the nutritionists have been surprised to find such health and growth as presupposes adequacy of diet" [*Cultural Patterns and Technical Change: Cross-cultural Studies of Technical Change* : (ed.) Margaret Mead: 1955: 198].

"In theory, all human-beings have essentially the same nutritional requirements and suffer in a similar way from the various kinds of deficiencies. In practice, however, immense numbers of human-beings all over the world remain healthy and vigorous on diets that are considered grossly deficient by nutritionists and would appear close to a famine ration for the American public. This paradoxical state of affairs can be explained in part by more efficient use of foodstuffs in underprivileged populations. As we have seen, many primitive people have developed empirical practices that permit them to find fairly adequate subsistence under conditions where food supplies are restricted" (Rene Dubos, 1965: 81-82).

It is obvious that Man had to find his food from the environment in the neighbourhood. Early man as collector of food and not as producer, like other living beings in nature, had to get his nutrition and food from the geographical area of his habitat. Man learnt the technique of collecting roots, tubers, fruits, leaves and game by processing it to make it edible. We do the same with bitter gourd, processing it with salt to make it less bitter. Even now, in the tribal belts, during rainy, monsoon season, several types of leafy and fruit vegetables are collected by the tribals as food. They know how to detoxify the 'harmful' products by water and other such treatments.

"Tubers of all sorts, grubs, ant eggs, bird nests, mushrooms, berries, and teas brewed from the buds of evergreen and other plants have supplied diets adequate in proteins and vitamins to countless generations of people who had acquired empirically a nutritional wisdom similar to that of wild animals. The diet of primitive people, quantitatively limited and monotonous as it may be, thus includes many items not recorded in textbooks of nutrition. ..... In many areas, empirical but useful culinary practices have been developed to improve the nutritive value of certain products. Despite the scarcity of meat and milk in most of China, each local community had worked out a diet of adequate nutritional value, with the proper amino acid composition, through the skilful mixture of plant products readily available in that particular region. The extensive use of sprouts—the germinated beans, peas, and lentils of China and India—also has nutritional merit, since essential amino acids, fats, and vitamins become more available in the sprouts as a result of germination" (Rene Dubos, 1965: 64).

"Dietary habits of populations in different regions of the world have been determined mainly by the availability of foods locally and local practices. Man has evolved his habitual dietary pattern to maintain good health, perhaps after a good deal of trial and error. Satisfaction of hunger is usually the primary criteria for adequate food intake" (C. Gopalan, *et al.*, ICMR, 1989: 1).

"The nutritive value of a mixture of two proteins need not be the arithmetic average of the individual value, but something higher than each value because of mutual supplementary effect. This is in illustrated case of protein efficiency ratio (PER) of wheat, pulse and a mixture of the two. This is because of mutual supplementary effect of the component amino acids. .... It has in fact been shown that protein value of cereals can be improved by the addition of leafy vegetables" (C. Gopalan, *et al.*, ICMR, 1989: 5).

Chapter 2
Poverty and Malnourishment

"Nutritional science developed at a time when the worst effects of malnutrition were caused by shortages of food, resulting in gross deficiency states. The most obvious manifestation of these nutritional defects was limitation of growth. ..... However, while measurement of growth rate constitutes an excellent and probably the most useful guide for improvement of nutrition in animal husbandry, this index is not sufficient for an evaluation of nutritional regimens in man. ..... The dietary factors most effective in the production of meat, milk, and eggs also bring about a rapid growth of children; but growth rates are not the most significant values of human life. Life span, resistance to disease, intellectual performance, emotional responsiveness and perceptiveness etc. are characteristics that cannot be measured on a weight scale (Rene Dubos, 1965: 85).

"Poverty and basic needs have more than one dimension, namely material, cultural and psychological. On the material *plane* basic needs are fundamental physical needs like adequate food, clothing and shelter, which are necessary to keep alive and maintain working capacity. On the other *planes* are basic social needs which are related to a sense of human dignity to the extent that their non-satisfaction prevents the concerned individuals/ families from following the established customs of the community and thereby alienates them from the rest of the society. While in developed countries an integrated view of all the above needs is adopted whereby human welfare is reckoned in terms of a full and fruitful life, in developing countries like India, only basic physical needs, which are objective in nature and thus easily amenable to physical measurement, are taken into account for determining the level of poverty" (Uma Datta Roy Choudhury, *et al*. in Tarlok Singh, 1990: 155-156).

Introduction

India presents a dichotomous situation whereby, we are self-sufficient in food on one hand, and large number of people suffering from malnutrition, in contrast. With good harvest, we cannot protect our food stocks from inclement weather threatening rotting, for want of warehouses. Supreme Court had directed the Government to give free food to needy people from the stocks which could decay and rot. "The cause is alleged to be the inefficient and ineffective implementation of, and huge leakage in, government's schemes meant to overcome hunger and malnutrition". The baseline survey in tribal communities across the State of Maharashtra as reported under AUK project give us the statistics that several tribal communities have no purchasing power even to lift the food available in PDS shops. Besides, low level of awareness about health and hygiene as well as about accessing entitlements and rights under the government's schemes/ resources and services compounds the problem. Centralisation of governance, resources, decision-making, and development action as well as concentration of productive assets, resources and wealth in a few hands further aggravates the problem. Lack of adequate political and social will is yet another cause. Although India is far better placed as regards availability and accessibility of data, lack of disaggregated data of district level and below up to Gram Panchayat (Village Council) level comes in the way of focused measures and efficient and effective monitoring, mapping and surveillance system. Actually, the administrative categories such as ST, SC, OBC and Others are not viable for planning and implementation at the micro-level, since there are wide disparities among ethnic groups as tribal communities and caste groups within the general categories. It is very unscientific that these general categories are used as research categories while analysing and presenting the data which could be used for budget planning, formulation of schemes and their implementation.

About 70 per cent of the population of India is rural, major part of which greatly suffers from poverty, hunger and malnutrition. Besides, major part of the urban population about 30 per cent, afflicted by poverty, hunger and malnutrition is actually rural that has migrated to urban areas and landed in urban slums while exploring employment and income opportunities. As is well known, India is a large and diverse country with disparities across various sections of the population, castes, classes, ethnic groups, gender and age as well as across the states and their constituents. Further down, it has about 600 districts, 5470 blocks/sub-districts, 2,30,000 Gram Panchayats, 6,40,867 villages and 1.4 million habitations. Similarly, there are 5161 large, medium and small towns in India. It is an uphill task to deliver efficiently and effectively anti-poverty schemes/resources and services to such a large, diverse and dispersed area, especially in a greatly centralised system, which, therefore, needs to be replaced with a well-monitored and well-managed participatory decentralised system already in place in form, but yet to be strengthened with content (functions, funds and functionaries).

"Numerous government measures to overcome hunger and malnutrition include National Food Security Mission, National Nutrition Mission, National Policy on Farmers, National Horticulture Mission, National Mission on Pulses and Oilseeds, National Rural Livelihoods Mission, Mahatma Gandhi National Rural Employment Guarantee Act/Scheme, National Rural Health Mission Integrated Child Development Services (ICDS) for children below 6 years to provide nutrition and pre-school education, Mid-Day-Meal (MDM) for children of 6-14 years, Public Distribution System, Janani Suraksha Yojana (Mothers' Protection Scheme) for pregnant/lactating mothers and Social Assistance to the poor/needy (subsidised food grains, pension, insurance etc.), besides the all-inclusive National Food Security Bill as mentioned earlier. Some of these critical measures are in the "mission mode" to ensure their efficient and effective planning and implementation with missionary zeal, but still leave much to be done and desired as regards their effective implementation. There are 1.1 million Anganwadi Centres (AWCs) across the rural India, catering functionally to the children of 3-6 years; while the need in terms of malnutrition is for the children up to 2 years, and pregnant/lactating mothers as also adolescent girls. Likewise, there are about 4,89,000 Fair Price Shops (FPSs) under the PDS to distribute subsidised food grains, sugar, kerosene oil etc. to the targeted poor households; but their functioning is ridden with huge leakage and corruption."

Former Prime Minister, Dr. Manmohan Singh regretted prevalence of malnourishment as National Shame. Around the same time, the Acceptance Speech delivered by the President of India immediately after his oath taking ceremony on 25th July, 2012 refers to poverty and malnutrition in India.

"Our national mission must continue to be what it was..... to eliminate the curse of poverty...... There is no humiliation more abusive than hunger...... We must lift those at the bottom so that poverty is erased from the dictionary of modern India."

Ref: Association of Voluntary Agencies for Rural Development (AVARD), New Delhi (pp. 11-14).

Arvind Panagariya who till recently was the first Vice-Chairman of NITI Ayog of India in Dr. C. Chandrasekaran Memorial Lecture at IIPS, Mumbai on November 8, 2012 spoken about "The Myth of Child Malnutrition in India", in the context of allegations of more malnutrition among the Indian children than most countries in Sub-Saharan Africa. Obviously, these are also methodological issues based on assumptions that "all differences between populations of children of given age and sex with respect to weight and height occur due to differences in nutrition."

Measurement of Poverty, Backwardness and Development

Prof. P.V. Sukhatme all his life measured poverty and development and initiated actions to predict the mitigation of poverty and herald development, more particularly rural development. But, he did not take action as a do-gooder or as a social activist but to test certain hypothesis in Biometry, which have a bearing on National/International policies.

Prof. Sukhatme was greatly influenced by a question from Pandit Madan Mohan Malviya who interviewed him for a position at Banares Hindu University, as to how his subject Statistics could be put to use of common man. His subsequent researches on Poverty, Protein deficiency, Malnutrition, Homeostatis and his action research in "community kitchen" and "improving living conditions in villages" have been acknowledged by Prof. Sukhatme to the question from Pandit Malviya.

The central concerns of human society appear to be longevity and productivity. Towards these ends, we have health care and nutrition programmes. Poverty has been measured in terms of food security over the year, and amount available or accessible for consumption, to provide enough energy for increased productivity. Poverty has been expressed in terms of malnutrition, mostly relating to sufficiency and quality of protein, or undernutrition, referring to calorie deficiencies. The issues about over-nutrition were later added for comparative analysis of health and productivity. Sukhatme has discussed all these.

Coming back, we are looking at poverty in terms of capacity to buy food to give calories for optimum health, i.e. optimum productive capacity. But, how many calories are needed for optimum productivity? Sukhatme has discussed this in terms of productivity of women working in the community kitchen. He has talked about intra-individual variability. These concepts of variability based on measurement actually correspond to Ayurvedic concepts of *Prakriti* and Charak's recommendation about food intake, which is based on empirical and clinical observations.

"The ability to adapt to a wide range of environments is of course not peculiar to man. Adaptability is found throughout life and is perhaps the one attribute that distinguishes most clearly the world of life from the world of inanimate matter. Living organisms never submit passively to the impact of environmental forces; however, primitive they may be, all of them attempt to respond adaptively to these forces, each in its own manner. .... Homeostasis implies that the body can function well only to the extent that it can rapidly make the necessary adjustments so that its internal composition remains within limits precisely defined for each organism. On the other hand, the responses to environmental changes made by each individual organism must be such that ideally they help it to function adequately under the changed conditions. These two demands are equally essential for the success of life. ....The complementary concepts of Homeostasis and adaptation are, therefore, valid at all levels of biological organization; they apply to social groups as well as to unicellular or multicellular organisms" (Rene Dubos, 1965: 256-257).

These discussions lead to the questions of what is poverty line? How much food the country needs to feed the people and what type of food? So, the policies about agricultural production, public distribution system, wage labour are to be based on the measurement of poverty.

It is said, man does not live by bread alone. So, poverty discussion does not restrict itself to nutritional poverty or income poverty alone.

Another pertinent question is : What do the common people think of poverty? How do they measure it? We asked women in a village not far from Pune? They said, the rich could buy food for the whole year, the poor had to purchase everyday. In the tribal areas in Maharashtra and Orissa, we were told that the food could last till *Diwali* (October), *Sankrant* (mid-January) and *Holi* (March), in different families or tribal groups, depending upon the ownership of land and land productivity. The frequency of meal from three times could reduce to twice a day or once. Also the menu could change, from rice to rice gruel. Expenditure patterns on food and non-food items would also bring out the difference between rich and poor. All these responses could be transformed into measurements.

The Western affluent World where food security or nutritional poverty is not a prime concern, (although people search food in garbage bins, or sleep in cardboard boxes) poverty includes non-economic considerations also. Human Development Reports since 1990 have defined human development as the process of enlarging people's choices, most critical being long and healthy life, to be educated, and enjoy a decent standard of living. Other choices refer to political freedom, human rights and self-respect etc. Some of these as we know engulf the disprivileged people and gender issues. It is thus obvious that if human development refers to these choices, denial of these refer to poverty. When we include, access to safe drinking water and health care services as parameters for measuring poverty, we may have a gradation where women and old suffer relatively more. Prof. Sukhatme as we know included personal hygiene, sanitation and safe drinking water as parameters of village development since they prevented infections to counter the so called ill effects of nutritional poverty. While discussing child growth, he put more emphasis on recurrent infections due to bad sanitation, lack of personal hygiene, degrading environment and contaminated water in contrast with nutritional supplements on which at least Rs. 100 crores were spent every year in India.

While discussing India's development and poverty alleviation efforts, Human Development Report 1997 brings out the variations in various indicators across the geographical boundaries of States ranging from impressive record of Kerala to bad situation in Uttar Pradesh, Madhya Pradesh and Bihar. Although Haryana's per capita income is one of the highest in the country, gender ratio is one of the lowest 865 females to 1000 males and infant mortality at 68 per 1000 live births. This raises the issues of what is development?

If children were reportedly sold in Kalahandi in Orissa, or so-called malnourishment deaths of children occurring in tribal areas in Maharashtra, how do we measure poverty? It is not uncommon to see young girls in the established flesh market localities, in the rooms, having been sold by their parents, particularly the father.

A journalist from Dholpur had 'purchased' a bride with a pseudo-name, Kamala for Rs. 1500 which raised a storm in the Parliament. Soon after, while I revisited (after 1958) my research study village on Gwalior-Jhansi road in 1981 I asked the villagers, whom I had a very good anthropological rapport, as to why they indulged in female infanticide while they considered unmarried (probably pre-puberty) girls (*Kanya*) representing Mother-Goddess, and touched their feet also. In several religious ceremonies and rituals, in honour of Mother-Goddess, across the country, teenage girls are treated with respect and great affection, and fed with special food while gifts are showered on them. As expected, with meek denial, I asked the villagers again as to how they coped with scarcity of women, for marriage. They showed me from the window of 'Choupal' two women crossing the field, whom they had purchased for Rs. 300 each. Is this not poverty?

In *Mahabharata*, Queen Draupadi was a pawn to be staked while the King lost everything including himself and his brothers in a game of dice. There is documentation that while some nomads had nothing to pledge against a loan from a money lender, they pledged their wives, whom they recovered, sometimes with a child, after the repayment of loan. How do we define poverty ?

In all these discussions about nutritional or income poverty, going beyond survival poverty, and more particularly, while discussing human poverty involving human rights, self-esteem and gender issues, the concept of mind assumes significance. Role of mind in health has always been accepted in Ayurveda and Unani, which is now being accepted in the West, although role of mind and the concepts of soul have been discussed in all religious theologies. Prof. Sukhatme has discussed about mind-brain interaction.

"The voluntary modifications of pulse rate and blood pressure by the *yogis*, the well-documented cases of death by suggestion, and the unquestionable effects of the will to live or its converse constitute further examples of the complex interrelationships between the **mind and body functions**..... Ignorance of the mechanisms through which the **mind acts on the body** does not decrease the importance of the role that psychic phenomena play in the responses of man to his total environment. The neural reactions integrated at the highest level do condition most of the processes that relate man to the physico-chemical world, and it is for this reason that the response to a given stimulus can be either protective or destructive, depending upon the person affected and the circumstances" (Rene Dubos, Man Adapting, 1965: 267-268).

Certification about Mother Teresa's miracle healing is an example of acceptance of mind-body interaction.

India is referred to as a developing nation, and figures about different kinds of poverty are given in International Reports. Within India, apart from geographical variations, there are variations in different caste-community groups. While democracy is accepted as a value in itself, true democracy does not lie only in casting a vote, but what was referred while discussing human development, as enlarging peoples' choices. In other words, it refers to sharing state power or in a family, woman having a share in decision-making in regard to all matters. Sharing state power means having access to the State's resources, natural, technological, educational and relating to health.

In India, due to age old caste hierarchies, there has been hierarchical inequality leading to inequity. The poor who are also socially disprivileged have less access to food, drinking water and health care facilities. The Constitution of India while championing the values of equality has professed protective discrimination to the socially disprivileged for a limited period, since equality cannot be achieved amongst the unequals. A child cannot be equal to an adult. An untouchable cannot be equal to a Brahmin. The policy of reservations for SC and ST and now extended to OBC which in Maharashtra includes VJ/ NT, and now a new category Special Backward Classes (SBC). As we know the category of reservation for economic backwardness proposed by the then Prime Minister, Narasimha Rao was unacceptable to the Supreme Court and it was struck down. Earlier Kaka Kalelkar Committee Report of a similar nature was not accepted by the Government of India. It is generally accepted that social and economic backwardness are coterminous in India. In India, poverty is a group phenomena, not an individual or family concern. As a consequence of 50 per cent reservations in public service and public institutions, there has been a competition to be labelled as backward. It is difficult to find out who is a real backward and who is a pseudo-backward. How do we measure backwardness?

However, the fact remains that in matters of bringing people from different social categories on the level of equality, India has adopted human development priorities such as basic health, basic education, safe drinking water and special attention for socially disadvantaged groups. Thus, the official policies for eradicating poverty focus on human development approach.

Coming back to measurement of backwardness for the purpose of reservation, SC included those groups which suffered centuries of untouchability while ST were those tribal groups who led an isolated life in forests, valleys or hill tops as *Adivasi*. In Maharashtra, VJ have been those who were notified as criminal communities during British Rule and NT have been the constant nomads, the family moving from place to place, the classical picture being non-remembrance of the place where children were born. OBC in Maharashtra have been largely the artisan caste groups such as carpenter, ironsmith, or service groups such as barber and washerman who fall into the *Shudra* category of *Varna* hierarchy. These are all traditional, cultural, qualitative indicators for bestowing benefits of reservation on castes/communities. Now there is clamouring to become more backward: non-OBC to OBC, OBC to NT, ST but not SC or VJ. Scheduled Caste is associated with stigma of untouchability, while *Vimukta* or denotified tribe/caste is associated with British records of criminality. British Raj included all those groups who rebelled against them as criminal groups.

Mandal Commission tried to standardize quantitative indicators and included such categories as male and female literacy, age at marriage of girls, females as workforce in wage labour, rates of school drop-out, proportion of matriculates, houses constructed of local material (*kutcha*), source of drinking water and distance, consumption pattern per family, landless labour etc.

Some other qualitative indicators included by us refer to the kinds of deities worshipped, local, regional or national and the distance of traditional pilgrimage centres; range of marital ties, geographical area of interaction etc.

A Backward Classes Committee appointed by the State Government, under my Chairmanship, had suggested scoring scale for each family whereby caste would be one of the indicators and not the only one, since class has developed within a caste and the creamy layers have emerged in all backward classes, on lines of non-backward.

At what stage should backward be declared non-backward? Should it be a caste or a family? Answers to these questions need measurement of indicators. In the days of vote banks, no political party is in a mood to look at these issues objectively.

Poverty, backwardness and development are economic and political agenda linked with vote banks. General socio-economic development by increasing productivity with the help of technology and pro-poor policies, seem to be the answer. Gender reservation is likely to set a new revolution in India which should be measured in terms of reproductive health, including infant/maternal mortality and improvement in status of woman. However, gender reservation in legislatures and parliament is still not in sight.

Research is considered necessary for generating data to be used for planning and implementation. The basics in community research as conducted on the ground by academics are—we do research about them, according to our agenda, what in anthropology is termed as etic approach. Westerners study us, we study other people—poor, slum dwellers, rural, tribal etc. We devise parameters and indicators to test our hypotheses and answer our research questions, treating people as laboratory subjects. What would happen if we ask people, train them to do research about themselves—participatory research. Will their parameters and indicators be the same as devised by us? Similarly, community management of development programmes would prove useful to address poverty issues.

How can we reduce the distance between we and they? Sukhatme innovated community kitchen as "Poor helping the Poor". The women from poor families were cooking food which was affordable to poor wage labour. Several times, we used community kitchen meals for our tribal seminars at Pune. The expenditure for wholesome, clean and simple food was less than the breakfast snacks purchased from the market. Some labour organisations got motivated to start such kitchens in the market yard area for the casual labour working in vegetable and grain market.

In summary, the issues of measurement of poverty, backwardness and development are complex. As the Human Development Report admits, it is difficult to develop universally applicable Indices. People live their lives amongst their respective kin groups and peer groups. They tolerate the conditions of their living within their respective worlds.

Prof P.V. Sukhatme in his paper on "Relationship between Malnutrition and Poverty" has argued:

> There are two beliefs which have influenced national policy on eradicating poverty. The first is that food is the most stark element in the deprivation of the people, so much so that some 40 per cent of the rural and 50 per cent of the urban population do not get enough of what they eat to meet the minimum energy needs for a healthy active life; in other words, some 250 to 300 million people are undernourished* for want of adequate income. The second belief is that because these people are undernourished, they are unemployable in that their work performance is low and that it does not pay to employ them* [Sukhatme in Tarlok Singh (ed.) 1990: 247].

Extent of Undernutrition and Poverty

"Measurement of poverty and undernutrition have been a subject of intensive debate in recent years, particularly between Sukhatme and Dandekar (1981, 1982). Dandekar has argued that poverty and undernutrition are two different phenomena. This is true. But at the same time it is also true that although different, they are related in the sense that average requirement is an integral part of the procedure for calculating the poverty line. The fact, however, is that

---

* An undernourished individual is usually malnourished though the reverse may not be true. In this paper I shall use the term 'malnutrition' primarily in the sense of under-nutrition.

man can maintain body weight and carry out assigned tasks on a range of intakes. In the circumstances, the question remains as to why should we aim to calculate the poverty line which corresponds to the average energy need when a man can meet his physiological needs on lower intakes. To use average energy requirement for calculating the incidence of poverty, is to suggest, by implication, that average requirement is the minimum need of man and is tantamount to assuming that intra-individual variation in energy balance in man maintaining body weight and doing assigned tasks is zero, which we know it is not and cannot be." (Sukhatme, *Newer Concepts in Nutrition and their Implications for Policy*).

"Food supplementation cannot be effective for improving health and stature as long as hygiene and sanitation are what they are, housing is inadequate, water for drinking is unavailable and education is lacking. By exaggerating poverty we merely help the non-poor to capture the benefits of official programmes, leaving the poor where they are or worse off."

Sukhatme's argument is that nutrition by western values are not the sole parameters of health, which would encourage people to work their assigned roles to optimum efficiency. Particularly, for children, any bout of infection causing diarrhoea or respiratory problem, leading to morbidity would affect food intake and nutrition. Water and sanitation are important public health issues to prevent frequent infections and morbidity, which cannot be corrected by nutrition.

Sukhatme undertook an intervention research programme, whereby latrines were introduced in villages to provide easy access, day and night. Drinking water wells were chlorinated every day. People accepted that the morbidity had appreciably reduced as compared to previous years. The geriatric age group told that their general health improved due to availability of latrine in the backyard, relieving them from risk of orthopaedic accident by going to the fields at night. As a result, they resumed normal diet at night, improving their health. The cryptic quote about the impact of latrine programme in the village was, "Old persons added age to their lives."

In the tribal world, supplementary food without improvement in water and sanitation, is not likely to arrest malnutrition amongst children effectively. Maybe, further intervention research projects on these public health issues are required.

Chapter 3
Emic Perspective: Going Native

University level training in Anthropology in India mandates fieldwork by following Malinowskian tradition of "Going Native" both in tribal and peasant villages. A single field investigator lives in a family. A group of students with teachers reside in the village settlement as close to people as possible.

I joined as a Lecturer in Cultural/Social Anthropology at the Pune University (now Savitribai Phule Pune University), Department of Sociology and Anthropology at Deccan College in July 1960, with Prof. Irawati Karve as the Head of the Department. In November 1962, I and my colleague R.K. Gulati, Lecturer in Physical Anthropology went to Dhadgaon (Akrani) and Akkalkuwa Tehsils in Dhule District (now Nandurbar District) in Deccan College jeep with a trailer, to collect tribal artifacts, to develop a tribal museum at the Department.

In ghat section on way to Dhadgaon from Shahada, with *kutcha*, muddy roads, we saw a vehicle which had met with an accident resulting in deaths of four persons. Those were government staff who had gone on *Diwali* vacation to the plains and returning back to join their duties. They were caught in rain which made the roads very slippery. One of the injured persons was a PHC doctor at Dhadgaon whom we carried in our jeep. We had great concern and difficulty in driving the vehicle with a trailer, on the slushy and muddy road by our elderly driver, Francis. From Dhadgaon, we had to put our jeep at the service of the police and BDO for *Panchnama* and other such services. Since there was no petrol pump at Dhadgaon, we were assured of petrol by the local authorities, since we had helped them in emergency, to use our official vehicle.

We met with Shri Janardan Valvi, Ex-MLA who was the first person to start schools in that part of the tribal area. He helped us to visit the villages and houses of tribal families, including search of *'potmala'* (Big storage space between bamboo ceiling and thatched/ tiled roof) for the original tribal artefacts kept along with the paddy baskets. We collected among other things, the necklaces made of smooth micro-stones used by elderly women. In the town market we purchased the ornaments made of German silver material worn by *Bhil* and *Pawra* women. The shop-keepers told us that they sold those ornaments to tribal women at one and half times the price that they charged us, against a receipt required by us for audit.

Field Trips: Gadchiroli and Bastar

Bifurcating from a combined course of Sociology and Anthropology with a Master's degree in Sociology, the separate Post-Graduate Anthropology teaching programme was started at Pune University in July 1963. Anthropology as a field science requires the students to undertake fieldwork training in a remote tribal area. The culture shock of observing alien cultures develops objectivity and capacity to observe details of living. Since the students are expected to live with the people in the midst of village settlement, if not in the families, by "going native" they get to know the emic perspectives of the people.

The first training field excursion of the students was undertaken in the interior tribal area at Laheri village, ahead of Bhamragad in Chanda District (renamed as Chandrapur and now a part of newly created Gadchiroli District) in the last week of December 1963. We were accompanied by Shri A.V. Bodhankar, the first Chief Research Officer of the newly established Tribal Research and Training Institute (TRTI) of the Government of Maharashtra in 1962. He had his training in Anthropology at Osmania University, Hyderabad under Prof. Haimendorf.

After reaching Chanda by train from Pune, we had a Government vehicle, an old bus to take us in the interior, which had a break-down at Bhamragad. After staying overnight at forest guest house at Bhamragad, we walked down to Laheri village, about 14 kms, next day, while carrying our beds, utensils and cooking provisions in the bullock-cart. We reached the village by evening. In the village we stayed in a partially constructed single room primary school. The bamboo walls of the school had yet to be plastered with mud and cow dung, thus exposing us to cold breeze. However, there was no dearth of firewood to protect from winter. The school kids had their class in the sunlight in the compound of the school. We were quite surprised that each one of them had seen a live tiger and a bear in the neighbourhood forest. We were advised not to go too deep in the woods for open defecation for fear of wild life. Every day, early morning, we used to hear the roaring of tigers.

We were shocked to see early morning, the cattle in the open, with dew-drops on their bodies in severe winter. We were wondering why they were not in the cattle shade, until we found the families including babies, sleeping around fire in the open. We were also surprised and embarrassed to see all women topless and barely a piece of cloth covering the thighs. All men were wearing only *langoti*, a piece of cloth covering the genital and anus. There were three or four families of *Hindu Teli* (oil pressers) caste who were peasants. The Madia village headman, Gaita, visited us everyday morning for a cup of black tea. We were carrying powder milk since the tribal people did not milch their cows. According to them, as mother's milk is meant for the babies, cow's milk is meant for the calves. The Gaita never carried any water for going for field defecation, but used the tree leaves as tissue paper. He would stop for a cup of tea on way back from the morning chores.

One of the days, I went for ritual hunting with the villagers to the forest on the hill. All the tribal residents of the village including the babes in arm went for hunting. Very old persons and women in menstrual period did not go for hunting. The villagers had carried the snare-nets and spears to the forest to trap the deer. On the way, I was shown the paw-marks and dung of tiger and bear. Although deer were spotted, they could not be trapped. Simultaneously, the women were collecting the tubers, leaves of trees, skin of some trees and firewood. I thought people would be unhappy since they could not trap any deer. However, their belief was, if they got a hunt, somebody had played black magic on them which was to be mitigated by sacrificing the animal as a ritual involving the priest. Since they did not get any hunt, according to them, no black magic was played on them. At the end of the day, all men and women from the village were carrying some forest produce on their heads except me.

Among the Madia, separate huts are provided behind the main house for women in menstrual cycle to live for four days. Similar custom has been reported among the American Indians.

"Menstruating women usually occupied a separate lodge, had a special diet, and were relieved of work during their periods" (Virgil J. Vogel, 1970: 237).

Once, I asked a Madia, as to what would happen if a married woman took another lover and deserted the husband, a practice not very uncommon among the tribals, particularly if she had no baby from her husband. He said the Panchayat would resolve the matter by asking the lover to pay back a part of the bride price to the husband. On intense questioning, as to what would happen, if he did not comply, he thought, that was a hypothetical inquiry, but replied that the husband would play black magic on the defaulter and that would work, since it was to uphold the custom.

Catching field rats was quite a sport for Madia children. They would follow and frighten a fatty rat, until the rat entered a hole in the field. Then they would smoke the pit by burning pieces of small wood sticks. As the rat would come out in a dazed condition, one of the boys would catch it in a hand. The rat would be roasted on open fire to be eaten like a roasted corn.

We had carried food provisions from Chanda. However, the stock was exhausted within few days due to the visits of Government Officers with their attendants and drivers. These officers had visited the field first time which was under their jurisdiction. The Range Forest Officer (RFO) from Bhamragad managed to give us coarse rice at a price of 25 *Paisa* (four *Anas*) per kg. We collected the greens as vegetables wherever available in the field.

I also went with some tribals to another village where I was housed in *Ghotul*, a youth dormitory, also used as a guest house. I was shown the paw-marks of tiger on the village road. Apparently, the tiger had passed through the village previous night, but did not attack any animal, since according to them, he may not be hungry. They also had tied the "charmed stones" at the village boundary with the belief that the tiger spirit would not harm the villagers. We were also warned that the tiger could relax around the fire or in the open sun for warmth in the winter, particularly in the morning hours.

While entering the tribal area for Laheri, we had a brief meeting with the *Raja* (ex-King) of Aheri Shri Vishweshwarrao who also happened to be Member of Parliament. He was not favourably disposed to the construction of roads in the tribal areas since he thought those roads would be more used by the exploiters to enter the tribal area than otherwise. He was aware about the writings of Verrier Elwin whose books he had in his personal library.

On another occasion, we had a field trip at Burgi not far from Allapalli. Few days before our planned field excursion, there was a Cholera epidemic in the village with seven deaths. We were assured by the district health authorities that the village well, supplying drinking water, was thoroughly disinfected and was safe. Burgi was known for drummers, about 21 in number. We were embarrassed to ask for a drummers' performance in view of the deaths. Towards the end of our trip we hesitatingly mentioned to the village Sarpanch about this matter. He said, *"Mele Gele"* (dead are gone). As a result, drum performance was organized.

We experienced that the tribal people (Madia) maintained a social distance from the ex-untouchables (SC). We invited the Sarpanch for meals on several occasions. He agreed but never turned up. I realized that a local attendant employed by our team to fetch water from the well was an ex-untouchable. One of the days, we sent him on leave and I personally drew the water from the well. The Sarpanch came for meals on that day. On another occasion, we saw a Gram Panchayat meeting in operation under a tree. The Sarpanch was occupying a chair which had three legs and the fourth leg was formed by the bricks. The other tribal members were sitting on the string cots. The two ex-untouchable members were sitting on the stone blocks.

We had another students' field trip in Bastar in Madhya Pradesh (now Chhattisgarh) in 1977. Then, Bastar was a single district, geographically larger than the State of Kerala. Bastar is connected to Gadchiroli through Abhujmar, Kua-kodi and Laheri. There were four Conservators of Forest against a lone Deputy Director of Tribal Welfare to look after the interests of the tribals. Bastar was in the news due to the Collector, Dr. B.D. Sharma who opened a crusade against the exploitation of tribal women by the officers posted at the newly functioning iron ore mines at Kirandul, ahead of Jagdalpur, the district capital of Bastar. Dr. B.D. Sharma later became Scheduled Tribes Commissioner with Government of India and after retirement, an activist.

We decided to go to Jagdalpur *via* Visakhapatnam, by train. At the Pune Railway Station, we were informed by the railway authorities that there was no such train. After reaching Visakhapatnam, the Commercial Superintendent of the Railway informed us that there was no passenger train to Jagdalpur. However, in the goods train, carrying iron ore from Kirandul mines *via* Jagdalpur to Visakhapatnam Port, for shipping the ore to Japan, there was one passenger bogey meant for the railway staff of the small stations on the way. He was willing to allow us to use that bogey for going to Jagdalpur. While travelling, we passed through beautiful Araku valley with around hundred tunnels. Now, a passenger train has been introduced between Visakhapatnam and Jagdalpur. In Bastar we crossed the boisterous Indravati river in dug-out canoes, to reach the interior villages. We cooked food in two earthen pots, one for rice and another for chicken curry.

On another occasion, I visited Bastar as a member of a joint team of senior forest and dam irrigation officials of erstwhile Madhya Pradesh and Maharashtra, to study the possible impact of proposed hydro-electric project by Madhya Pradesh Electricity Board in Bastar, on dehabilitation of the tribal people and destruction of the *Sal* forest. The forest officials toured the would-be affected area in jeeps, to study the *Sal* trees, carrying a cook and food provisions. Although they offered the same facilities to us to visit the tribal villages, I decided to walk down a distance of twenty kilometres to reach out to the last village threatened with dehabilitation. I invited my colleague from the Pune, Department of Anthropology, Dr. B.V. Bhanu, to give me company and make a team of two members. On the way, we interacted with the tribals in several villages, to assess their reactions about the project, had meal with them and observed the interesting cock fights with baiting. Home made rice beer was available at the site of cock fights. Every single tribal at the cock fight site including children had a cock or a chic held in their arm-pit. One of the winners from a village on our way invited us for lunch at his residence.

In Bastar as also in Laheri village in Gadchiroli, there has always been a shortage problem of common salt particularly during monsoon. It was reported that the traders sold salt at the price of paddy, putting salt in one pan of the scale and paddy of equivalent weight in another. Otherwise red ants were added to vegetables or made as chutney-paste of it to eat as supplement.

On way, we came across a primary school with fourth standard classes. We were surprised to see Anganwadi age group children in class fourth. The teacher informed us that the elder siblings of these children had gone to the forest with village cattle, and the villagers had deputed these children in exchange. The village headman informed us that the teacher required students to retain his job. So, we provided him with students. We had no use of this school education.

The tribals who faced the risk of dehabilitation, in case, the hydroelectric project of Madhya Pradesh Electricity Board (MPEB) dam was constructed, were opposed to the dam. They were emotionally attached to the land, to the house and to the trees which were planted by their ancestors. When we talked to the engineers, we realized that they were not concerned about the rehabilitation issues. They were willing to compensate by cash payment. A model rehabilitation site was shown to us, erected by the contractors, by way of housing and land levelling, which was too expensive and dysfunctional, from tribal perspective. The houses were too small as compared to those erected by the tribals. We pointed out to the engineers that the tribals were capable of erecting their houses and undertake land levelling manually as a cooperative endeavour. They could be provided with wood for housing and wages, instead of giving money to contractors. Our group of forest officials and we ourselves gave a report against the construction of the dam which would have also destroyed the precious *Sal* forest. As a result of several government committees, mainly from Forest Institutes, giving reports against the project, to save the precious *Sal* forest, the hydro-electric project was called off.

Field Trips—Nandurbar District

In Akrani Mahal (Dhadgaon) in Dhule District (now Nandurbar) we had a students' field trip in 1970 helped by Shri Janardan Maharaj Valvi, the pioneer educationist of Dhadgaon. We travelled from Shahada in the plains to a distance of 20 kms in the hills on muddy road in a truck carrying the provisions of Sarvodaya Seva Mandal. We were so much with dust on us that we had to take bath in the river at Dhadgaon at 11 p.m. We camped at Jamana Ashram School of the Sarvodaya Seva Mandal about 15 kms from

Dhadgaon. We had to walk that distance with Janardan Maharaj through hills. We passed through Mundalwad, his village where his family lived in a hamlet called Maharaj Pada. In the house of his sister, we found all cooking utensils of earthen ware. On a small hill, there was a church and a school where Janardan Maharaj had his early schooling.

During a ritual festival coinciding with *Diwali,* three goats were sacrificed to propitiate their deities. As a part of the ritual the deities were worshiped by a representative of each hamlet of the village Jamana. We students with teachers were also treated as a distinct hamlet for the purpose of offering worship. The mutton was cooked in three earthen pots by the side of the river on slow fire with only turmeric and salt as spices. Surprisingly, the non-tribal manager of the Ashram School who was residing in the village for 16 years was not invited to participate in the ritual as also in the village feast. We had stayed in the village for six days, but were invited for full participation at all stages. Our two girl students were not allowed to come close to the ritual site, but were allowed to observe from a distance. At the end of the two week field tour, the entire village bid us good-bye at the village boundary visibly showing the emotions on both sides.

Some other time we participated at the famous *Holi* Festival at Kathi which was a capital of a princely State in the hills of Dhadgaon—Akkalkuva. Not less than ten to fifteen thousand *Bhils* and *Pawra* danced whole night in their respective groups bedecked with traditional ornaments, peacock feathers, *ghungroo* (small dancing bells), and non-edible musical bottle gourds, also used for carrying or drinking water. The sloping hill is used as a natural stadium at the foothill of which *Holi* pyre is ignited in the early morning. Within few minutes after the ritual fire is ignited, the entire crowd disappears very peacefully. There are shops of petty traders selling trinkets and small oranges to quench the thirst of water whole night. It is noteworthy that not a single policeman is required to organize the crowds. There are no complaints of any stealing or molestation. When our project of Adivasi Utthan Karyakram was started, we provided drinking water to all the people free of cost by hiring water tankers. People were surprised that all the previous years, neither the government nor elected representatives thought of providing drinking water to people.

During our first visit to Dhadgaon in 1962, there was not a

single shop in the town. There was an old lady who was providing food in her house for the government personnel who were posted in Dhadgaon and lived singly. We could get our food, i.e. *Jwari Bhakar* and *Pithala* (cooked gram floor) for Re 1. After about 40 years, we found a regular market with several shops and roadside food stalls. One of the food stalls is owned by the grandson of the old lady. When asked about the nature of change during forty years, people said, "there used to be a weekly market in 1962, now there is a daily market with several shops". Custard apple is a forest fruit and is collected and sold to the traders in the planes. *Chironji* (charoli) a dry fruit is a cash crop available in the forest which need to be grown on a big scale. The commonest prevalent diseases are Goiter and Sickle cell anaemia.

During the first field trip of the students of School of Health Sciences of Pune University in Ranipur village, during January 1995, there were three child deaths in about ten days. During the preceding two years, 39 children died in the village, of which 11 were neonatal deaths and 4 in the age group of 1-6 years. Common causes of reported deaths were diarrohea, dysentery, measles and malaria. During 1994 about 9 per cent deliveries were conducted by a doctor and the rest were conducted by a *dai,* usually in the kitchen. It has been a common practice that if a baby during birthing did not cry, umbilical cord was touched to a hot *Tawa* (iron pan), which made the baby cry. The *Vaidu* in Ranipur had good knowledge of the herbal medicinal plants in the nearby forest. For improving lactation, 5 *laddus* (balls) made of roasted earthworm mixed with wheat flour, ground nut, fenugreek seeds, millet-*Bajra* (all roasted), sugar and edible oil were given to a new mother.

Janardan Maharaj was greatly respected by one and all. Many tribal leaders have been the students trained in his schools. The school at Dhadgaon has now become a degree college affiliated to a university. We had several field trips in Dhadgaon-Akkalkua region facilitated by Janardan Maharaj. I always stayed with him during field trips for AUK work. If he was alone visiting Pune, he stayed with me on the university campus. He was also the President of MAAS for ten years.

As per custom, he paid the bride price to brides' families for his two sons' marriages. The male and female doctors at the Dhadgaon PHC were a tribal couple. The male doctor had paid the bride price for his marriage to the lady doctor.

Field Trips—Palghar District

I had my first visit to Mokhada in 1970, immediately after *Holi* at the festival of colours, *Rangpanchami* in Thane (now Palghar) District, which continues to be one of the most backward taluks in Maharashtra. On the next day, the taluka town of Mokhada was full of crowds to witness *Bhovada* whereby there were processions depicting scenes from Hindu mythology showing ten *'avatars'* (incarnations) of Hindu God. There are prominent scenes from *Ramayana* showing the abduction of Sita and Ram-Ravana war. The *Bhovada* is later enacted in several villages by local actors. *'Bhovada'* is a classic example of great tradition getting transmitted as little tradition.

The interior villages in Mokhada had a Primary Health Centre (PHC) at Sakharshet. On several occasions I stayed at Kortad village which was headed by a dynamic tribal leader Sonu Kondu Govind popularly known as Sonu Patil belonging to *Thakar* tribe. He was a prosperous farmer growing paddy on irrigated land which originally belonged to a Parsi (Zoroastrian). He had a two storied house in which I stayed. Senior villagers keep on reminding that I was the first outsider to visit and live in the village. Subsequently, we had several students field trips in the villages in the neighbourhood facilitated by Sonu Patil. He and both his sons had two wives each, which is a sign of prosperity, since bride price had to be paid in each case. The labour intensive economy required more manpower in case of ownership of more cultivable land. Bride price has been rationalised as a consideration to bride's father losing working hands, according to some anthropologists. While Sonu Patil's son married second time, son's first wife went to her parents in protest. On inquiry, I was told that she had expected a marriage present of a good saree, as a token compensation for bringing a co-wife. During my trips to Kortad, I always stayed with the family.

Later, Sonu Patil became the chairman of the social welfare committee of Thane Zilla Parishad (Z.P.) and had an official ambassador car. After him, his daughter-in-law became the chairman of Mother-Child Welfare Committee of Thane Z.P.

There was a Saturday weekly market, couple of kilometres from Kortad, where we could see an old woman selling three brinjals or two-three fish on a leaf for barter sell. Sonu Patil showed me at a shop in a nearby town as to how the tribals were exploited. A woman would come with some millet such as *Ragi* (*nachani-nagali*), *Varai* on her head in a piece of cloth, give it to the trader and asked for some salt or chilli powder or turmeric which she required. There was no consideration or discussion about the cost of her grain or of what she purchased. We have seen a tribal walking five kilometres to a weekly market to purchase two tablespoonful of edible oil. At Daskot village, we saw the tribals leaving their cattle in a nearby forest on the hill during entire summer. They would bring them back only after the onset of monsoon.

We found a tribal with a hurt shoulder due to a branch of a tree fallen on his shoulder. I offered him to bring the PHC doctor from a distance of couple of kms. to treat him. However, he sent a message to an old tribal *Vaidu* in the next village to treat him. We found the *Vaidu* making cuts at the shoulder with a blade. He fixed a horn of a cow/bullock with a hole, sucked the blue blood and sealed the horn with tar for some time. After removing the horn, the oozing blue-greenish blood was removed. The tribal fully recovered and joined the youth dance next day evening.

During our stay, there was a case of molestation of a tribal (*Thakar*) girl by a petty trader commonly known as *Kachhi* (from Kutch area) in Jawhar area. Sonu Patil got a pamphlet printed asking the people of the area to organize a *Morcha* (rally) in Jawhar town to protest molestation of *Thakar* girl. I advised him to replace the word '*Adivasi*' in place of '*Thakar*' since only *Thakar* community was likely to participate in *Morcha*. With this change there was a huge *Morcha* of not less than a thousand *Adivasis* with sticks and axes on their shoulders. The police officials invited Sonu Patil for talks at the police station in Jawhar leaving the *Morcha*. I advised him that he could send the local educated tribal MLA for talks since Sonu Patil's absence could disrupt the *Morcha*. Some persons also shouted slogans such as *Pakistan Zindabad* obviously to disrupt the *Morcha*. *Morcha* ended in the meeting in the nearby Mango grove.

In village Kortad, there has been a shrine and the wooden idol with the facial shape of a calf male buffalo which is called Kodtoba. A separate bamboo structure with tiles has been created around Kodtoba. Once a year, there is a *Jatra* (religious fair) at the site. All families in the village contribute for the festival. Since we were living in the village, with our students on field trip, we requested to be treated as a distinct family and contribute our donation. In earlier days, a *Redka* (small male buffalo) was sacrificed on this occasion. However, the goat has been replaced for *Redka*. Other food items include rice, millet *bhakari* and greens from the forest. For each family, a leaf of a tree is laid on the ground. On each leaf, a portion of each food product is kept. The parts of the sacrificial goat are evenly distributed. This is one visible example of the cooperative life of the tribal people. We also received a number of such leaves since we were large in number than a normal family.

We witnessed *Jagran* (whole night vigil) in the house of the priest of Kodtaba shrine to propitiate the evil spirits to treat his ailing son, who was on the lap of the father whole night. There were too many people in a small hut, full of smoke. The child died after few days.

In a village Daskot in the neighbourhood of Kortad, the tribals leave their cattle to graze on the hill forest in summer and collect them back at the onset of monsoon. There is no wild life in that area.

This area though in close proximity to Jawhar town was a part of Mokhada taluka. After the construction of road linking Sakharshet (having a PHC) to the villages, Vavar and Vangni up the hills, 135 children from these villages perished in an epidemic of measles. The Chief Minister of Maharashtra visited these villages and annexed this area to Jawhar taluka.

At Suryamal village in Mokhada, Mangibai *Thakar* woman did bone setting on sheep, cattle and humans. She would use a bamboo stick and tie the bones after setting and would also give internal medicine for which she charged Rs. 10 per case. Patients from nearby non-tribal urban areas also came for treatment.

At least one member from 50-70 per cent families migrated for work during November to March. Returning briefly for marriage season, they would migrate again to return back during monsoon. During November 1976, we organised a fieldwork training workshop in Chalatwad area of about 40 college teachers in social sciences from all over Maharashtra about collecting primary data on education. The data was analysed in the field and presented in a seminar at Jawhar town in the neighbourhood, attended by some of the tribal villagers. Prin Dabholkar, Vice-Chancellor of Pune University, Prof. I.P. Desai, a prominent sociologist from Surat and Prof. G.B. Sardar, a respected thinker in Maharashtra were present.

Other Field Issues

In village Junuthi in Peth Tehsil of Nasik District, I found Aware-Guruji discussing about 600 medicinal plants with two other herbalists (*Vaidu*) and their actual site in the neighbourhood. At a village dominated by CPM, the villagers remarked that horticulture projects which required more irrigation put additional burden on women since they had to fetch water from the river in pots to irrigate the plants.

In all our students' field trips, we carried the milk powder for making tea since the tribals did not milch their cows. They expressed "Mother's milk is meant for the babies and cow's milk for the calves". When we found a tribal having a cow and a bull used for ploughing, we expressed surprise at the cow being used. The tribal expressed "when my wife works on the field why not the cow?"

There is no doubt an issue about the spirit world. Once we had a chance to occupy a newly constructed hut since it was abandoned due to the death of the owner, surmising that the hut was under the influence of evil spirit. Another example relates to a village which was electrified, that means some bulbs were put as street lights by the electricity board. When I asked the tribals, as to what change it brought, they said, "the spirits and ghosts had disappeared".

We find in the tribal villages some houses are abandoned since it was believed that the evil spirits were responsible for tragedies in the house. Even in the mainstream Hindu society, *Vastu Shanti* is performed with the belief that the *Vastupurush* would provide protection and prosperity to the family occupying the house.

In case of epidemics, all the tribal villagers go out of the village and stay in a forest for a few days or outside the village and come back after performing some rituals ending in a formal village feast at the site.

In Amravati District, in Dharani Block in the villages close to Tiger Reserve, there used to be instances when the tiger would lift the cattle from the villages for which the government had agreed to pay compensation. On one occasion, the Governor of the State who happened to visit the Chikhaldara Reserved Forest area also visited Dharani and offered few gunny bags full of rice to villagers from one affected village. The villagers insisted that there were four villages which were affected and as such, the rice should be distributed in four villages. Since the government did not comply with the wishes of the people, after Governor's exit, the villagers invited their peers from other three villages and redistributed the rice given to them.

At Dharani fieldwork, we invited the district level officers to interact with the students after presenting the data from a single village. They were expected to relate the village data with the district level aggregate data to understand the ground level reality.

Field Trips—Odisha

During fieldwork in Odisha in Raygada District among the Dongariya and Kutia Konds, the stark difference between the two communities became visible. All the children among Kutia Konds had bloated bellies obviously showing the degree of malnutrition. Shifting cultivation called *'Podu'* was followed by burning the land patches in the forest. Eighteen kinds of crops were grown on this acquired land and the produce was distributed equally among all the families, including for the old women, who could not participate in the agricultural activities. Dongariya Kond Development Authority (DKDA) promoted the cultivation of horticulture such as banana and pineapple, and cash crops like ginger and turmeric. However, the marketing of these products was done by the Scheduled Caste Communities staying in the area, thereby earning more prosperity than the Scheduled Tribes, which was obvious from the material goods in their respective houses.

It was a sight in tribal villages in the hills to see all houses taking electricity from the main wires by putting hooks on it, obviously without official electric connections. There were mobile PDS vans for which the tribals kept on waiting for hours together.

Fieldwork was undertaken in Daringwadi, Tumdibandh and Belghar among the Desia Kond, Dongariya Kond and Kutia Kond. We could see trees of mango, jackfruit, bamboo, cashew nuts, *mahua*; guava and turmeric. The Dongariya Kond Development Authority has allowed the tribals to use revenue and forest lands for horticulture development.

Field Visits for Adjudication

Besides anthropology student's fieldwork training excursions, I had occasions to undertake fieldwork for adjudicating the issues of pseudo-tribals claiming ST status as per Article 342 of the Constitution of India. Prominent among them has been the Halba–Halba Koshti dispute whereby the Halba Koshti, a sub-caste of weaver Koshti caste were claiming to be Halba ST, in Vidarbha region of Maharashtra. The clan structure, life cycle rituals, deities, pilgrimage centres, ceremonies and festivals, of both the communities are so widely divergent. The female clan/phratry deities of Halba are kept in earthen pitchers while the Halba Koshti temples have prominent masonry structure with all the regalia that is seen in Hindu temples. Some of the deities of Halba, like Thakurdeo, Dagadideo, Jungledeo and Shikaridevi are located in the fields and worshiped after the harvest.

Another prominent dispute has been about the Gowaries, the grazing caste in Vidarbha claiming to be Gond Gowaries who are enlisted as ST. It is said that the Gowaries who were grazing the cattle of ruling Gonds had live-in relations with the Gonds, in historical times, which gave rise to the sub-tribe Gond Gowaries. They continue to live in the vicinity of Gonds. The women from the three communities, that is Gonds, Gowaries and Gond Gowaries showed us the different pattern of their *pallu of sarees* covering the head. The issue became prominent since 125 Gowari, mainly women and children died in stampede in front of the legislative assembly (Vidhan Sabha) at Nagpur while they had participated in a procession to claim the Gond Gowari status.

Currently, the Jarawas in Andaman islands have been in the international media. The tourist companies were seen taking the tourists to Jarawa reserves to show them the Jarawas as normally the children are taken to zoo to show the animals. There have been cases of sexual exploitation of the Jarawas. The Jarawa seem to be the living exhibits about the symbiosis with nature. The Supreme Court of India and the British Government banned such tourist activity in the Jarawa reserves. The Jarawa probably provide us with an example of how the human communities lived in ancient times, from where the social and cultural evolution has developed from hunting, collecting, pastoral stage to river valley agricultural civilizations. *Mahabharata* provides an example of prosperous pastoral society. There are no references to crops and agriculture in *Mahabharata*, save a plough as a weapon of Balram, Lord Krishna's brother.

To summarize, the tribal communities are distinct from the mainstream caste—Hindu peasantry. This has been recognized in the Constitution of India. There are affirmative clauses in the Constitution to bring them up to the level of other people using the principle of Equity. There is a separate tribal sub-plan, a distinct Tribal Development Department and special powers to the Governor of the State to take appropriate decisions, if needed, by superimposing the decisions of the respective State Governments.

We have to understand the issues of tribal health and malnourishment in the context of distinct tribal cultures, their relationship with the environment, and governance by the State.

In Maharashtra, the tribal problem is about large scale migration of the tribal people to earn their livelihood during summer. In Odisha main problem is about shifting cultivation, i.e. migration of plantation.

Summing up

Fieldwork tradition is important in anthropology. Comparative method enjoins cross-cultural field excursions to understand the universals and variations in different cultures. The macro decisions about tribal development schemes are counter-productive, which are based on etic perspectives. No schemes could be successful without community involvement and community management. Understanding of emic perspectives, therefore, is of prime importance for micro-planning and effective implementation. It helps to understand the concerns and issues of different ethnic tribal groups. Tribal health and malnutrition may be a general tribal issue. We cannot generalise that all ethnic tribal groups have the same proportion of malnutrition, across the country or in all tribe dominant regions of the State. Field investigation is, therefore, required to devise area and tribe specific schemes for health and development.

Chapter 4
Tribal Health and Development: Maharashtra

"Medicine and public health do not develop or function in a social void. They provide the social adaptive mechanisms that complement the biological adaptive responses to the conditions of life at a given time. They can fulfil their purpose, to improve the people's health, only if they are fitted to the needs and resources of the community as well as to the special conditions created by the total environment" (Rene Dubos, 1965: 456).

Introduction

Maharashtra State was formed on May 1, 1960. In Maharashtra, the Tribal Welfare Department was separated from the Social Welfare Department in 1975-76, while Dr. V.B. Mandlekar was appointed Secretary-*cum*-Tribal Commissioner to head the Department. He accepted to be the first President of Maharashtra Association of Anthropological Sciences, the NGO who with CRHP developed a model for addressing issues of tribal child nutrition presented in Chapter 5. The Tribal Research and Training Institute of the State Government was established in 1962 with a Chief Research Officer working under the Director, Social Welfare. Tribal Development was a part of the Community Development Programme with some multipurpose Tribal Development Blocks forming part of the programme. One of the major hurdles in tribal development and the sore point for the people has been the deteriorating relationship of tribal people with the forest department. The common portfolio of forest and tribal welfare under a single Minister did not improve the relationship. Cultivation of forest lands by tribals has been labelled as 'encroachment' and has been the major source of agitation by the tribals.

Maharashtra has the second largest Scheduled Tribe population in India, totalling about 9 per cent of the total ST population, next to Madhya Pradesh. In 2011, the ST population was 10.5 million constituting 9.35 per cent of the total population of the State; while it was 8.85 per cent in 2001. The decadal growth of ST raises the doubts about pseudo-tribals procuring ST certificates. As can be seen from the map of Maharashtra, tribal areas constitute the border areas of the State on the boundaries of Gujarat, Madhya Pradesh, Chhattisgarh and Andhra Pradesh (undivided). There are 47 tribal groups, the major ones being the Bhil, Gond, Mahadeo Koli, Kokana Pawra, *Thakar* and Warli. Katkari, Maria Gond and Kolam are the three Particularly Vulnerable Tribal Groups (PVTG, earlier PTG).

Tribal Areas : Redeeming the Promise

"The tribal people constitute the most deprived and neglected section of the population in the State. Broadly, they live in three inaccessible hilly and remote forest regions of the State; in the Sahyadris, the Satpudas and Eastern Gondwana. Prominent in the Sahyadri group are Mahadeo Koli, Kokna, Varli, *Thakar,* Katkari, Malhar Koli and Dhor Koli. Satpuda group is dominated by Bhil and Korku, while Gondwana group has preponderance of Gonds, Andh, Kolam and Halba. Anthropological literature and *Maharashtra State Gazetteers* (Karve, 1968) mention Andh, Mahadeo Koli and Kokna, as numerically preponderant Scheduled Tribes sharing several similarities with the Kunbi caste. *Bhil* and *Gond* tribal groups are also spread over in the neighbouring states such as *Bhil* in Gujarat and Rajasthan and *Gond* in Madhya Pradesh, Chhattisgarh, Andhra Pradesh and Orissa."

"These habitats fall along the periphery of the State. The deprivation of tribal people thus starts with geographic marginalization. Secondly, the communities are scattered in 15 districts and more than 80 talukas. Though they have inhabited these contiguous tracts historically, in the recent years they have become a minority in several of these areas. Thirdly, the marginalization and exploitation of tribal people has historical links. During the colonial period, the British deprived them of their ancestral domains and forest rights. After independence, although, the Constitution of India provided various safe-guards and guarantees, the tribals were victims of administrative neglect and exploitation by non-tribal people. Fourth, their culture and languages are threatened by the modern urban-industrial juggernaut" (Kelkar Committee Report, 2015: 209).

The tribal communities in India are commonly understood as forest dwelling or people living in the hills. There are references to tribal communities even in the mythological scriptures, *Ramayana* and *Mahabharata*. The most common term used for these communities is *Adivasi*, which literally means original inhabitants or dwellers of the land, which is objected to by those who prefer to call them *Vanvasi*, meaning dwellers of forest. Other terms such as *Adim Jati* and *Girijan* were also discussed in the Constituent Assembly debates before Independence.

According to Article 342 in the Constitution of India, the Scheduled Tribes are "the tribes or tribal communities or parts of or groups within tribes or tribal communities", which the President may specify by public notification. Parliament has the Constitutional authority to include or exclude from the list of Scheduled Tribes, specified in the notification, any tribe or tribal community thereof. For the purpose of Article 342, for a group to be included as Scheduled Tribe, Government of India has recommended the following broad parameters: (a) Primitive traits, (b) Distinct culture, (c) Geographical isolation, (d) Distinct dialect, (e) Animism, (f) Clan system, (g) Shyness of nature, and (h) Backwardness. These parameters conform to the characteristic features of a typical or theoretically ideal tribal society (also referred to as ideal folk society) described by anthropologists on the basis of sustained studies of tribal communities all over the world.

Due to geographical isolation for ages and experience of exploitation by outsiders, tribal communities have lived in protective shells becoming timid, shy and non-communicative with the outsiders. In consequence, they have remained in relative "time-freeze" and backward from our perspective. They have historically lived in a symbiotic relationship with the environment and developed coping mechanisms to meet with any distress as a cooperative community. Backwardness of tribal people has to be understood in terms of lack of motivation and vision to seize the existing opportunities of development, let alone demand them or lobby for capturing them in the democratic political set up. Operationally, this signifies a lack of capacity to utilize the development infrastructure facilities to improve their quality of life.

A benchmark survey carried out by the Tribal Research and Training Institute (TRTI), (Government of Maharashtra, 2000) generated data about village and hamlet population, road connectivity, distance of public amenities from villages and hamlets, land use in relation to forest areas, landholding and landlessness, migration, and beneficiaries of government schemes. The data indicate that there are not enough anganwadis, schools, ashram schools, primary health centres (PHC) and sub-centres in tribal districts and blocks, which reduces the physical accessibility of these institutions to the people. Many positions in these institutions also continue to be vacant and there is marginal use of these facilities by the people. Health care facilities and other infrastructure facilities in tribal areas need not be located according to population norm, but according to the time and distance required for the tribals to access it, with the use of locally available public transport or on foot.

The major health concerns of tribal communities are infant and child mortality and malnutrition. These problems persist despite the institutions and personnel such as the anganwadi, primary health centres, sub-centres, pada workers and now ASHA. As per the benchmark survey carried out by the TRTI, a majority of tribal people in Maharashtra are in the below poverty line (BPL) category. Food security is a major concern among tribal people, with the most deprived not having the means to utilise the public distribution system even under subsidized BPL rates. Schemes such as the Nav Sanjeevan Yojana and Matrutva Anudan Yojana do not show any visible impact. The techno-centric solution of admitting the children in Grade III and Grade IV on the anganwadi scale to PHCs would fail to provide a lasting solution to malnutrition and mortality, as the same children could revert back to severe malnutrition once they are discharged from the PHC.

Given the low age at marriage, there needs to be a focus on

addressing the health of adolescent girls who would become mothers within few years. The special nutrition needs of pregnant and lactating mothers also need to be addressed. Livelihood opportunities need to be provided nearer their homes, which would prevent seasonal migration. This could be by way of work such as developing nurseries or kitchen gardens in a scheme such as EGS or MNREGA. The sex-ratio in tribal communities is known to be in favour of women, which reflects a better status for tribal women as compared to women in caste peasant communities. There is no female infanticide or foeticide in tribal communities, which is probably due to practice of bride price and the value of female labour in the household production activities.

Malnutrition and Child Health amongst Tribals in Maharashtra: A Case Study

To investigate and study the causes of persistent malnutrition amongst children, especially tribal children, in Maharashtra, an in-depth analysis of the impact of the socio-cultural and economic environment of tribals on the nutritional status and health of children was carried out by Sonowal (2010). Some of the main inferences from this study which have important policy lessons are highlighted here. The loss of right to access forests and forest produce (fruits, green shoots, tubers etc., which are the main source of natural nutrients for tribals) and the degradation of forest land coupled with rising population have led to changes in the dietary composition of tribals as well as their economic condition. Seasonal migration of tribal families to neighbouring states such as Gujarat for wage labour is found to have a debilitating effect on the health and nutritional status of tribal children. The study clearly states that the number of households with malnourished children increases sharply when wage labour is the primary source of income. With both parents working, the smaller children and babies are found to be exposed to dust, heat, insects and dirt. Breastfed babies are reported to be more prone to infections and illness as mothers are unable to feed them often whilst working. The study reports a strong negative relationship between mother's work participation and a child's health and nutrition, which is an important finding as it is contrary to general belief that higher family incomes should lead to better child health. Female literacy, age at marriage, small gap between two births and poor diets of pregnant mothers are found to have an important bearing on children's health and nutrition. The study finds that low female literacy amongst tribals (as low as 21% in Gadchiroli for the sample households studied) could be a possible reason for programmes related to health awareness not being very successful. With as many as 80 per cent of girls getting married before the age of 17 in the households surveyed, and subsequent early pregnancies, the study finds a negative relationship between age at marriage and child malnourishment. The close relation between the treatment of diseases and the socio-cultural perceptions of tribals influences the extent of health care availed by them. Reasons found for the low utilization of available PHC facilities for antenatal care and childbirth practices include long distances from PHCs and the inability to rush expectant mothers there, loss in household work and wages due to regular visits required to PHCs, the need to stay away from home when engaging in contract work even during pregnancy and the need to observe some religious rites during pregnancy and delivery (MHDR, 2012: 100).

Anganwadi and Ashram School

Anganwadi is an important institution in tribal areas. It, however, attracts children above three years of age while the real problem of mortality and malnutrition is up to the age of two years. Unless the mothers of children upto two years are drawn to anganwadi and are provided with home based supplementation for improving the lactation, anganwadi will continue to be the balwadi of yesteryears. Anganwadi could be developed as a nodal institution for women and children's health care under the management of women members of village Gram Panchayat. Anganwadi should function for the whole day as a nodal centre for women and children focusing on health, pre-school and adult education and as child care centre. Every hamlet must have a mini-anganwadi with a local woman, even if illiterate, to serve as *Sevika*. Anganwadi should be brought under the purview of Gram Panchayat, so that local monitoring would be effective.

The traditional herbalists (*Vaidu*) who have good knowledge of herbal medicine and the traditional *dais*, who provide health services to the people need to be trained for up scaling their knowledge and skills. At the local level, the functionaries in the public sector and the traditional sector are ANM at the sub-centre, anganwadi worker, pada health worker, ASHA, Gram Panchayat members, *patwari/talathi*, forest guard, teachers, *dai*, *bhagat* and *vaidu*, and educated youth seeking work and employment. Their capacity building to work with the local community would go a long way in addressing issues of human development. As a confidence building activity the government needs to reach out to the people to address their concerns of morbidity, infant mortality and starvation at their doorstep.

The educational levels of tribal people are known to be much lower compared to the average educational levels in society. The aim of education imparted in tribal areas should be to transform the traditional, inward looking people into an outward looking confident community ready to compete with the non-tribal, caste-peasantry neighbourhood in accessing and demanding the development infrastructure offered by tribal sub-plan. The perceptions regarding education among tribal people are directly linked to their livelihood concerns. It is, therefore, necessary to include vocational education in the curriculum after the primary school stage itself. Education is looked upon as an instrument of getting a job and ensuring a fixed monthly income through the mechanism of reservation. Entry into industrial training institutes (ITIs) requires completion of matriculation, however, many tribal children fail to complete their matriculation. As a result it is often observed that benefits meant for tribal children after matriculation in institutions such as ITIs are not utilized by genuine tribals but by pseudo tribals or non-tribals. Unless vocational courses are introduced at the completion of primary school, tribal children may not be able to get the advantage of growth in service sector.

In tribal areas, ashram school is an important institution for education, personality development, and for acquiring skills useful for livelihood. The purpose of ashram schools in tribal areas should be viewed differently from that of conventional schools in the mainstream society. The ashram school needs to be viewed as one of the nodal institutions for tribal development, rather than only performing the functions of a conventional school. Wandrekar Committee in 1949 had made recommendations about the establishment of residential ashram schools. The ashram schools are expected to possess at least eleven acres of cultivable land for training in agriculture, however, this is rarely observed in practice.

It is observed that there is tremendous disparity in the infrastructure of ashram schools managed by voluntary institutions, which are perennially starved of grants receivable from the government, and those ashram schools managed under the Integrated Tribal Development Project (ITDP). It is also observed that in ashram schools, food sometimes gets ascendancy over quality of education. One of the major functions of the Project Officer of ITDP on the ground appears to be to supervise the ashram schools. However, there also needs to be local participation of Panchayati Raj Institutions (PRIs) in the affairs of the schools. Ashram school can be developed as an information centre to facilitate the utilisation of government schemes by the people who are unaware of the schemes, and how to benefit from them, which requires paper work and documentation to be completed.

Education of tribal girls and female illiteracy provides a dismal picture. Adolescent girls require sanitation facilities and sex security for their schooling whether in the day schools or in ashram schools. Girls require special training in maternity and reproductive practices and knowledge of child rearing to prevent child mortality and malnutrition. They also need special training in nutrition and food processing. A mini-curriculum to meet these needs could be developed for girls.

Cultural identity expressed through folk literature, folk songs, dance and traditional youth institutions through '*ghotuls*' as among the Madia Gond provide self-esteem and self-confidence. Ashram schools could foster these identity parameters. *Ghotul* is an excellent traditional youth club not only for dance, music and fellowship but for taking the responsibilities of development in tribal villages. Similarly, among the Kolam in Yavatmal, identity is expressed through a common meeting place '*chawdi*', which distinguishes them from Gonds living in the same village.

Ashram school and anganwadi are the important functioning institutions in tribal areas. These institutions should address the multiple dimensions of tribal development and need to be strengthened as nodal agencies of development at hamlet and village level.

Livelihood

The issues of tribal livelihoods are inseparably linked to land-forest issues. In tribal belts much of the land, as in the most backward Dhadgaon and Akkalkuwa talukas in Nandurbar district, is under the ownership of Forest Department. This kind of ownership does not signify that the forest land has tree cover on it. Much of the land is also probably under inferior cultivation of the tribal people due to low quality of land, but is labelled as encroachment, which leads to disputes between the people and the government.

Although the Forest Rights Act has been promulgated, there seems to be primacy on individual rights as compared to community forest rights. It is reported from the field that the forest department in Maharashtra is reluctant to accept the ownership of *gram sabha* over minor forest produce, especially the bamboo and *tendu* leaves. Forest department is supposed to help the *gram sabha* in preparing bye laws and work plans in respect of community forest rights. The need to restructure the joint forest management committees in Maharashtra is being emphasized at the level of Ministry of Environment and Forests, Government of India.

As collectors of food from forest, the tribals have traditionally not shown primary interest in land as a productive asset, as a property. However, in view of regulatory use of forest limiting the use of forest resources by tribals and in view of acquisition of tribal lands by non-tribals, there have been several legislations to safeguard the interest of backward communities in land. The Bombay Land Revenue Code, 1879 as Amended in 1901 prohibited transfer of land in certain tracts or villages without the permission of the Collector. Maharashtra Land Revenue Code, 1966 prohibited transfer of tribal land to non-tribals. However, since the tribals are unaware of these legislations they do not appeal for restoration of their land rights and the land continues to get transferred due to loopholes in such legislations. Subsequently, the Maharashtra Land Revenue Code and Tenancy Laws and the Maharashtra Restoration of Lands to Scheduled Tribes Act, 1974 were promulgated. However, in spite of such legislations, tribal land continues to get transferred on a large scale for developing hill stations or farm houses etc., since proactive action by the revenue officials is not taken. Tribal lands around the mega city like Mumbai are usurped by builders declaring the tribals as non-tribals.

Tribal people have been the worst affected due to development induced displacement and the process of economic globalization. Due to hilly terrain in some tribal belts, construction of dams in such areas is considered as cost effective and useful. However, several tribal villages get inundated in the process, although the tribal communities do not receive water for irrigation nor hydro-electricity. It is common experience that the rehabilitation of displaced families does not take place to the satisfaction of dehabilitated people. There is a tendency to compensate in one time cash payment, which does not address the concerns of sustainable livelihood of the tribal people. If the tribals are resettled outside the Scheduled Area, they do not get the benefits meant for Scheduled Area.

Hill stations for the neo-rich are also being constructed on tribal lands circumventing the prevention of land alienation laws. The SEZs are not coming up exclusively in tribal areas, but due to scarce population, tribal areas are often more preferred sites. It is now obligatory to get environment impact assessment done by the Ministry of Environment and Forests of the Government of India and obtain clearance. However, keeping in view the social and cultural impact on the communities, Ministry of Culture, Government of India, is in the process of finalizing a social and cultural impact assessment module with the assistance of Anthropological Survey of India.

The communities who own land and are engaged in agricultural operations for a major part of the year are relatively better off as compared to marginal cultivators or the landless. However, mere ownership of land on paper is not a reliable indicator of economic level in tribal areas due to hilly terrains and uncultivable land. Seasonal migration to work on brick kilns, construction sites and as agricultural labour are the only alternatives for the landless and marginal land holders. The Bharatiya Agro Industries Foundation (BAIF) has successfully demonstrated through its 'Wadi' project that horticulture could reduce migration considerably. Innovative programmes like medicinal plant cultivation, processing of locally available fruits like mango, custard apple, *amla* could provide livelihood in tribal areas. As mentioned earlier, livelihood schemes for women could be located in the village itself or around the house, including development of nursery and kitchen garden. The PRI will have to be given authority to facilitate these programmes.

Khadi Village Industries Commission (KVIC) and Boards need to play a proactive role in providing work to tribal people. No serious attempt has been made to the use of amber charkha in tribal pockets, as a vocation. Honey, minor forest produce, processed fruits and dry fruits are some of the areas which KVIC could promote in collaboration with NABARD. For sanitation, soap making is another skill, which could be taken up by tribal SHGs.

There are differences in socio-economic level among Scheduled Tribe communities. Ethnic groups such as Kokna, Mahadeo Koli, Raj Gond seem to be relatively better off as compared to other tribal communities. The Katkaris in Raigad and Thane districts, the Kolams in Yavatmal and Nanded districts and the Madia Gonds in the Bhamragad area of Gadchiroli district have been declared as "primitive tribal groups (PTGs)" or "particularly vulnerable tribal groups (PVTGs)" by the government and special central assistance is sanctioned every year by the Central Government for their development. Among these, the Katkari are a predominantly landless community and are probably the most deprived ethnic group even within the PTG category in Maharashtra.

Health Concerns of Tribals

A Case Study of the Katkari Tribe

"Inclusive growth and human development needs to address the multiple dimensions of deprivation faced by primitive tribal communities. R.K. Mutatkar (2007) details in his case study of the Katkari tribe (Jawhar block, Thane district) the various constraints faced by this socially backward tribal community in accessing health care. The Katkaris are regarded as the lowest in the social hierarchy among the ST ethnic groups and the demographic composition of the village they live in shows their hamlets to be excluded, with limited interaction with other groups. The living conditions of the Katkari are found to be very simple and minimal, comprising either *pucca* dwellings or *kutcha* houses constructed through government schemes, with no sanitation facilities in their hamlets and dependence on wells or public taps for drinking water.

They are mainly landless, and dependent largely on wage labour for their livelihoods. Seasonal migration along with women and children is found to take place between the cultivation and harvesting seasons and in the post-agricultural season. Their food consumption patterns highlight the extreme deprivation faced by them. Food purchases are made in piecemeal quantities just before every meal. The Katkaris depend mainly on the public distribution system for food grains. To cope with food shortages they resort to liquefying and grinding the food, consuming wildly grown food or borrowing food. Anthropometric indicators reveal severe under nourishment among Katkari children (aged 0–6 years). Morbidity is found to be the highest in the monsoon period, which is also the agricultural season when absence from work due to any illness results in loss of daily wages. Work-related injuries due to labour-intensive stone breaking also lead to a vicious cycle of ill health and loss of wages. There are no health-care facilities in the region studied, especially in terms of specialized care for women and children" (MHDR, 2012: 93-94).

Pseudo-Tribalism

The decadal growth rate of Scheduled Tribe population in Maharashtra and of certain Scheduled Tribe communities seems to indicate that the growth is not as a result of biological growth alone, but due to a large number of pseudo-tribals claiming Scheduled Tribe status successfully. The claims by non-tribal communities claiming Scheduled Tribe status citing similarity in nomenclature with minor variations in suffixes or affixes has led to the appointment of many expert committees by the State Government to ascertain these claims and make recommendations. Tribal certificates are required by aspirants who want to get entry in higher educational or technical educational institutions as also public sector jobs by getting the constitutional benefits of reservations for Scheduled Tribes. The Tribal Research and Training Institute has been reduced to an appellate authority for validation and issuance of tribal certificates, to the detriment of not being able to focus on development research issues of tribal people.

Pseudo-Tribalism has largely increased after the "area restriction" about tribal affinity was withdrawn. The major claims and disputes in Maharashtra with regard to false claims have been about Halba-Halba Koshti, Govari-Gond Govari and Koli-Mahadeo Koli. The expert committees in this regard made recommendations to reject the false claims. There have been mobilized efforts by communities to claim Scheduled Tribe status. For example, it is documented that the Halba-Koshti organisations had issued a circular to all members of the community to report themselves as Halba Scheduled Tribe to the census enumerators. It is common knowledge as was reported in the media that in an unfortunate incident in 1994, more than 100 people, mostly women and children, from the Govari community, had perished in a stampede at Nagpur where they had travelled from rural areas in large numbers to claim Gond-Govari Scheduled Tribe status during the State Assembly session.

Those pseudo-tribals who are successful in getting the Scheduled Tribe status are depriving the genuine backward tribals from getting the benefits of reservation in education and public employment. The pseudo-tribal issue has also been in the limelight in other states. For example, the Gujjars in Rajasthan have been staking their claims to be labelled as Scheduled Tribe citing the examples of the Meena in Rajasthan, who are enumerated as Scheduled Tribe.

Tribal Development

Dr. Verrier Elwin in his report in 1960 on special multipurpose tribal blocks acknowledged Nehru's Five Fundamental Principles —"*Panchsheel*" as providing the basis of what should be the government's policy approach to tribal development.

1. People should develop along the lines of their own genius and we should avoid imposing anything on them. We should try to encourage in every way their own traditional arts and culture.
2. Tribal rights in land and forest should be respected.
3. We should try to train and build up a team of their own people to do the work of administration and development. Some technical personnel from outside will no doubt be needed, especially in the beginning. But, we should avoid introducing too many outsiders into tribal territory.
4. We should not over administer these areas or overwhelm

them with a multiplicity of schemes. We should rather work through, and not in rivalry to their own social and cultural institutions.

5. We should judge results, not by statistics or the amount of money spent, but by the quality of human character that is evolved.

The governments at the Centre and State have shown sensitivity to tribal development issues by formulating distinct tribal sub-plans (TSP), and by having separate Ministries and Departments for Tribal Development. In Maharashtra, the budgetary outlay for TSP is 9 per cent of the State Budget commensurate with the 9 per cent ST population in the State. The objectives of the tribal sub-plan are: (a) to narrow the gap between the levels of development in the tribal areas and the other areas of the State; (b) to improve the standard of living of the tribal population in the State; (c) to tackle important problems facing the tribal people; and (d) to speed up the process of socio-economic development of the tribals.

As directed by the Government of India, in 1975-76, the villages with more than 50 per cent tribal population were constituted into integrated tribal development projects (ITDP). Subsequently, the villages with marginally less than 50 per cent were incorporated in ITDP as additional tribal sub-plan (ATSP) blocks. There were small concentrations of tribal population just outside ITDP. It was, therefore, directed that a group of villages having population about 10,000 and having more than 50 per cent tribals be brought under modified area development approach (MADA). Similarly, two or three villages having total population of 5000 with more than 50 per cent tribals could be constituted as min-MADA clusters. In Maharashtra, there are 24 ITDPs, 43 MADA pockets and 24 mini-MADAs. About half the tribal population of the State resides in the ITDP area including MADA and mini-MADA and the remaining half of the population lives outside these areas. Those outside the ITDP can benefit from schemes for individuals and families like stipends, scholarships etc.

Out of the 24 ITDPs in Maharashtra, 11 ITDPs have been identified as more vulnerable areas. They are expected to be governed by the IAS, IFS (Forest) and Maharashtra Forest Service Class 1 Cadre Officers, combining the powers of Additional

Collectors and CEOs, thus having both regulatory and developmental responsibilities to ensure single line administration. However, this has not yet been fully implemented.

In order to understand and improve the methodology for preparing tribal sub-plan and its implementation and to focus on the role of Tribal Development Department in this process, the State Government had appointed a committee under the chairmanship of Shri D.M. Sukhtankar whose report of 1992 was accepted. The Committee found that the Planning Department left it to the individual departments as per their own discretion and priorities to decide about the schemes under TSP. The departments giving priority to area development, implemented large development projects such as in irrigation and electricity using TSP money. As a result, the budget provisions under TSP were exhausted without making any impact on tribal development and the lives of tribal people. The Committee, therefore, recommended that the Tribal Development Department should act as the planning department for tribal development and to put the major budget at the level of district plans. It was also recommended that 75 per cent of the budget be provided for the development of tribals in ITDP project area and 25 per cent for tribals outside the project area.

It was thus recommended that the Tribal Development Department should finalize the TSP in consultation with the concerned departments with the mandatory principle that the provision for TSP area cannot be diverted for utilization outside the sub-plan area. The Committee recommended evaluation of TSP schemes by non-governmental agency. There is also a recommendation to motivate and encourage voluntary organizations in tribal development. The recommendations of Sukhtankar Committee had been accepted by the State Government. It needs to be assessed as to what extent the recommendations are being implemented. As per the recommendations, the Tribal Development Department now makes the tribal sub-plan in consultation with the sector departments. However, the Tribal Development Department has no authority to monitor the usage of funds which are sanctioned to the sector departments. The TRTI of the State Government is also expected to undertake evaluation of TSP schemes. But the TRTI is too much preoccupied with supervising the validity procedures of issuance of tribe verification certificates.

Tribal Development Department

Tribal Development Commissioner with four Additional Tribal Commissioners and 24 Project Officers of ITDP are the implementing authority for tribal sub-plan. The coordination between the office of the District Collector, CEO of Zilla Parishad and Project Officer of ITDP is not workable under the hierarchical structure of civil services. The recommendation to appoint Project Officer from civil services has not yet been implemented properly. It would be desirable to have a high official of the level of Joint Director or Deputy Director from each sector department posted with the Commissioner and Additional Tribal Commissioner's offices to supervise, monitor and take appropriate action of the functioning of sector departments in tribal blocks. The position of Principal Secretary, Tribal Development also needs to be equivalent to that of Additional Chief Secretary of the State to facilitate coordination at the Secretary level of sector departments.

PESA and Governance

The PRI are supposed to continue the tradition of self-governance as a result of 73rd Constitution Amendment and the Panchayats Extension to Scheduled Areas (PESA) Act. However, there are certain structural issues about the village, hamlets and the PRI in tribal areas. Tribal communities live in hamlets which are grouped together as revenue villages. Several such revenue villages are put together as a multi-village group Gram Panchayat. For example, in the hilly Dhadgaon tehsil of Nandurbar district, there are merely twenty-five Gram Panchayats for 163 villages and 260 well-defined hamlets. Moreover, it is often observed that one Gram Sevak or Secretary of Gram Panchayat looks after more than one group Gram Panchayat. It is important that hamlet should be taken to be the unit of social action and development effort, not the revenue village, which is an administrative unit to facilitate the functioning of revenue personnel. This recommendation was also made almost four decades ago in 1972, by an expert committee chaired by the eminent anthropologist Prof. S.C. Dube. The least that should be done by way of structural changes in the PRI is to have one village-one Gram Panchayat-one Gram Sevak, irrespective of the population of the village and provide for representation of each viable hamlet on the Gram Panchayat.

The Central Government PESA Act accords recognition to traditional organisation of people living in hamlets or settlements in groups of huts, as a Gram Sabha which may consist of 150 to 300 voters. However, there is a wide variation between the Central Government PESA Act and the Maharashtra government PESA Act, which continues to follow the Gram Panchayat Act of 1958 recognising the revenue village as a unit of action. The Central Government Act recognises the right of gram sabha over all kinds of minor forest produce including bamboo and *tendu* leaves, while in Maharashtra *tendu* and bamboo have been dropped from the list of minor forest produce and are under the control of the Tribal Development Corporation. The Central Government Act has also accorded authority to Gram Sabha in respect of small scale mining, transfer of tribal lands, water supply, controlling money lending, procurement of land for development, rehabilitation of tribals in a village, monitoring the work of voluntary institutions in the area, selection of beneficiaries and approval of Gram Panchayat budget etc. Gram Sabha is expected to prepare village/hamlet plans of development in a micro-planning exercise. However, in Maharashtra in many of these respects, the old Acts continue to be in operation.

Government of India has been concerned about the governance issues in tribal areas. Naxalite problems are debated as development issues leading to law and order situations. The 5th Schedule to the Constitution has assigned special responsibilities to the Governor regarding the administration of Scheduled Areas. To assist the Governor in discharging his constitutional responsibilities a Tribal Cell has been set up recently in the Governor's office in Maharashtra.

The Tribal Cell has to coordinate with Tribal Development Department about submission of Annual Reports to the President of India regarding health, education, livelihood etc. among the tribal communities. It also seeks reports about restoration of land to the tribals under Recognition of Forest Rights Act, 2006 and suggest policy interventions at the legislative and executive levels.

The Tribal Cell assists the Governor to monitor and modify the composition and functioning of the Tribes Advisory Council. Briefly, it has to prepare proposals for the Governor's directives to the State for peace and good governance of the Scheduled Areas. The activation of the Constitutional authority of the Governor about Scheduled Tribes is an indication of the concerns of the Central and State Government about the status of these backward communities (Mutatkar: *Background Paper for the MHDR 2012: Backward Communities in Maharashtra*).

Action Strategy

Anthropological research approach is based on winning the confidence of the people by sharing their lives and concerns for about a year, which is a unit of life. This helps to understand the culture and concerns of the people from their perspective. The programmes of change and development have, therefore, to provide experience of results to the people, such as curing the morbidities of women and children. People change their attitudes and participate in development efforts if the programmes address to their concerns and provide experience of solution to their problems.

Sustainable tribal development and culture change is achievable only by strengthening the people's sector involving Panchayati Raj institutions (democratically elected bodies at village, sub-district and district levels) and the people. The basic approach to tribal development, therefore, lies in capacity building of the people, which essentially becomes a programme of human resource development.

Also, it is very important to educate the community through Information Education Communication (IEC) efforts in health and development issues. Educated boys and girls from tribal areas could be motivated to form *Mahila Mandals* (women's groups), youth groups, self-help groups (SHGs) for which they could be remunerated with a very modest activity based honorarium.

NGO-Government Collaboration

Tribal Development Department (TDD) is providing funds to other departments like health, education, agriculture etc. for special schemes in tribal areas. TDD has no mechanism to monitor the use of these funds and to assess the efficiency of the programmes. There is lack of co-ordination between the TDD and other departments at the State, district and sub-district level due to hierarchical bureaucratic structure. NGO-Government

Organizations (OGs) committees at State, district and sub-district level could be formed to monitor the implementation of development schemes.

NGOs like Comprehensive Rural Health Project (CRHP), Jamkhed, Maharashtra and Maharashtra Association of Anthropological Sciences (MAAS), Pune, Maharashtra have been able to upgrade the knowledge and skills of illiterate village level women workers—Traditional Birth Attendants (TBAs) and workers of the Integrated Child Development Scheme (ICDS). The *Bhagat* has good knowledge of medicinal herbs available locally. If he is given proper respect as a health functionary, he could be weaned away from some of the exploitative and superstitious magico-religious practices. Similarly, Bharatiya Agro Industries Foundation (BAIF), which is the largest NGO in India dealing with livelihood issues, has already started utilizing the indigenous knowledge of *Bhagat* in providing health care to the people.

Competent and available NGOs could be allocated a geographical area in tribal regions, about twenty villages comprising about ten to fifteen thousand population to implement schemes of Tribal Development Department in order to develop a model in each geographical region.

Due to the commitment of national leaders like Mahatma Gandhi and Nehru and also due to political expediency of elective democratic structure from village to national level with adult franchise, the schemes of tribal development and the budgets provided are not meagre. However, as the data on health and socio-economic indicators clearly bring out the continuing gap between the ST, SC, OBC and others, that is open categories in Indian Caste System. The head count ratio of poverty confirms this gap obviously. The MDG cannot be achieved in India without addressing to these gaps. The SC/ST needs to reach at least to the level of OBC.

Some of the honest attempts about tribal development like developing Tribal Sub-Plan, Integrated Tribal Development Programme, separate tribal Ministry and initiating a debate on developing a National Tribal Policy do not meet with desired success. Health issues are often misunderstood as ill health or disease management, by the use of technology developed for global use. The disease control or population management/control programmes are administered uniformly across the country with failures in the tribal belt. The techno-managers never reach out to the people. They expect the people to seek them, their technical expertise, listen to them, and comply with the advice so as to get rid of their disease conditions. There is contempt for "indigenous knowledge and wisdom and the local herbalists are rejected as quackery, superstition and exploitative due to magico-religious procedures". Unless the local medicine man is respected and co-opted in the health care system, people will not develop confidence in health care delivery provided by the government. The private sector is hardly existent in tribal belt since the people have no money to feed the private sector.

Research is, therefore, needed in programme implementation and the NGO experiments in model building. The extent of intersectoral co-ordination and the efforts of gaps in tribal development need to be documented. Attempts have been made to orient the tribal medicine men about health issues and update their herbal information and knowledge, which could be evaluated. Some of the new institutions like Anganwadi and Ashram School have contributed and have the potential to be the nodal agencies of health care, information and development. These need to be further studied and recommendations made accordingly. Work and employment are the key concerns of people. Research in alternative production sector/non-farm sector or forest based production is needed. The indigenous knowledge of Andaman Island tribal communities, who with their knowledge of ecology could cope up with the Tsunami tidal waves, needs to be studied. Similarly, the cultural factors which obstruct/impede female foeticide unlike the mainstream India is a researchable issue.

Bottlenecks

The failure to bring about a distinct change in the tribal situation is probably the result of differing perceptions of administration and the people. The administration has floated multiple schemes of development for tribal people and tribal regions. But, about 80 per cent of tribal people in the region have no knowledge of development schemes except education, and those who do have knowledge cannot fulfil procedures to access them (GoM, 2000). Centuries of geographical isolation and experience of exploitation by outsiders has resulted in the tribal community becoming suspicious of external contact. People do not have the experience of government schemes addressing their concerns. As a result, people have not gained confidence in the development administration system. Even where the development infrastructure exists, tribal people lack the capacity to utilize it to improve their quality of life. This is an indicator of backwardness in the tribal context and necessitates reaching out to the tribal people for their capacity building and confidence building.

Mechanisms to plan, implement and monitor tribal development programmes suffer from a lack of inter-sectoral coordination at the State, District and Tehsil levels. The creation of the Tribal Development Department, based on an integrated approach to tribal development, in practice, is functioning like a conduit to distribute budgets to sectoral departments, without any workable monitoring system. The most recent attempt to integrate various schemes has been the "Nav Sanjeevan Yojana" (NSY) addressed to issues of malnutrition and health.

The Sukhtankar Committee's recommendation to shift 75 per cent of the ITDP outlay to the district plans is a welcome step in decentralization and devolution of financial authority to the Panchayati Raj Administration. However, the Panchayati Raj Institutions at the Tehsil and Gram Panchayat level have yet to be functionally involved in planning, monitoring and orienting development programmes to local situations, addressing to the concerns of local community.

The crucial issue is to address the concerns of the people in terms of policies, implementation and logistics, to gain and instill confidence among them in the government system. These concerns are most explicit in issues of subsistence and morbidity, which relate to issues of "health" and not only those of "health care". Health refers to the total fitness of an individual, which would ensure performance of social roles to his optimum efficiency. Thus, health refers to inter-sectoral development, while health care involves sectoral issues under the purview of the health department.

Inappropriate and Inaccessible Health Care

"The health status of tribal people (nutrition, child mortality, infections like malaria) and access to health care are much worse than the State average. The major reason is that the present health care system is not designed to suit the specific social and geographic context and the needs of tribal people. Critical health issues are not addressed; standard and generalized patterns of health care are applied, tribal-specific ailments and diseases are not prioritized and the insufficiency of health personnel is not rectified.... Hence, access to health care remains extremely inadequate. This has been brought out by repeated episodes of malnutrition and child deaths in Melghat, Nandurbar and Thane and in the several public interest litigations as well as the *suo motu* cases in the High Court. Hence what tribal areas need is actually well-functioning and accessible health care appropriates to the needs and the features of tribal areas" (Kelkar Committee Report, 2015: 218).

The prime health concerns of the tribal people are :

(a) Safe delivery having implications for maternal mortality.
(b) Child survival/preventing infant and child mortality.
(c) Food Security closely linked with migration.

How are existing schemes and institutional infrastructure addressing these concerns? What are people's experiences about livelihood, health, mortality and morbidity, which have shaped their attitudes and coping mechanisms? People would prefer infant mortality to maternal mortality. Babies cannot be saved where the terrain is hostile, transport not available and referral hospitals lack facilities and specialists like pediatrician, obstetrician and anesthetists. Impractical schemes like Maternity benefit (*Matrutva Anudan Yojana*) whereby a pregnant woman is to be provided tonics, vitamin syrups, and a cash incentive, which is seized by the husband; instead of pulses (*dal*) as proteins and cooking oil as fat, cannot deliver desired results. Our concerns of increasing the birth weight of babies by providing nutritional supplements may not match the concerns of the people, who may prefer low birth weight babies for safe delivery, avoiding risk of maternal mortality.

The following initiatives on the part of TDD would be meaningful :

1. Health institutions to be located in terms of time required for the people to reach on foot, not in terms of population coverage or distance in kilometres.

2. Local health functionaries like *Dai, Bhagat, Anganwadi* worker, hamlet health worker to get continuous training.
3. Inter-sectoral coordination at the State, District and Sub-district level under the initiatives of Tribal Development Department.
4. Effective IEC in health by CBOs and NGOs with the help of local functionaries and PRI.
5. Public-Private coordination for health care, particularly the specialist care not available under public health system.
6. NGOs in health and livelihood to be organized for implementing and monitoring development programmes under the leadership of reputed NGOs.

Special Scheme for Tribals : Nav Sanjeevan Yojana (NSY)

According to the Hon. Minister of Tribal Development, Maharashtra State, Nav Sanjeevan Yojana has been instituted with a focus on reducing the prevalence of infant and child mortality in tribal areas. The NSY includes the following main components:

1. *Matrutva Anudan Yojana (Maternity benefit scheme)*: A tribal pregnant woman is given Rs. 400 in cash when she reports for ANC and Rs. 400 by way of medicines, which are mostly tonics in syrup form.
2. *Dai training*: *Dais* conducting the delivery are given a one day orientation every three months and are paid Rs. 50 per training day.
3. *Pada health worker*: A community member mostly male is appointed during monsoon to undertake water disinfection, distribute chloroquin and ORS to patients and report outbreak of epidemic to PHC. He is paid Rs. 300 per month.
4. Compensation for loss of wages to the parents of Grade 3 and Grade 4 malnourished children for treatment at the PHC or rural hospital.

Besides, there is provision for appointment of honorary doctors for health check up of mother and child in every *pada*/ village and examining children at Anganwadi. The ICDS, EGS, Grain bank schemes have also been brought under NSY. The collector of the district under TSP area acts as the chief implementing officer assisted by CEO, DHO and PO of ITDP. (*Ref.* Nandurbar Report. pp. 33-34).

Strategic Operational Recommendations

(A) *Government Sector*

1. Secretaries of various departments could co-ordinate only under the authority of the Chief Secretary. It may, therefore, be necessary to have an Additional Chief Secretary to co-ordinate development efforts in tribal areas.
2. Tribal Commissioner and Additional Tribal Commissioner's office should have either external subject experts and consultants, or officers from various departments on deputation to monitor the development programmes by the respective departments in ITDP areas, under the authority of Tribal Development Department. Currently, the schemes are implemented and monitored by the respective sector departments on the same lines as in non-tribal areas, without accountability to the Tribal Development Department, which provides the budget.
3. NGO-Government committees at the State, District and Tehsil levels could be formed for monitoring. NGOs could implement schemes in a limited geographical area ranging from five to twenty villages in a Tehsil.
4. Powers and authority of the Project Officer (ITDP), CEO of the Zilla Parishad and Collector need to be clear about tribal development. Project Officer should be the Convener/Secretary of the coordination committee.

(B) *Panchayati Raj Institutions and Community*

1. Further multiplication of government functionaries in development is not necessary. Local health functionaries like *Dai*, *Bhagat*, Anganwadi worker, *Pada* health worker should receive continuous updated training.
2. Community based organizations like Mahila Mandal, Self-Help Groups, Youth and Farmers clubs need to be involved in monitoring and implementation.
3. Schemes like ICDS and Maternity benefit could be handed over to Gram Panchayat for implementation.

4. Women members of Gram Panchayats and Taluka Panchayat Samiti need to be oriented to health issues and given authority to audit health care.
5. Every village should have a village health committee headed by a woman.

(C) Health Services

1. Since plural systems of medicine are functioning in India with government recognition, no discrimination should be made between MBBS and BAMS doctors etc. They may be reoriented to meet the specific needs and resources available. BAMS doctors have better communication with the people and local health functionaries and have knowledge of herbal medicine but lack in surgery.
2. Health care facilities need not be located according to population norm, but according to the time and distance required for the tribals to access it.
3. Mobile clinics have to be functional without breakdown, at least two in each Tehsil.
4. Rural hospitals need to be fully equipped in all Tehsil places. In case of non-availability of specialists, private sector needs to be hired on payment.
5. Medical interns and post-graduates in the district colleges, from all systems of medicine, need to be posted for internship and housemanship to tribal PHC and Rural hospital.
6. Nav Sanjeevan Yojana needs to be faithfully implemented with proper co-ordination between the Collector, CEO – Zilla Parishad and Project Officer (ITDP). The monitoring committee in Nandurbar should include the tribal MP, MLAs, and Zilla Parishad, Taluka Panchayat and Gram Panchayat women members at the appropriate levels.

Unnecessary controversies have been raised about the status of MBBS and BAMS degree holders. Both of them undergo about 5 years of medical college training, both joining medical education from the stream of biology. In both colleges they dissect the human bodies as part of anatomy and physiology training. There is no reason why MBBS should be appointed in Class II grade and BAMS in Class III grade service. It is always mentioned that BAMS are appointed in case of non-availability of MBBS, thus inflicting direct insult to the Indian Systems of Medicine. India has a National ISM policy and so has the WHO policy on traditional systems of medicine. Actually the MBBS in tribal area admitted that there was no difference between them and BAMS except that BAMS were not confident with surgical procedures. In view of the knowledge of BAMS about herbal medicine and home remedies, which are rooted in Ayurveda, BAMS should be preferred for posing in tribal area. Similarly, the medical interns from medical colleges of all systems of medicine should get internship postings in tribal area.

Wherever specialists are not available for referral services from public sector, the private specialists could be hired on prorata basis. They may also enjoy different experience in the interior tribal area.

(D) *Structural Issues*

1. There are few revenue villages, which have large number of hamlets and lesser multi-village Gram Panchayats. They need to be restructured taking hamlet as a functioning unit with more villages and more Gram Panchayats for proper functioning of Gram Sabha according to 73rd Constitutional Amendment. Population need not be the criterion for identifying a village or a Gram Panchayat. Logistic functioning beneficial to the people needs to be the indicator.
2. Anganwadi/Mini-Anganwadi managed by local women, and for women and children, needs to be the nodal institution for health and health care at hamlet level.
3. Ashram School, as a prime academic institution, needs to be the nodal centre for initiating change and should not be narrowed down as a scheme or responsibility of the education department alone. As an information centre for government schemes, vocational guidance centre and a place for training and experiments in agricultural technology, it has to be a public institution catering to several villages. Students in Ashram Schools coming from several neighbouring villages could disseminate information in their respective villages. Capacity building

of Ashram Schools in the government and voluntary sector may require more investments.

(E) *Livelihood and Health*

1. Issues of food scarcity force migration, endangering health due to poor nutrition, insanitary conditions and lack of health care facilities at the site of migration. Bharatiya Agro Industries Foundation (BAIF) has changed lives of tribal families, who volunteered for accepting horticulture technology and wasteland development known as Wadi project. The project has checked migration.
2. Issues of property rights to tribals in forest land in their possession need to be expedited.
3. Cultivation of medicinal plants, processing of herbal drugs locally and cooperative or buy back marketing has to develop as a commercially viable proposition to be managed by NGOs and Ayurvedic pharmaceutical concerns. The Forest Department and Tribal Development Corporation could be the partners in the programme.

Role of Panchayati Raj Institutions in Public Health

In case of primary health care decentralization will bring decision-making close to the community as also to field level service providers, leading to balanced adjustments of demand and supply of health care.

To develop a community based health care system, following issues need to be addressed at Gram Panchayat, Tehsil and District level. PHC and subcentre could be taken as units for action plan:

(i) Preparation of a tehsil/district-wise inventory of existing institutions, Government, private providers and NGOs/ CBOs and assessment of their reach, strengths and weaknesses.

(ii) Preparation of a district-wise inventory of community based resource persons, viz. traditional birth attendants, women groups, active youth groups, savings and credit groups, co-operative societies and women Sarpanch etc.

(iii) Tehsil/District-wise mapping of existing resources to

identify gaps as well as resource rich pockets for competency building of community based functionaries.

(iv) Tehsil/District-wise strategy building for utilization of services of the resources, institutions and human resource. This may include training need assessment and capacity building plans, strategy and resource planning and a comprehensive system for monitoring and feedback.

Nodal points about PRI participation in Health Sector

- 73rd Amendment about Panchayats and 74th Amendment about Municipalities provide increasing decentralisation.
- Emergence of CBOs like SHG and Mahila Mandal could strengthen Gram Sabha.
- Composition of health and other committees at village level for wider participation, not to be replaced by development committee. Representation for women.
- Training of PRI members on powers, responsibilities, strategies and finance with focus on convergence/ intersectoral coordination.
- Increasing accountability of ANM, MPW, Gram Swasthya Rakshak, PHC staff to PRI, at village, taluk level.
- Focus on RCH, Girl child, adolescent health and aged including role of ISM.
- Strength of PRI: Intersectoral coordination, local level planning, monitoring and implementation.
- Involvement of CBOs and other development functionaries in health related matters.
- IEC to focus on promoting local health traditions, which are not harmful according to modern medicine and validated by ISM.
- Decentralised management functions to be finalised for each taluk and district.
- 74th Amendment about urban area would need logistic recommendations about finance, budget planning and involvement of private sector.

There has to be a clear-cut delegation of powers and responsibilities at the Gram Panchayat, Panchayat Samiti and Zilla

Parishad levels in regard to management issues about public health activities. These would be in the areas of :

(a) *Financial resources*—Source of financing, level of expenditure, budget structure, spending flexibility and control.

(b) *Human resource*—Selection procedure at various levels in favour of women, with more involvement of women members in PRI. Payments and accountability to PRI and not with government functionaries, except in technical supervision and assessment.

Networking of development and health personnel has to be supervised by PRI such as the functions of AWW, ANM, *Dai*, Gram Swasthya Rakshak have to be linked and monitored for maximizing productivity.

Feedback-*cum*-continuous training is required for all categories of primary health care workers.

Role of health education/IEC/BCC cannot be underestimated for developing human resources. However, for want of budgetary allocation and performance assessment, the activities have not been undertaken. Health education campaigns have been disease or issue specific to enlist recruitment of people in the targeted programmes.

(c) *Equipment and Infrastructure*—Maintenance of equipment, vehicles and building has proved to be a big road block in poor performance of public health facilities. Sub-centre buildings have been the crying need. The PRI could monitor such activities. There has to be a PRI control over the use and repair of vehicles, which could be effected faster at local level. The needy and poor patients have to get transport at affordable rates for emergency referral services.

Panchayat Samiti and Zilla Parishad need to be have finances and powers and availability of expert advice to build the referral system and have equipment and transport in functioning condition.

(d) *Drugs and Supplies*—There needs to be decentralization about assessment of need, demand and procurement, which could be helped by PRI.

(e) *Health Information System*—At the village, taluka and

district level, information has to be compiled and analysed which could provide epidemiological picture to help need assessment. Data on registration of births, deaths, abortions, chronic diseases and seasonal communicable diseases, ANC, post-partum care etc. would be useful for decentralized planning up to village level. Gram Panchayat could be involved in this activity, which would empower them for planning at the village level.

The involvement of PRI in health care also includes involvement of CBOs like, SHGs, Mahila Mandals, Youth groups and the local NGOs who are functioning at the village, taluka and district levels.

Community Participation

"In order to strengthen democracy, 73rd Amendment of the Constitution provided more authority to Panchayati Raj Institutions and to the Gram Sabha, particularly in tribal areas. It is envisaged that some programmes like maternity benefit scheme and ICDS could be implemented by the Gram Panchayats with adequate financial powers to do so. Every Gram Sabha could have a health agenda and the Bhagat as expert member of the community could be oriented to play an important role in health monitoring. There has to be a village health committee. Panchayat members, other village level functionaries could be oriented to health issues and made aware about the traditional and modern knowledge, which would help to develop plural health care system at the village level" (Nandurbar Report: 49-52).

Government Sector

Tribal Development Department is providing funds to other departments like health, education, agriculture etc. for special schemes in tribal areas. TDD has no mechanism to monitor the use of these funds and to assess the efficiency of the programmes. There is lack of coordination between the TDD and other departments at the State, district and taluka level. Secretaries of various departments could coordinate only under the authority of the Chief Secretary. It may, therefore, be necessary to have an

Additional Chief Secretary to coordinate development efforts in tribal areas. An effective arrangement at the District level involving the Collector, CEO and Project Officer of ITDP has to be developed.

Tribal Commissioner and Additional Tribal Commissioner's office should have either external subject experts and consultants, or officers from various departments on deputation to monitor the development programmes by the respective departments in ITDP areas.

NGO-GO committees at State, district and taluka level have to be formed to monitor the implementation of development schemes.

Competent and available NGOs should be given a geographical area about twenty villages comprising about ten to fifteen thousand population to implement schemes of Tribal Development Department to provide a model in each geographical area. NGOs were successfully involved in leprosy elimination programmes by the Central and State Governments. In Nandurbar district it is possible to identify the NGOs to monitor the health and development schemes of the government in partnership with TDD.

Summary of Recommendations

Action Strategies for tribal development would be applicable in all tribal pockets in Maharashtra. In districts like Thane, Yavatmal, Amravati, Gadchiroli, Raigad, Nasik and others, there are tehsils and pockets with a high concentration of tribals. The aggregate population of tribals would be less in these districts, but as high as in Nandurbar district in the selected tehsils and pockets. In Nandurbar district also, the tribal population varies in different tehsils, with varying degrees of levels of backwardness and prospects for development. In various ethnic group of tribals such as Mahadeo Koli, Kokna, Raj Gond, Pawra, Bhil, Thakar, Warli, Katkari, Halba, Maria Gond, the capacity to develop varies as also in the caste society with differences in OBC, nomadic and *vimukta jati* and amongst the various Scheduled Caste communities.

Integrated tribal development programme recognizes the geographical variability and also recognizes some tribal communities as more primitive with special schemes of development.

Tribal people being backward, not having the capacity, drive and initiative to utilize the schemes of development, the government and NGOs have to be proactive and reach out to the people at their doorstep to equip them for demand generation capacity. In such situations, the local level logistics become as significant as the district or State level strategies. The worldview of the tribals being very narrow, their concerns and satisfaction levels are also very narrow. "Think not for the morrow" is their philosophy of life.

It is necessary to train more women in reproductive child health practices. Actually all women Gram Panchayat members, all women teachers, all girl students from Ashram schools, particularly, Girls Ashram schools in the age group of 12 and above could be trained in RCH. If we really care for women's health, all women volunteers from villages and hamlets could be trained in obstetric, paediatric and gynaec issues, in batches. Women are the custodians of family health in general and children's health in particular. Household therapies are also practiced by women under the guidance of elderly women, *Bhagats* and peer advice. The information about health and health care has to be more directed to women according to the principles of modern medicine and Ayurveda. Tribal health culture will change only if women accept the modern scientific methods of health care, while following the time tested positive traditions of Ethno-science.

The local professionals, the *Bhagats* should not be ignored since they are part of the local community available all the time to the people. They would welcome training in Ayurvedic principles and would be willing to learn processing of local herbs into medicine since the folk knowledge and practices are the little traditions, which have synthesized in the great textual tradition of Ayurveda. The BAMS doctors can communicate with the *Bhagats*, more effectively unlike the MBBS doctors.

ICDS scheme is very good but the worker is burdened with too many records and registers. Anganwadi workers have shown good output in all their work as volunteers. Traditional midwife is another useful category. New volunteers could be recruited in this category and hamlet howsoever small may be her work area.

There are no programmes of nutrition education. Promotion of poultry, fisheries which are dear to tribals could final favour with tribals, which would supplement nutritious diet. People who go for work in Navapur tribal area were seen on road carrying food in tiffin containers. They could also be motivated to carry water. It was an experience to see several cases of adult diarrohea in PHCs and RH since the farmers took water from ponds close to their fields in monsoon.

As mentioned earlier, issues of food security, livelihood, migration and child deaths or morbidity during migration are interconnected phenomena. It is for this reason that Tribal Development Department and ITDP/TSP have been formed. However, the Sectoral Administration is not sensitive to the distinct and integrative nature of tribal issues. The State Government has yet to act fully on Sukhtankar Committee recommendations in empowering the TDD for planning, monitoring and evaluating the comprehensive development schemes of tribal development.

The High Level Committee on Socio-Economic, Health and Educational Status of Tribal Communities of India, Ministry of Tribal Affairs, Government of India, (May, 2014) has made following observations about tribal health issues.

> "A reason for the inappropriately designed and poorly managed health care in Scheduled Areas is the near complete absence of participation of Scheduled Tribe people or their representatives in shaping policies, making plans or implementing services in the health sector. This is true from the village level to the national level. Even though the PESA gives Gram Sabhas the right and the role of influencing social sector schemes, which include health, there are no mechanisms in place for such participation or oversight at the village level. Similar situation is observed at the ITDP, district and the State levels. At the Central level, the Ministry of Health and Family Welfare has no separate body to shape policies or monitor programmes in Scheduled Areas. This is in complete disregard to the promise of the Constitution and the *Panchsheel* guidelines." (243)
>
> "Traditional healers and *Dais* play an important role in the indigenous health care. Instead of alienating or rejecting them, a sensitive way of including them or getting their cooperation in health care, must be explored. Traditional herbal medicines should be protected through community ownership. The ownership and intellectual

property rights of tribal community over their own herbal medicines and practices should be ensured."

"Apart from the physical distance, a huge cultural distance separates the tribal population from others. Health care delivery to the Scheduled Tribe population should be culture-sensitive and in the local language in order to overcome this distance." (246)

"*Human Resource for Health* : The well-known difficulties in deploying doctors, nurses and other technical personnel from outside into Scheduled Areas have made the problem of human resources the Achilles' heel of health care in Scheduled Areas. We recommend that, instead of making futile efforts to import unwilling and unstable personnel from outside, the most feasible and effective long term solution will be to select, train and deploy local Scheduled Tribe candidates."

This should be done at the following levels:

- The Accredited Social Health Activists (ASHAs) and Anganwadi workers—from the same village or the hamlet.
- The ANMs and paramedic workers—from the same block.
- The doctors and public health programme managers —to a large extent, from the same district.

The candidates must be local, belong to Scheduled Tribes, be fluent in local tribal dialects, be selected on merit and should be committed to serve in the local Scheduled Area for at least ten years."

"The ASHA workers, Anganwadi workers and ANMs will continue to be the mainstay of health care in rural and tribal areas. Due to the physical isolation of tribal communities, compounded by a lack of doctors, it will be pragmatic to train, equip and empower the three 'As'—ASHA workers, Anganwadi workers and ANMs—in tribal areas to a higher level." (247)

It is hoped that these observations and recommendation would be translated in health action plans. A distinct tribal health policy is the need of the day.

Conceptual Approach to Action Strategy

Tribal development strategies cannot be the same as that of development of the mainstream society. Tribal cultures due to historical and geographical reasons are distinct cultures and are more closely integrated wholes. Theory of culture, integration of culture and its implications for change indicate that change in one aspect of culture cannot be implemented with success without understanding the implications of change in other aspects. More closely the integrated cultures like the traditional tribal cultures, more difficult they are amenable to change with conventional sectoral interventions. Tribal cultures are labelled as primitive and backward since they do not change easily in spite of establishment of development infrastructure.

The Symington report of 1938 about chronic poverty, exploitation and backwardness of the tribal pockets, which comprise the present day Nandurbar district holds true even after sixty-five years.

There are perennial debates whether tribal poverty is distinct from rural poverty in general. Since tribal cultures are close-knit integrated systems, the issues of livelihood, health and education cannot be separated for designing action strategies for development. The holistic approach to development, which is also called comprehensive development, envisages different action strategies.

World Health Organization's "Health for All" declaration (Alma Ata, 1978) is based on the primary health care approach highlighting inter-sectoral coordination, whereby interventions in non-health development sectors such as education, transport, communication, electricity, food and water would ensure better health to the people.

In Maharashtra, "Jamkhed approach" of comprehensive development with health as an entry point has been internationally acclaimed and pursued in several developing countries. Bharatiya Agro-Industries Foundation (BAIF) also follows the holistic 'Wadi' approach to comprehensive development, focusing on tribal livelihoods thereby ensuring food security and reversing migration.

Anthropological research approach is based on winning the confidence of the people by sharing their lives and concerns for about a year, which is a unit of life. This helps understand the culture and concerns of the people from their perspective. The programmes of change and development have, therefore, to provide experience of results to the people, such as curing the morbidities of women and children. People change their attitudes and participate in development efforts if the programmes address to their concerns and provide experience of solution to their problems.

The strategies for tribal development do not visualize a multiplication of the government sector. Sustainable tribal development and culture change is achievable only by strengthening the people's sector involving Panchayati Raj Institutions and people. The basic approach to tribal development, therefore, lies in capacity building of the people, which essentially becomes a programme of human resource development.

A. TRIBAL PALGHAR

It is strongly argued that the communicable diseases disappeared from the West as a result of general socio-economic development much before the drugs were found for the cure of these diseases. In order to test this hypothesis, BAIF decided to introduce development inputs; in the poverty stricken tribal areas in Thane (now Palghar) District. With an experience of improving the quality of life among tribals, as a result of general development efforts, BAIF has been the most suitable agency to undertake such a task, initiated by the late Shri Manibhai Desai.

Scientific testing of hypothesis of this nature needs proper evaluation of the project estimating the improvement in health status as a result of development inputs. Baseline study conducted by MAAS is a first step towards this objective. Subsequently, concurrent evaluation of the health and development relationship could be undertaken at periodic intervals.

The village profiles of study village, ethnography of tribal group detailing the economic organization, religion organization and status of women, besides data on nutrition, anthropometry, health behaviour, morbidity, mortality, disease burden and issues concerning maternal and child health have been presented. The baseline study was designed to help planning of intervention packages and consequent evaluation. These presentations of methodology, data and its analysis would undoubtedly help voluntary organizations in planning and executing similar studies.

Discussion of malnutrition of tribal children in Maharashtra has become a political issue and the measures taken are episodic and sporadic. The study team has reported 30 per cent infant mortality in the study year. Food security beyond January and March-April is widespread, forcing migration of tribals to urban areas to work at construction sites. The Wadi project initiated by BAIF is a step in the correct direction to increase food security and provide avenues of income on their own land or wasteland. The impact of Wadi project on their culture including health is a matter for assessment.

Summary

The baseline study of the culture of the tribals in selected villages in Jawhar Taluka of Thane (now Palghar) district, Maharashtra was undertaken to prepare a scientific base for designing intervention packages so as to study its impact on development in few years time. The study was meant to help to devise process documentation and evaluation in areas where quantitative indicators were found difficult.

The villages range from 20 to 40 kms from the Taluka place Jawhar, connected mostly by *Kachha* roads with seasonal public transport available. The nearest permanent market, bank, veterinary dispensary and police station are equally distant from study villages. The Primary Health Centre or the Primary Health Unit are, however, within reach, although its utilization is not ideal. Distance of police station would indicate functioning local systems which ensure law and order and do not warrant external controls. The level of illiteracy ranges from tribe-wise variations of 54 to 77 per cent excluding the age group upto 5 years, but including those attending Balwadi. Over the years, village Sakharshet has developed some facilities like grocery shops and the flour mills, besides having a PHC.

The major tribal groups ranging in population size are respectively Wadi, Kokna and Thakar, while other tribals include Dhor Koli, Malhar Koli and others. However, on the basis of literacy and economic indicators, the ranking is in the descending order of Kokna, Thakar, Warli and other groups. The Wadi acceptors as at present range in the order of Kokna, closely followed by Warli and *Thakar* and others lagging behind.

Tribal economy is a subsistence economy. Kokna possesses more land, more than 5 and 10 acres followed by *Thakar* and Warli, while more Warlis are landless. The tribals do not report starvation, a small percentage report missing one meal out of three during summer. However, the proportion of migration for work and borrowing in cash and kind for meeting food scarcity are indicators of shortfall in agricultural production. Wardli top in borrowing in general, and specifically to meet food shortages, while Kokna borrow for managing sickness and to meet marriage expenditure. 43 per cent of the loans are taken from financial institutions while 57 per cent are drawn from informal sector like friends, relatives and money lenders.

Out migration for work is as high as 82 per cent in the total population, meaning the migration of at least one male member per family. Predictably Warli and Thakar migrate more than the Kokna.

The cash economy has entered tribal belt by way of wages earned in migratory jobs. Local payments continue to be made in grain. At weekly markets, purchase of food items and vegetables continue to be exchanged in barter.

The data on morbidity in the month of December, 1993 which is usually labelled as healthy season, brings out 43 per cent cases of total morbidity under 5 children, females leading the males. Of these, fever tops the list followed by diarrhoea and other intestinal problems. The utilization of government facilities of health care is good, around 59 per cent while around 20 per cent people have contacted *Bhagat* as the first or second contact. They have their own classification as to the diseases like diarrhoea and fevers being controlled by doctors while the *Bhagats* ward off evils due to spirit and ghosts and ensure preventive care of health and increased production.

Infant mortality under 12 months show more mortality under 1 month, males out numbering females in all ages. The major causes of infant deaths appear to be measles, followed by diarrhoea and low birth weight. The number of deaths in the first month are same as that from 1 month to 1 year. Diarrhoea has also been killer under 5 population during the last two years, again male out numbering the weaker sex in mortality. There has been only one maternal death.

People are aware about the relationship of diarrhoea with water and believes that medicine put in water may prevent its occurrence. In diarrhoea blood gets converted to water according to them and body becomes cold.

Due to the custom of bride price, tribal women enjoy better status than the caste Hindu women. Divorce and widow remarriage are easy. In the patriarchal society of tribals, boys are preferred to girls, although girls are not shunned. In case of divorce, usually sons are left with father to get share in property while the girls go with the mother. Desertion of women is a non-issue in tribal society.

Women enjoy greater autonomy in decision-making to the extent of exercising rights over self-earned income and the expenditure. Levirate and Soroate marriages are accepted, but the custom is on the decline. A woman deserts a man in case of sterility and marries another to prove her fertility. However, a woman has no position in religious matters on account of pollution due to menstruation. A woman enjoys no special privileges in terms of special diet or restrictions on her work during pregnancy. After child birth, there are restrictions on diet for a month. Colostrums is given immediately after birth.

Contrary to many regions in India vasectomy is preferred to tubectomy among the tribals. Consumption of milk by mulching the cows is very uncommon as cow's milk is meant for the calves. Tribals, both man and women are given to alcohol which has become an inseparable part of social and religious rituals. People are generally aware about the importance of personal hygiene, there is no strong motivation or facilities to take remedial action in the matter.

The acceptance of Wadi technology though in its early stages has brought about changes in attitudes. They have learnt the importance of caring for plants and close monitoring. They are more busy on the land than ever before and are willing to sacrifice such traditional recreation as dance. However, there is a big gap between awareness and acceptance, particularly of new varieties of crops such as wheat. Marketing of vegetables is a problem since transport is expensive to reach vegetables to the town market. There is growing awareness about the acceptance of Wadi. But meagre land used for Paddy and Nagli cannot be converted into wadi for fear of shortfall in food production necessary for subsistence. Care will have to be taken that acceptance of Wadi by local "Haves" does not lead to widening gaps between "subsistence haves" and "starvation have nots".

Looking at the proportion of waste land, there is scope for

waste land development and improving the land yield from cultivated fields. Gender bias not being a strong culture pattern can be used for promoting women development schemes. It appears necessary to take up special surveys on child morbidity and mortality and provide relief from diarrhoea and measles which have been the major killers. The nearest town market is Jawhar which unless tapped may not provide real income to the people, in spite of increased production. Programmes like dairy development will need change in behaviour and faith in the production of healthy bulls, ensuring their survival, since people are not used to consumption of milk in the interest of health of the calves. There is scope for poultry and fisheries development even for increased consumption. People may respond well to technology for increased Nagli and Paddy production.

In the background of total nakedness among children in Vavar village in the hills in month of December, quality of life could be measured in terms of the children being clothed by their parents to protect them from inclement winter.

Jawhar Baseline Study

Introduction

Primary Health Care approach has strengthened the philosophy of intersectoral coordination, emphasizing the role of non-conventional health inputs in health development. The impact of general socio-economic development on health and disease control in Western countries has been accepted as a proved hypothesis. To study the impact of development on health can, therefore, be a researchable area by undertaking a prospective study.

BAIF has undertaken poverty alleviation programmes using wasteland development schemes as an entry point popularly known as Wadi project. The studies in Vansda in Gujarat clearly indicate the improvement in the quality of life by improvement in the economic status with the spin off effects on other aspects of life.

If a prospective intervention study on impact of development on health has to be undertaken, it becomes necessary to build the monitoring and evaluation system in the study itself. Since BAIF is in the process of introducing development inputs as Wadi project in the tribal areas of Jawhar tehsil, Thane district in the State of

Maharashtra, it was found necessary to undertake a baseline study which would help in the monitoring and subsequent evaluation at periodic intervals.

The baseline survey was to include both the qualitative and quantitative indicators, such as, village survey, family survey, socio-cultural profile, nutrition and diet survey, including anthropometry of under fives, health and ethno-medicine, status of women, and economic and agricultural activities.

Methodology

The data were collected with the used of both qualitative and quantitative research tools. The villages were selected by purposive selection, i.e. the villages selected by BAIF for Wadi project. The families selected as acceptors of Wadi project were taken in the sample for study. Similarly, Wadi non-participant families were also selected to serve as control for future studies. Since the Wadi project has just begun, no difference was anticipated in the Wadi acceptors and non-Wadi tribals at the baseline study.

The following villages were selected :

1. Sakharshet-Umbarvihir,
2. Vavar-Behedpada,
3. Kharonda-Hedichapada,
4. Chambharshet, and
5. Akra.

BAIF had provided a list of families included in the Wadi project. The control families were selected at random in the neighbourhood of Wadi families.

A team of 23 researchers was selected for undertaking essentially the collection of quantitative data. Of these, about 8 researchers were to stay back for collecting exclusively qualitative data.

A one day workshop was organized of these researchers on 8 January, 1994 to discuss nature and canvas of fieldwork. Detailed discussion was held of the Schedules for family data, nutritional survey, morbidity survey and the qualitative data collection about health and health behaviour and the status of women. The traditional methods of collecting ethnographic information covering all aspects of culture were also highlighted.

The research teams stayed in villages, amongst the people, hiring a hut or a part of it. Local hands were hired to cook food. There were problems about cooking utensils. The local cooks brought utensils from their homes which were very insufficient.

The following tools and techniques were used for the collection of primary data:

1. *Village Profile* : A guide was prepared to collect the following information:
   (a) Population and land,
   (b) Transport and communication,
   (c) Public amenities and facilities, and
   (d) Developmental activities.
2. *Household Schedule* : A structured schedule to collect the following data:
   (a) Family census, and
   (b) Economic data including land holding, cattle, house types and material artifacts, income, expenditure, credit, food security and migration. This also included morbidity, mortality data and diet survey.
3. Data were collected on the following on the basis of semi-structured guidelines:
   (a) Diet of children,
   (b) Diet of lactating mothers,
   (c) Morbidity history of children under 5, and
   (d) History of most recent pregnancy and delivery.
4. Nutritional assessment, diet survey by weighment method and Anthropometry.
5. Semi-structured interview guide to collect information on health behaviour.

Informal interviews to collect ethnographic data, data about status of women and health behaviour. (*Ref*: BAIF Study).

Ethnography

Detailed ethnography covering the individual life cycle and the ritual cycle has been narrated in a descriptive manner. The changes in the culture during the last twenty-five years or so as mentioned by the informants have also been presented. With economic and technological advancement, certain aspects of culture, particularly the material aspects of culture undergo change.

Individual Life Cycle-Birth

No ceremony is held when a married woman conceives for the first time. The '*Dai*' said that a married woman who gets menses may get pregnant after having sexual contact with her husband. It is the God who gives birth to a foetus. It all depends on him. Initially the foetus is in the form of a lump of flesh. Hands and legs develop gradually and then it goes on increasing. A good, healthy child is not born until the period of 9 months 9 days is complete. A woman is believed to be pregnant if she does not menstruate for 3 to 4 months. Since a woman sits in isolation during menstruation, all family members come to know about her pregnancy. A Kokna woman said that they go to the '*Dai*' to confirm pregnancy. There are no special rituals or ceremonies associated with pregnancy. A pregnant woman performs all her routine works like cooking, fetching water, grinding, pounding, forest work, farm work etc. The *Dai* said that all sorts of work should be performed during pregnancy. Only after a woman completes 9 months, she does not go to the distant place for work, in the forest, if it is far away from the house.

Women do not go anywhere for check-up. Only if they have some problem, they consult '*Dai*'. If an ANM happen to visit the village, she gives some tablets and injection to a pregnant woman. If there is abdominal pain after fetching and lifting pots of water, women go to the '*Dai*'. The *Dai* then holds her lower abdomen and moves the foetus towards the upper direction. Kokna women said that they did not undertake heavy work. During pregnancy there is no special diet as such. It is the same daily dietary pattern— *Bhakri, Dal* and Rice. However, following things are avoided, differing from tribe-to-tribe.

Diet Restrictions for Pregnant Woman

Thakar

A *Thakar* woman said that the pregnant women did not eat fish, sticky substances like Mangoes, Karvanda and avoided because if eaten white spots appear on the body of the child. All oily foods are avoided so also coconut, since it is oily.

Kokna

No specific diet. Only Papaya is avoided, the reason is not known. Eggs and alcohol are also avoided.

Warli

No specific diet restriction, can eat everything.

Delivery

The *'Dai'* after checking gives tentative dates of delivery. *Dai* is called to the house when the labour pains start, and the delivery takes place at home. There is no special room in the house for delivery. Generally, it is done in a room which is nearer to the cowshed. At Vavar, in one of the Warli houses, the delivery took place in the kitchen, in spite of having other rooms. Three *dais* are required for the delivery, one for holding the stomach, one experienced *dai* for taking out the child and one for assisting her. Even a single *dai* can also conduct the delivery. Then the other women in the house assist her. Delivery is done in the sleeping position.

All the deliveries, including the first one, take place at husbands house. Only amongst certain Kokna of Sakharshet the first delivery of a woman takes place at her parents' house. Amongst the Vavar-Kokna, it takes place at the husband's house. Regarding the disposal of placenta a Kokna woman said that the placenta is buried in the room whenever delivery takes place. At Vavar, in one of the Warli houses we found that the delivery took place in kitchen and the placenta was buried there itself.

A Thakar *Dai* said that the placenta is buried in the cowshed. Placenta is not thrown out but buried so that the crows do not touch it or take it away. Placenta is not taken out, but left on its own to come out. If the placenta does not come out, it moves upwards, i.e. towards heart and gets stuck up there, causing the death of the woman, said *Dai*.

The umbilical cord is cut by a razor blade. Only the trained

Dais of Umbarvihir said that the blade was boiled in the water and then used. If there is no blade, a sickle is used. Since blade is much thinner than a sickle, it is very convenient to use, said *Dai*. She said that the cord comes out along with the baby. It is to be cut while it is still beating and is cut at a distance of 3 inches measured by fingers from the navel. Its portion left over on the baby's navel is then immediately tied by a cloth so that the air from the baby's stomach does not go not. The dung of the goat is burnt along with the dried leaves of Tamarind and ash prepared is applied to the cord so that it gets dried and falls on its own. A Kokna woman said that earlier they used to tie the cord with black thread and apply *Sindur* (vermilion). Now-a-days, they apply medicinal powder so that it gets dried on its own and falls down.

After delivery, both the mother and the baby are given bath immediately, after which the mother starts breast feeding the baby. For the first 5 days, mother's diet consists of Warli gruel only. If the solid foods are eaten by the mother the stomach of the baby bulges out. In certain houses, these days Rice gruel is given instead of Warai. This may be because whatever Warli is produced is sold as it fetches good price. After the fifth day ceremony (*pachvi*) mother can eat dal, Jowar Bhakri and Rice. Fifth day ceremony which was observed in a Warli house at Vavar where the woman got delivered in the kitchen and the placenta was buried there itself. On the wall of the room, the *Dai* had plastered a square using cow dung. The floor of the house and the hearth were also plastered/cleansed. The baby was given bath by the *Dai*. No oil was applied. She prepared very small packets of *Haldi, Kumkum, Gulal, Sindur, Bukka* and the powder made out of the burnt wood from the hearth.

Dai tied pieces of 'Vekhand' on the baby's left hand and around mother's neck. She said that the baby should be given the taste of that piece if baby cried. On the plastered wall 2 lines of 10 dots each of *Haldi, Kumkum, Gulal, Sindur,* and *Bukka* were drawn in the ascending order. And 6 dots of *Bukka* were put on the sides, which meant that the God had been put into puzzle (*Devalakandi*). On the winnowing pan a figure of a woman carrying a baby on her left side, was drawn. And to her right side the *Dai* kept 5 fistful of rice after worshipping the lamp and the wall. An earthen lamp was lit on one side of the pan. Twenty five paise coin was kept on each fist of rice. The baby was then put in the cradle usually made of cloth (*Jholi*). The baby was passed to the mother from the lower side of the cradle, after which the mother had put the baby in the cradle and this was repeated 5 times. Those who had held the cradle were given 10 paise each. After this the liquor was first served to the *Dai*, in the *'drona'* (leaf cup). She put 5 drops of it on the ground by taking the names of all Gods. The liquor was again put back into the bottle and then given in the *drona* to all those who drink. Each one touched the feet of the person serving the liquor, before taking it and then all of them drank the whole in one sip. Rice and boiled lentils (*Turichya Ghugrya*) were distributed in the *'palas'* leaves to all those present.

The ritual of the 5th day is same amongst the Warli and Kokna. In addition, amongst the Kokna the mother and the child are taken near the hearth meaning thereby that after the 5th day she can start attending to all household work except fetching water. Black coloured thread or just a string of black beads is put in the baby's hands in order to save him from evil eye. Amongst the Thakar, it is slightly different. On the 5th day a stone is placed by the *Dai* in the cowshed where the placenta is buried, to which she applies *Haladi, Kumkum, Gulal, Sindur, Bukka* and it is worshipped. An earthen lamp is lit. In offering, a coconut is broken and the baby is put into the cradle. The *dai* serves the mother and the baby for 5 days.

During these 5 days the *Dai* applies oil to the baby and gives bath. She also gives bath to the mother, but no oil is applied to her body. After the 5th day's ceremony gets over the elderly woman in the house gives bath to the mother and the baby up to 5 weeks. For the first 5 days after delivery the *Dai* is responsible for mother's and baby's health care. For conducting delivery the *Dai* is paid in cash and kind. Rs. 25-30, one bottle of liquor and one basket full of Rice (approx. 2.5 to 3 kg.).

Pollution period after delivery is observed for 12 days. Ceremony is held on the 12th day after which she is deemed purified. On the 12th day the delivered woman takes an empty pot to the well. Any stone available nearby is placed near the well. *'Sindur'* is applied to the stone, an *agarbatti* is lit. Five types of grains like *Udid,* Rice, *Nagli, Warai* and *Khurasani* or any other that is available is put near the well and on it water is poured 5 times. The well is worshipped and fetching of water begins.

Diet and other Restrictions after Delivery

After delivery the mother is on a dietary restriction for a month:

1. *Udid dal, Nagli* or *Jowar bhakri,* spicy food, jiggery is prohibited because it disturbs the baby's stomach. It bulges out and the child suffers from constipation.
2. Onion, garlic, oily food, meat of cock and goat are avoided as it affects the lactation. However, uncooked raw oil is allowed, if poured on the vegetable.
3. Eggs are prohibited. When asked, they said that hen did not give milk, so it is not good for the mother.
4. The edges of the *bhakri* are not eaten as they are hard and also affect the quality of the milk. Milk gets diluted.

Breast-feeding starts immediately after delivery. It is continued till the woman becomes pregnant again.

Other Restrictions

Sexual contact is avoided for 2 months after delivery otherwise the woman dies.

Prescribed Food

Warai porridge is important. It is easily digestible and nutritive, and is considered light. The white roots of the forest beans are amashed and its fluid is given. As a result of consumption of beans the quantity of milk gets increased and the quality is also good.

When a child starts holding neck, usually in the 3rd month, maternal uncle cuts the hair of the child. Amongst the Kokna and *Thakar,* Monday is the auspicious day for hair cut, while amongst the Warli, Wednesday, Friday and Sunday are considered auspicious. Amongst the Kokna, the maternal uncle cut the baby's hair with the help of blade once only. Remaining hair are cut by the barber. By any chance if the baby girl's hair cutting is not performed, the girls is given a golden ornament. This rule is not applicable to the boys because the boy's hair are always cut. Mother's brother is presented a handkerchief amongst the Kokna and a coconut amongst the *Thakar.*

There is no particular naming ceremony of the child. The child is named at any time. Some of them ask the Anganwadi teacher for naming the child. After naming, it is reported to the health worker. When the child starts drinking water and eating food on his own, then onwards the child is given rice and *bhakri* of *nagli*.

A barren women is called as "decayed wife" (*Sadi Bayko*). It is believed that the causes of bareness are formation of ball of flesh in the body of the woman or evil eye.

Still birth is believed to take place when there is sexual contact during the latter period of pregnancy. It is believed that a man can marry at any age since he does not become infertile. While a woman cannot marry since she losses her fertility after menopause.

Shidwa: It is a cultural remedy for multiple problems, like barrenness, abortion, still birth, infant death and if the child becomes sick, the *Bhagat* is consulted. He spreads rice on a winnowing pan ('*Diva Pahane*') and gives medicine according to calculation of even or odd number of grains. He prepares amulets with rice locked in it and after chanting *mantras* ties around the mother's and baby's neck. After recovery (*sukhi alyavar*) the family members and the *Bhagat* go to the forest and the *Peti* is broken (*Shidwa Utarawane*) and as suggested by *Bhagat* a goat or a cock is cut and all eat food there.

Menstruation

(Terms used : '*Dhanphul*'—Kokna, *Dhan*—Thakar, *Palwi*—Warli)

When a girl attains puberty and starts menstruating, she starts wearing half *saree* up to knee, blouse and a piece of cloth is taken over the head or is used as a *dupatta*. On the onset of menarche she holds the wooden beam that supports the roof with her hands, as it is believed that after holding it, she would not have heavy bleeding in future. No other ceremonies or rituals take place.

A girl comes to know about the menstruation from her friends. While they are together in the forest or on the farm. They also get knowledge from the discussions of the elderly women and from their observance of pollution. During menstruation period no special clothes are used. However, recently, very few women have started using clothes which they wash daily and wear it again. The women not using special clothes, on experiencing heavy bleeding, change their *saree* twice in a day, or take the cloth surrounding the waist in doubles. Bath is taken daily. Head bath is taken on the day bleeding stops. During their monthly periods women observe pollution by isolating themselves in a corner of the house, especially away from the hearth. During these days cooking, fetching water, working on the threshing ground, and touching others is not allowed. Working on the farm is permissible, but not on the threshing ground, because it is a sacred place and they believe that the agricultural yield decreases in the succeeding year if the norms are violated. Serving food to husband and other men is also not allowed, since men take part in the rituals and they should not get polluted.

Nutritional Status

In India malnutrition, especially that affecting young children, is one of the important public health problems. Assessment of Nutritional status should be continuous process aimed at evaluating and extending such activities to the most needy communities whenever resources will permit. The nutritional assessment can be carried out by using the following methods:

1. Anthropometry or body measurements,
2. Clinical examination for nutritional deficiencies,
3. Diet survey,
4. Biochemical tests, and
5. Vital statistics such as mortality and morbidity rates.

For the present study method numbers 1, 3 and 5 have been used to assess the nutritional status.

I. Anthropometry

Growth retardation may be the first response of the body towards nutritional deficiencies while appearance of clinical signs may be the final stage. From the public health point of view identification of sub-clinical forms of malnutrition is very important for planning programmes of nutrition intervention so as to prevent such milder cases going into severe forms with consequent risk of high mortality. Anthropometric measurements, i.e. body measurements are the most widely used means to assess nutritional status.

Use of anthropometric measurements usually depends upon two factors:

1. Accurate age assessment, and
2. Appropriate normal values for comparison

(a) Age Assessment

In the absence of documentary evidence of birth, the local calendar in the form of festivals and other local events become useful for the age assessment. Recently, however, due to the spread of education and Government propaganda on many developmental programmes the rural and tribal folk are becoming aware of the correct age statements. Such evidences, although less in appearance, particularly among the tribals of Jawhar area, are aware in the usefulness of "age". For the present study, however, the age assessment was done by the expert anthropometrists by the way of either recording the documentary evidences from school records and cross checking them with the interrogation method by asking a number of question etc. Hence, the age information of the present data would be fairly acceptable.

(b) Standard Values

The normal values referred to as growth standards or norms have been obtained, from "well off" healthy children of Hyderabad—the NNMB standard—and the NCHS and Harward standards, that are currently in use all over the country.

The most commonly used body measurements such as Height, Weight and Arm Circumference have been considered for the present project and these were recorded by the anthropometrists. The standard procedure and techniques of measurements have been followed besides the standard instruments such as Anthropometer rod and flexible tape, sliding and spreading calliper etc.

The extent of the problem of malnutrition in a community was assessed by calculating Body Mass Index (BMI) which is an index of two basic measurements, viz. Height and Weight and which is independent of age and sex. As a part of the analysis of data, besides BMI calculations, 50th percentile values of the communities have been compared with NCHS, Harward and well-off Hyderabad 50th percentile values. Usual statistical constants, such as mean, standard deviation, have also been calculated and presented in the tabular form. (*see* Table 4.1 to 4.4)

(c) Results of Analysis

The details of the study are as follows:

Villages covered: Kharonda, Vavar (Behedpada Hamlet), Umbarvihir, Sakharshet.

Tribal Groups covered: Warli, Thakar, Kokana and Koli.

Sample Size: 302 individuals taken together

Body Mass Index (BMI)

$$\text{Formula : BMI} = \frac{\text{Body Weight in Kg.}}{\text{Height in Metres}}$$

Table 4.1: BMI Gradation

Presumptive	*Diagnostic*	*Grades used*	*Index Values*
1	CED*	III	< 16.0
2	CED*	III	16.0–17.0
3	CED*	I	17.0–18.5
4	Low Weight Normal		18.5–20.0
5	Normal		20.0–25.0
6	Obese	I	25.0–30.0
7	Obese	II	> 30.0

* CED: Chronic Energy Deficiency.
Source: Field Survey by MASS.

Table 4.2: BMI Classification

BMI-Kharonda-Warli

Village : Kharonda Tribe : Warli

Presumptive Diagnosis	*Male*		*Female*		*Total*	
	N	*%*	*N*	*%*	*N*	*%*
CED Grade III	3	11.1	8	34.8	11	22.0
CED Grade II	9	33.3	9	39.1	18	36.0
CED Grade I	10	37.0	3	13.1	13	26.0
L.W Normal	4	14.8	3	13.1	7	14.0
Normal	1	3.7	–	–	1	2.0
Obese Grade I	–	–	–	–	–	–
Obese Grade II	–	–	–	–	–	–
Total	**27**	**54.0**	**23**	**46.0**	**50**	**100.0**

Source: Field Survey by MASS.

Table 4.3: BMI: Vavar-Warli

Village: Vavar, Hamlet: Behedpada, Tribe: Warli

Presumptive Diagnosis	*Male*		*Female*		*Total*	
	N	*%*	*N*	*%*	*N*	*%*
CED Grade III	37	56.1	29	69.0	66	61.1
CED Grade II	8	12.1	4	9.5	12	11.1
CED Grade I	11	16.7	6	14.3	17	15.7
L.W Normal	7	10.6	2	4.8	9	8.3
Normal	3	4.5	1	2.4	4	3.7
Obese Grade I	—	—	—	—	—	—
Obese Grade II	—	—	—	—	—	—
Total	**66**	**100**	**42**	**100**	**108**	**99.9**

Source: Field Survey by MASS.

Analysis of these data of Warlis of Behedpada (Village: Vavar) reveals that nearly 88 per cent of the total cases belong to Grade I, II and III catagories of CED taken together. The percentage of the cases belonging to severe CED, i.e. Grade III is also considerable high (i.e. 61% of the total of 108 cases).

From among females nearly 93 per cent belong to Grade I, II and III catagories of CED taken together. And 29 (69%) out of the 42 females belong to Grade III (severe) CED condition. From the male figures 85 per cent belong to Grade I, II and III catagories of CED taken together and out of the 66 males, 37 (56.1%) belong to

Table 4.4: BMI: Umbarvihir-Thakar, Dhor-Koli

Village: Umbarvihir Tribe: Thakar, Dhor-koli

Presumptive Diagnosis	*Thakar*			*Dhor–Koli*		
	Male	*Female*	*Total*	*Male*	*Female*	*Total*
CED Grade III	9 (90)	14 (77.8)	23 (82.1)	12 (75)	7 (77.8)	19 (76)
CED Grade II	1 (10)	2 (11.1)	3 (10.8)	0	1 (11.1)	1 (4)
CED Grade I	0	2 (11.1)	2 (7.1)	2 (12.5)	1 (11.1)	3 (12)
L.W. Normal	–	–	–	2 (12.5)	–	2 (8)
Normal	–	–	–	–	–	–
Obese Grade I	–	–	–	–	–	–
Obese Grade II	–	–	–	–	–	–
Total	**10 (100)**	**18(100)**	**28 (100)**	**16 (100)**	**9 (100)**	**25 (100)**

*N.B. : Bracketed figures show percentages.

Source: Field Survey by MASS.

Grade III (severe) CED condition. These results also indicate predominant female malnutrition than males. Thus, overall malnutrition in Vavar is more than the Kharonda Warlis.

The data on Thakars and Dhorkolis of Umbervihir show that among Thakars 100 per cent of the cases belong to CED Grades I, II and III taken together. And the percentage of severe type of CED (Grade III) is also high, i.e. 82 per cent of the total cases.

The females also show 100 per cent of CED Grades I, II and III taken together and the severe type of CED is also high, i.e. 77.77 per cent of the total female cases. In all 100 per cent Thakar males belong to moderate (Gr. II) and severe (Gr. III) CED catagories. These results clearly indicate over all malnutrition, without any doubt.

Among Dhor Kolis 92 per cent belong to Grades I, II and III CED categories taken together. Whereas 76 per cent of all the cases, i.e. 25 belong to severe CED category.

One hundred per cent of female are malnourished out of which 77.77 per cent belong to severe CED category (i.e. Grade III). 87.5 if male belong to Gr. III and Gr. I catagories of CED out of which 85.7 per cent belong to severe category of CED. There are only 2, i.e. 8 per cent normal cases of males are with lower body Weight. These results again indicate Gross malnutrition.

Thakars show 80.76 per cent of total cases belong to Grade I, II and III categories of CED taken together. Bisexual variation is also observed indicating more female cases (i.e. 90.47%) belonging to Gr. I, II and III CED categories taken together than male cases (i.e. 74.19%)

Koknas show 82.76 per cent of all the cases belonging to Grade I, II and III categories of CED taken together. Whereas only 17.24 per cent cases are normal so far as the nutritional status is concerned. Numerically male and female cases belonging to Grade I, II and III taken together are the same but percentagewise females are relatively more malnourished than males. Hence, among Koknas the female appear to suffer more from malnourished condition than males.

The results of BMI, although used as a ready reckoner, should be employed with certain precautions as follows:

1. Body weight is a fluctuating measurement for which environmental factors such as diet health condition are more responsible than Genetic factors. Hence, BMI should

as far as possible be used as the indicator for determining "current nutritional status of the individual".

2. Although, it is independent of age and sex, it is always advisable to use it to understand bi-sexual variation because of more malnourished female cases for the obvious reasons.
3. The index can be used as a measure of starvation with reference to Grade condition in particular.
4. This is a quantitative measure of Nutritional status. These results should be supplemented by the qualitative measures such as dietary pattern and morbidity and mortality conditions.
5. Interpretation of the present results has a different angle.

The present survey was conducted in a "Plenty of" season. Hence, the people usually are getting relatively enough food to meet two ends of the day, than the "Scarcity" season. In view of this background extent of malnourishment appear to be exaggerated. If we relate the results with "Work out put" we may have different interpretation. During "Plenty of" season the work load in the fields and related activities in more and hence whatever excess calories are obtained than the scarcity season, are used for these work and hence the Body Weight—the fluctuating factor would remain more or less constant and consequently BMI. During "Scarcity" season relatively both the caloric intake and the work output is less. Hence it should not affect much on the Body weight and consequently BMI. This can be confirmed by the similar survey during "Scarcity season".

II. Diet Survey

Let us have a glance at the results of Diet Survey for further clarification. It is well recognised that in India malnutrition is primarily due to consumption of inadequate diet. Hence, assessment of diet of individuals becomes an important aspect. For the present survey two methods of diet survey have been employed.

These are:

(1) 24 hour recall method.
(2) Weighment method.

The Diet Survey has certain limitations in the sense that a single day's assessment does not represent the real consumption and the method is affected by the respondent's capacity to recall. The method is not really sensitive and need not be associated with the actual nutritional status of Individuals as measured by anthropometry or clinical examination. However, at the community level these could be used as to find out the extent of the problem so that policy makers can draw suitable plans to fill the gap. Nutrient intake depends upon a number of factors the most predominant of which are the seasonal variations, age, sex variation, availability of food; personal taste, individual capacity etc. Hence for effective nutritional assessment, on the basis of diet, longitudinal method is the best of all. However, for the present survey the cross-sectional method was adopted, where we may talk about the current diet and nutritional pattern and status.

People living in the study area have subsistence economy and not the surplus economy. Hence, whatever is cultivated in the fields is fully consumed by the family members and there remains nothing to sell in the market.

People are habituated to eat food 3 times a day whenever available, i.e. early morning before going to the fields, in the afternoon and in the evening. Early morning eating generally includes *Bhakari* made of *Ragi*, some *chatni* or sometimes *dal* whatever is available. Lunch includes *Ragi, Bhakri* and *Dal*. The Dinner usually consists of Rice and *Dal*. The consistency of *dal* is more thin in the evening than in the afternoon. This pattern is subject to availability of a particular item and hence subject to change also according to convenience.

In the study area availability or non-availability of foods play important role. Usually during or immediately after the summer there is shortage and sometimes acute shortage of food. Sometimes, they have meals once in a day or sometimes they may have to skip it.

Considering the above situation, the results of the study can be presented as follows:

> Recall method included about 154 individuals and the weighment method included 9 families. In all 260 households were contacted for such diet survey out of which the above 154 cases could be treated as having relatively authentic information. These cases included 79 males, 19 females, 15

Table 4.5: Results of Diet Survey

Villages	*Tribes*	*Sample Size*	*Per Capita Caloric Intake*		
			Family	*Male*	*Female*
Vavar	Kokna	3	—	—	—
	Warli	19	2405	2416	1970
Sakharshet	Thakar	20	2340	1626	2074
	Kokna	3	2183	1902	—
	Koli	5	2259	—	—
Kharonda	Kokna	31	—	1752	1518
	Warli	5	—	1980	—
	Koli	2	—	1405	1305
Chambharshet	Kokna	11	—	1643	1848
	Warli	40	—	1782	1381

Source: Field Survey by MASS.

pregnant and lactating mothers and 41 families. The weighment method is used at the family level only.

Average caloric intake:

Females (19) Intake = 1509 cal.
Males (79) Intake = 1804 cal.
Pregnant & lactating Mothers (15) Intake = 1518 cal.
(Figures in bracket indicates no. of individuals)

From the results of analysis it would be clear that there is no difference between the calories intake of Normal Women and Pregnant and Lactating Mothers. Generally, the energy requirement during pregnancy and for the lactating mother is higher by on an average of 300 and 500 calories. respectively. The inadequate caloric intake in the present study for pregnant and lactating mothers could be because of inadequate food supply which could be the prime factor.

Table 4.6 shows results of the weighment method. This exercise was carried out in 9 families of three different tribes in the study area. Raw food quantities required for a family for one day was measured and converted into calories with the help of standard values. Average intake for adult man was calculated by dividing it by number of consumption units in the family.

The average caloric intake for adult man in the study population by weighment method is 2153 kcal. per day. This average is high as compared with caloric intake by 24 hour recall method.

Results of the Weighment Method shown in Table 4.6:

Table 4.6: Caloric Intake by Weighment Method

Sl. No.	Tribes	Family Members			Consumption Units	Intake of Family K cal.	Avg. Intake for Adult Man K cal.
		M	F	T			
1.	Thakar	2	2	4	4.3	11460	2665
2.	Thakar	4	3	7	5.6	12472	2227
3.	Thakar	4	3	7	6.6	14592	2210
4.	Thakar	2	6	8	6.9	14016	2013
5.	Warli	2	4	6	5.4	12840	2377
6.	Warli	3	2	5	5.1	12108	2374
7.	Kokna	6	6	12	10.7	22988	2148
8.	Kokna	3	4	7	4.8	8796	1833
9.	Kokna	5	2	7	5.7	8626	1513

M—Male, F—Female, T—Total.
Source: Field Survey by MASS.

Reference Values and Comparison

Besides the analysis of nutritional status, the data were processed for preparing reference values of the various tribal groups under study for Height and Body Weight measurements and presented in the forms of statistical constants such as means and standard deviations. The restriction on the size of the sample from "Wadi respondents" and the "anticipated Wadi participants", is the controlling factor of less number of cases. The 50th percentile values were also calculated and compared with the same units to NCHS and Harward Standards. It would clearly be seen from these tables that the values of the tribals under study come closer to NCHS and Harward Standards around the age of ten year or so, indicating thereby that these tribals are retarded due to some other extraneous factors such as inadequate food supply and partial exploitation of the resources.

III. Vital Statistics on Morbidity and Mortality

Malnutrition influences morbidity rates, maternal mortality rates, life expectancy and other health statistics. A variety of vital statistics, therefore, may be used as indirect indicators of nutritional status of the community. Some type of malnutrition have a particularly high incidence at certain age so that the mortality rates at these specific age period have been used as indicator of the incidence of certain types of malnutrition. Numerous data are available to show that mortality rates of certain age groups—infant mortality rates and 1-4 years old mortality rates are higher in developing countries. These data indicate that malnutrition is either an underlining direct cause or associated cause in as high as 60 per cent of deaths in children under 2 years of age.

For the present project various measures used for indirect/ direct nutritional assessment for the support of anthropometric results have been as under:

1. Morbidity condition.
2. General mortality trend with probable causes.
3. Infant mortality trend with probable causes.
4. Incidence of Disability.

Analysis of the data with respect to these variables show the following results:

(a) Morbidity Condition

Malnutrition is an important contributory cause of morbidity and mortality in diseases such as diarrhoea, tuberculosis and measles, out of which diarrhoea is one of the principal causes of death particularly among young children. On a community basis incidence curves of malnutrition and diarrhoeal diseases run parallel with one another. Between the nutritional group, grade III parallels with diarrhoea. The duration of illness is also as important as the incidence. For the present project the salient features with respect to mortality and morbidity condition are as follows:

The incidence of illness during the last 1 month just before the survey was, 173 cases out of 1427 population, i.e. 12.12 per cent out of which female morbid cases were more (94 out of 173) than the male morbidity (79 out of 173). The morbidity appears to be more up to age 6 years and between the age groups 30 and 50 years. Village-wise morbidity distribution shows that Sakharshet area stand first, followed by Kharonda and then by Vavar in descending order.

Various disease types recorded in the survey are related to infections such as fever, malaria, measles, diarrhoea, pains and aches, injuries and wounds; dermatological and the other problems that includes gynaecological problems, urinary infection, B.P. etc. The incidence of fever is recorded with the highest frequency, followed by diarrhoea. The incidence is more related to the disorders of digestive system rather than the other ones. Besides, 12 cases of disabled individuals are noted related to the problems of eyes, deafness, dumbness, handicap, paralysis and mental illness (2 cases).

(b) Mortality

The proportion of infant mortality to the total population covered (and not number of births) appears to be very high, i.e. 24 cases of infant mortality during one year (1993) for 1427 population. Mortality for other age groups is 25 cases for 1427 population during last two years before survey, out of which 56 per cent contributed towards children below 5 years of age. The causes of mortality have also been noted such as fever, measles, diarrhoea, chicken pox, low birth weight and other minor causes for predominantly infant mortality.

Besides the CNSM Report, according to the ICDS Report, 2012 on tribal projects in Maharashtra, the following seven (tribal projects) areas had less than 60 per cent normal children.

Table 4.7: Tribal Projects Nurtitional Status March-12 Ranking

Sl. No.	*District*	*Block*	*Survey 0-6 Years*	*Weighted Children*	*Classification of Nutritional Status of 0 to 5 years Children*			*Normal % Rounded*
					Normal	*MUW*	*SUW*	
1.	Thane	Jawahar-2	10437	7993	3736	3391	866	47
2.	Nandurbar	Dhadgaon Khuntamohi	8115	5555	2830	2076	649	51
3.	Thane	Jawhar	7781	5922	3018	2325	579	51
4.	Nandurbar	Dhadgaon-2	11264	9007	4755	3495	757	52
5.	Nandurbar	Dhadgaon	11822	8836	4674	3169	993	52
6.	Nandurbar	Akkalkuwa-2	7124	5696	3074	2229	393	54
7.	Nashik	Harsul	12947	9749	5564	3307	878	57

Source: Field Survey by MASS.

Table 4.8: Tribal Projects Nutritional Status March-12 Ranking

Sl. No.	District	Block	Surveyed Children	Classification of Nutritional Status of 0 to 5 yearrs Children				Normal %
				Weighted Children	Normal	MUW	SUW	
1.	Thane	Jawahar	7811	5991	2683	2195	1113	44.78
2.	Thane	Jawahar-2	10466	8319	3954	3316	1049	47.53
3.	Nandurbar	Dhadgaon	11516	9052	4993	3032	1027	55.16
4.	Nandurbar	Dhadgaon Khuntamohi	8360	6434	3646	2165	623	56.67
5.	Thane	Mokhada	11531	8766	5024	3089	653	57.31
6.	Nandurbar	Dhadgaon-2	11856	9667	5600	3113	954	57.93
7.	Nandurbar	Akkalkuwa-2	7488	6144	3563	2139	442	57.99

Source: Field Survey by MASS.

ICDS report, 2014 reveals that out of the total number of children weighed (6265120 children), 89.35 per cent (5598037 children) were of normal weight, 9.25 per cent (579254 children) were moderately malnourished and 1.40 per cent (87829 children) were severely malnourished.

In August 2014, the status was as mentioned in Table 4.8:

In 2014, Harsul in Nasik district had made considerable progress in nutritional status (72.69% normal children) as compared to year 2012 (57.07% normal children). Mokhada which was not present in the first 7 ranking of poor performing block in 2012 (67.79% normal children) moved up the list of poor performing blocks in 2014 (57.31% of normal children).

The data clearly reflects that even today there are blocks where not even 60 per cent children are in normal category.

Reference: Malnutrition Status in Tribal Belts (An evaluation in 7 blocks in Rest of Maharashtra Region) (Prepared for Rest of the Maharashtra Statutory Development Board, 20th May, 2015).

Table 4.9: Expenditure Pattern Per Family, March 1996: Western Maharashtra

(in Rs.)

Items of Expenditure	*Kokna, Mahadeo Koli*	*Warli, Thakar, Katkari*
Food, other than cereals	15,000	4,000
Clothes	2,500	1,200
Medicine	500	100
Fuel, Electricity	600	250
Bus, transport	600	250
Alcohol	900	600
Tobacco	600	350
Holi	1,500	500
Diwali	1,200	200
Panchvi Ritual	100	100
Marriage	15,000	8,000
Death Rites	3,000	1,000

Source: Field Survey by MASS.

Table 4.9 clearly reflects the ethnic group disparities, probably among those who have lands and others landless or with marginal land.

AUK project focusing on tribal child nutrition during 2004-2013 had villages from Jawhar and Mokhada talukas, where interventions were made. BAIF had focused on livelihood issues with Wadi-horticulture project which was possible only with families having some land. The objective has been to prevent migration of the tribals. AUK had an immediate goal to reduce malnutrition, in response to *suo motu* injunction of the Bombay High Court. Palghar presents a picture of multiple tribal ethnic groups living in respective hamlets, showing the stark disparities and migration pattern for livelihood. Due to urban centres, not too far from tribal pockets offering work for survival, also present more exploitation of the tribals by non-tribals and land alienation by the builder lobby, as also farm-house culture.

B. TRIBAL NANDURBAR

Introduction

The Human Development Report, Maharashtra (MHDR), 2002, identified Nandurbar, Jalna and Yavatmal as three of the most backward districts in Maharashtra on the basis of their Human Development Index (HDI). As a follow-up to the MHDR, action research studies were proposed in these districts with a focus on three broad components of human development, viz. Livelihood, health and education.

Among these three districts, Nandurbar stands out because of its predominantly tribal population. The Maharashtra Association of Anthropological Sciences (MAAS) offered to undertake action research studies in Nandurbar due to familiarity with the tribal situation in that area. This report discusses health issues in Nandurbar district. The purpose of this report is to suggest action strategies, which would help improve human development of the tribal people of Nandurbar.

The report is based on anthropological, qualitative field study. The experience of four decades of field visits to Nandurbar district during the course of several research projects and as a member of government committees has helped to understand the tribal situation and make suggestions for development. Two long duration and intensive field visits were undertaken for the purpose of this study. There were interactions with the government officials at the district, tehsil and village level. The educational and health institutions were visited and discussions held with the health personnel, teachers and administrators. Meetings were also held with the leaders in the tribal communities, elected representatives at the tehsil, district, state and national levels as also the NGO managers. Some focused group discussions were held with the community members to understand their perceptions on health and educational issues.

Nandurbar: A Tribal District

Nandurbar district was carved out of Dhule district on 1st July, 1998. The composite Dhule district had 41 per cent tribal population. 1991 Census document mentioned Dhule as the "Tribal District", which ranked first in the State in Scheduled Tribe population. In the newly created Nandurbar district, 62 per cent of the total population and 75 per cent of the total rural population is tribal. Three of the six tehsils in Nandurbar district have more than 80 per cent tribal population. There are only five towns among six tehsils in Nandurbar. The demographic composition of Nandurbar indicates that development issues in the district are issues facing a predominantly tribal population and calls for a concentrated attention on tribal development. Indeed, the motive behind creating a separate district of Nandurbar was to create a tribal district. Some years ago, Gadchiroli was also carved out as a separate district for similar reasons. The division of Thane district has been on the agenda of the government for quite some time in order to focus attention on development of tribal people of Thane district.

Since Nandurbar has recently been formed as a separate district due to heavy tribal concentration and since the government effort is geared to the development of the tribal people of Nandurbar, it is necessary to understand the tribal situation and the government's approach, strategies and implementation machinery towards tribal development, including those related to health and educational issues. The governments during British Rule and after Independence appointed several committees and commissions to study tribal issues and make recommendations about their development. There is a distinct tribal administrative mechanism with exclusive budgets for tribal development. This report, therefore, first discusses the tribal issues in general. The special situations in the tribal district of Nandurbar are then reviewed before discussing the focused issues on health.

Symington Committee

With the formation of Provincial Governments around 1935, Sri B.G.

Kher, a Sarvodaya worker who headed Bombay government appointed a committee on partially excluded areas to improve the conditions of *Bhils* and other aboriginal tribes under the Chairmanship of D. Symington, ICS, Special Enquiry Officer who gave his report in 1938. The report is mainly based on the partially excluded area in West Khandesh, namely: (A) Nawapur Petha, (B) Nandurbar Taluka, (C) Shahada Taluka, (D) Taloda Taluka including Mewasi estates, (E) Akrani Mahal. These six constituent units are precisely the constituent tehsils of present day Nandurbar District formed sixty years ago after the Symington report. The Committee made recommendations about land, rural credit, wages, excise, education and local self-government and other administrative and public health matters. Symington's observations and approach for development given in 1938 are very poignant.

"Actually the problem of the aboriginal and hill tribes lies not in the isolation from but in their contacts with the main body of the community. Where their geographical position keeps them beyond the reach of the outside world, as in the Akranimahal, they are happy and independent; but in the places, now all too many, where they are in constant contact with more educated people, they are degraded, timid and exploited. Since the time of the cession of the Peshwa's territories, successive governments have been occupied in the pacification of the country, the creation of a land revenue system, the introduction of civil and criminal codes of law, the development of communications and irrigation, and other measures for the progress of the province. In the course of such major activities no government appears to have asked itself or at any rate to have answered, the question: whether the Presidency's large tribal areas required any special treatment? These areas have not been totally neglected, it is true, but it has hitherto been usually assumed that whatever measures were suitable for the country at large were suitable also for the tribal areas. This assumption is now being queried, and I submit that the conspectus of these areas contained in the following report will show that, in point of fact, the common law of the land is in many respects highly unsuitable for the tribal areas and produces serious oppression and exploitation. The thought underlying all the proposals which follow is that the State ought now to take an entirely new view of the problem of the aboriginal and instead of relying on the forces of time and example, should adopt active measures designed both to free him from the tentacles of his exploiters and to educate him up to becoming an intelligent and useful member of the community. My position is that, at any rate for the next generation, we must regard the aboriginal as being in the nursery. Like a child he must be protected from outside interference and victimization and like a child he must be taught how to hold his own. In short, the State's attitude must be parental."

The observations and approach of the Symington Committee are still valid and relevant for policy planning even after 65 years.

Nandurbar District Profile

Despite heavy concentration of tribal population, a separate tribal district of Nandurbar was created only recently in 1998. In Dhule district, the tribal population was 41 per cent of the total population. In Nandurbar district, the tribal population is 62 per cent of the total population of the district and 75 per cent of the total rural population. There are 5 towns in Nandurbar district among six tehsils.

Nandurbar district comprises six tehsils, viz. Nandurbar, Navapur, Shahada, Taloda, Akkalkuwa and Dhadgaon (Akrani). Main tribal groups in the district are: Bhils, Dhankas and Gamits, and Kokna in Nandurbar ITDP. Now, Dhule district comprises four tehsils, namely Dhule, Sakri, Sindhkheda and Shirpur.

In Nandurbar district, there are two ITDPs:

1. Taloda covering the tehsils of Taloda, Akkalkuwa, Akrani and Shahada of which all the villages in first three tehsils are under main ITDP.
2. Nandurbar ITDP has two tehsils, namely Nawapur and Nandurbar form Nandurbar District, and the four tehsils from erstwhile Dhule district, namely the tehsils of Dhule, Sakri, Shirpur and Sindhkhed. In Nawapur, all the villages are under main ITDP.

Some other characteristics of the Nandurbar district in comparison with the State and its ranking given in Table 4.10.

It needs to be noted that ST form 75 per cent of the rural population in Nandurbar district, the same as the percentage of BPL families.

The district has poorly developed road infrastructure. Out of the total 947 villages 671 villages (72%) have connectivity by an

Table 4.10: Nandurbar District in Comparison with the State and its Ranking

Indicator		*Nandurbar*	*Maharashtra*	*Rank*
Literacy Rate		56%	77%	35
Drop out rate —	7th std.	45%	31%	29
	10th std.	56%	53%	17
BPL families		75.43%	34.55%	
Human Development Index		0.20	0.58	35
Per capita district domestic product (Rs.)		8195	15804	34

Source: *Human Development Report of Maharashtra 2002* – Table Nos. 21, 111, 112).

all weather road. Remaining 262 villages (28%) get cut off during monsoon months. Total length of roads in the district is 4338 km., out of which 2063 (47.5%) are *kachha* village roads.

Thus, it is clear from the above statistics that the district occupies the lowest position in the State on the development scale and is the most backward district. There is an utmost need to make concerted efforts towards development and improve the standard of living of the tribals.

Summary

Nandurbar district is rural with only 5 towns, rural population varying from 68 to 100 per cent and rural tribal population varies from 52 to 93 per cent in six tehsils. Total tribal population of the district is 62 per cent while the rural tribal population is 75 per cent.

Villages are small and medium size, 11 to 15 per cent with less than 200 population, 26-42 per cent between 200 and 500 population, 54 to 77 per cent between 500 and 2000 population and 8 per cent, 10 per cent and 16 per cent villages in the three tehsils between 2000 to 5000 population. The geographical area of four tehsils is 100 per cent tribal, for two it is 86 per cent and for one tehsil it is 56 per cent. Similarly, four tehsils have 100 per cent tribal viilages, two 91 per cent and 94 per cent and one comprising 70 per cent tribal villages. Out of 932 villages in the district, 83 are not connected by road and out of 770 hamlets, 248 are not connected by road. However, the data on number of *Pada* is not reliable since *Pada* is not defined properly. According to some records, in the hilly tehsils of Akrani and Akkalkuwa, there are

1180 cluster of huts, which commonly are referred to as *Pada*. Majority of the villages have common amenities and facilities like public bus, telephone, post office, veterinary dispensary, PHC etc. beyond 5 to 10 km.

Looking into livelihood issues, about 50 per cent families own land and are formally pursuing agriculture as the main occupation, the other 50 per cent being landless and 56 per cent as agricultural labourer. However, many tribals cultivate land in forest area as illegal encroachments. Income from agriculture varies from Rs. 5000-6000 per annum per family while from service it ranges from Rs. 22,000 to Rs. 26,000 per annum. There are more migrants from the plain areas than from hilly regions. As for the development schemes of the government, 80 per cent people do not know the schemes except education. About 70 per cent of people have reported to have benefited from educational facilities. In the year 1997-98, 75 per cent of the families in the district were categorized under BPL (MHDR, 2002), while the largest tribal group *Bhils*, are about 94 per cent under BPL category in Taloda ITDP and 93 per cent in Nandurbar ITDP (GoM, 2000).

It is thus very clear than Nandurbar is a predominantly tribal district. The issues relating to backwardness are the tribal issues in hilly as well as plain area. Human development in Nandurbar district is clearly an issue of Tribal Development.

Tribal health issues are inseparable from livelihood issues. Their food, nutrition, water, obstetric practices, disease care systems are a part of their adjustment with local environment. Universal value systems of humanity and civil society expect us to help them to live longer, leading a creative life, to enjoy the freedom of choices in life. All societies including our own suffered from high mortality, epidemics and communicable diseases. Scientific advancement made it possible to reduce mortality and enhanced life expectancy in the world and in India.

Since Nandurbar is predominantly tribal, the issues of Nandurbar district have become the issues of tribal health. The livelihood problems of tribals promote ill health, and the paucity of modern health care facilities accelerate morbidity and mortality.

Health and Health Care in Nandurbar

The tribal people in Nandurbar interact closely with local healers, the spirit world and use herbs for treatment and cure. Due to improved roads and transport, communicable diseases get transmitted to erstwhile virgin areas that have led to epidemics of measles resulting in child mortality. Due to depletion of forests, depriving the tribals of roots, tubers and animal life, nutrition standards have decreased. Primitive subsistence economy posing problems of survival has resulted in seasonal migration. The malnutrition and under-nutrition, and lack of health care facilities result in increased morbidity and mortality. Child deaths due to malnutrition in recent years has become an explosive issue in tribal health.

Government of Maharashtra accepted deaths of 1034 children in the age group of 0-6 years in the tribal area of Nandurbar district from March 2000 to February 2001, 594 being children under 1 year of age. 76 per cent of the siblings of dead children were found to be malnourished, indicating malnourishment as the cause of death, although 35 per cent of dead children were reported suffering from diarrhoea and vomiting according to mothers.

The Tribal Research and Training Institute, Pune, Government of Maharashtra, conducted a study under the direction of Government of India to investigate the causes of deaths of tribal children in large numbers and suggest remedial measures. Accordingly, 158 child deaths from 143 families below the age of 6 years in 24 villages in Akrani, Akkalkuwa and Navapur tehsils of Nandurbar district were investigated.

The fact finding study reported that 78 per cent of the households had a food deficit of 6 months or more and had less than 3 acres of land and about 40 per cent had less than 1 acre land or were landless. Faults were identified in the EGS and in reaching the health care to the people, particularly to pregnant women. Recommendations have also been made in the report on agricultural rehabilitation, on employment, public health and participatory planning etc. The studies have identified very frequent transfers of PHC doctors, indebtedness due to procurement of food as predisposing factors besides lack of nourishment to pregnant women (GoM, 2002 B).

In Nandurbar, many health facilities have been created under ITDP, but fall short of requirements. Basically, the coordination between health department and Tribal Development Department is lacking. The schemes are drawn by health department, being labelled as technical in nature. A case in point is the maternity benefit scheme whereby a pregnant tribal woman on getting registered for ANC gets Rs. 400 in cash in installments and Rs. 400 in kind by way of iron, calcium and protein rich syrups and tonics. Actually all the ANC women are provided with iron and calcium all over the State. There is no reason why ITDP funds should be diverted for routine disbursement of tablets. What pregnant tribal women require are the pulses, lentils and cooking oil. Moreover, the medicine during pregnancy is discarded particularly by tribal women for fear of enlargement of size and weight of foetus, which would make labour difficult endangering woman's life. In a difficult terrain with hamlets and villages, not connected by roads, and absence of public transport, unless safe delivery is ensured, women and the community would have no incentive to take measures to increase the weight of foetus. LBW is preferred for low maternal mortality.

There are no gynaecologists, paediatricians, anesthetists or blood bank in Nandurbar district. It would be desirable to have these specialists in every rural hospital; at least one in a tehsil. Measurement of distance by kilometre is illusory. What is realistic is the time taken to reach the health facility. There are certain norms of one PHC, one sub-centre etc. for certain number of population.

The referral systems in Nandurbar are very poorly equipped. The field observations revealed, there are motivated ANMs and nurses. There are young tribal doctors, doctor couples who are committed. They need to be encouraged to share their experiences with their peers from the metropolitan cities. They would feel satisfied by opportunities to go for update training to attend seminars and conferences. They also need exposure. As one BDO mentioned tribal postings if treated as punishment postings inflict punishment on the people by sending unwanted and unmotivated personnel. One additional increment for 3 years of service in tribal belt is recommended by local officials.

According to the study by the Gokhale Institute of Politics and Economics (Draft Report, MHDR follow-up project), there is a discrepancy in the number of beneficiaries as reported in district health records, which is especially wide in the case of the maternity benefit scheme.

Field observations of all research teams (IGIDR studies after MHDR, 2002) clearly bring out the severity of malnourishment among tribal children from the admissions to malnourishment wards at the PHCs and cottage/rural hospitals. Although, there is an improvement in the malnourishment grade in the hospitals, the cases recur after the discharge from the hospitals. It is common knowledge that the tribal girls marry immediately after attending menarche and the birth order is very frequent with less spacing. The practice of not giving kilometres to new born children and the low birth weight babies lead to infant and child mortality. In spite of the maternity benefit scheme, ANC is not considered important. The visiting health functionaries do not find the women at home during field visits for ANC.

The DHO accepted that the welfare schemes for tribals were not run efficiently due to implementation problems and varying local conditions. Particularly in difficult terrain, all children do not go to Anganwadi. The road connectivity is very poor in such areas and there is absence of transport facilities. An ANM also finds it difficult to reach scores of small hamlet settlements on foot, which are under her charge.

Another major cause of child morbidity and mortality is large-scale seasonal migration to Gujarat. The tribals are trapped in the vicious circle of having taken loans from the contractor and to work for him for repayment year after year.

The Bharat Vaidyak Sanstha, Nasik in its study (Draft Report, MHDR follow-up project) of infant deaths in Nandurbar from April to August 2003 reported a progressive rise in infant deaths in that period. Of the total infant deaths, 33 per cent were early neo-natal deaths, 18 per cent were late neo-natal deaths and 49 per cent were other infant deaths. Shahada (101), Akkalkuwa (109) and Dhadgaon (143) together had the highest number of deaths (353 out of 581 in the district). About half of infant deaths were within the first month of life and within these deaths, 33 per cent in the first week. One-third of total infant deaths were early neo-natal deaths. BVS has also reported SBR for the district at 26.8 (2001-02) and 17.33 (2002-03). The ICDS data on child mortality (U-6) in Nandurbar district for the period April-August 2003 indicated 395 deaths. Of these, Shahada, Akkalkuwa and Dhadgaon account for 63 per cent deaths, each taluka sharing equal burden. 53 per cent deaths were under one year age, 31 per cent between one to three years and 16 per cent account for three to six years of age.

The BVS report on child mortality considers still births on account of unmanaged ANC. There were no health care facilities of any significance in Nandurbar for risk management in childbirth. The antecedents of child mortality are low age at marriage, women's nutrition, and spacing of pregnancies, poverty, migration, and literacy. The ICDS scheme does not function at some *padas* and there is under-reporting of child deaths by health staff for fear of investigations.

Field Observations

1. The basic equipment in Rural Hospitals has been in functioning order. Some competent ANMs are running the PHCs and RH with confidence. Tribal doctors, doctor couple and BAMS doctor are motivated. They need to be given incentives about post-graduation and out of turn increments or seniority. They demand more occasional participation in the knowledge update programmes offered in seminars, workshops and conferences.
2. There have been patients of adult diarrhoea in wards due to drinking water from pits near the fields. Water stored in home and schools has been safer. Some schools trained children to use chlorine drops at home. Use of copper vessels, if affordable and drum stick seed could be used for cleaning water at household level.
3. Condition of referred services has been poor in Nandurbar district. There is no blood bank, anaesthetist and gynaecologist in the district in the public sector while paediatrician and gynaecologist are required in each Rural Hospital.
4. BAMS doctors are found useful due to knowledge of herbs except that they are not trained for minor surgeries.
5. There is a large army of para-health workers at grassroots level: Anganwadi, Mini-anganwadi teachers and helpers, trained *dais*, and *pada* workers appointed for monsoon season as "*sandeshwahak*" to report epidemic risk or emergencies. There are no mobile clinics. Referral services for obstetric care or surgery are not satisfactory even at Nandurbar civil hospital.

   Mature women instead of adolescent boys and girls need to be appointed as *pada* workers for whole year, trained by CRHP village women trainers.

6. Post-graduate Medical students from Allopathy and Ayurveda could be posted at RH and civil hospital for the respective specialities.
   Medical interns could be posted at PHCs.
7. Local herbalist, *Bhagat, dais* and Anganwadi women could be co-opted for health care by providing periodic training and feedback sessions.
   Every village needs to have a health committee monitored by women Gram Panchayat members and mobile clinic team.
8. Paid health worker should not be transferred for at least one year and be rewarded for continuous service for three years.
9. Community must get the experience of safe delivery and pediatric care to enlist their co-operation. Better transport, communication (phones) and mobile teams and referrals at a distance of 1 to 2 hour travel time are necessary.
10. Parameter for infrastructure facilities need not be kilometre distance or population, but the time required to cover the distance on foot or by available mechanized transport.

Other Observations

1. There are few revenue villages and fewer Gram Panchayats in proportion to the large number of hamlets, which are units of social action. There are only 25 Gram Panchayats for 163 villages and 260 *pada* in Akrani tehsil. How could a village or Gram Sabha function effectively as per 73rd Constitution Amendment? The parametres for separate status of a revenue village and Gram Panchayat need to be flexible according to the terrain and infrastructure in an area.
2. The powers and authority of P.O.-ITDP, Collector and CEO are not clear about tribal development. What is the mechanism of their co-ordination? How does ITDP monitor sectoral programmes? Education department feels that health department has more authority in supervision of their sector in tribal area.
3. It was recommended by BDO that EGS could be provided

on one's own field like land levelling and bunding.

4. Postings need not be punishment postings in tribal area as it resulted in punishment to the community. Staff in the age group of 50+ lack physical energy to work in difficult tribal pockets.
5. *Pada* should be taken as unit for EGS like making an approach road, digging well, sanitation etc.
6. Forest department has to be tribal friendly. Tribals have looked after forests through centuries on a non-commercial basis.
7. Concerted efforts are required to form Mahila Mandals, Youth Groups and Farmers clubs.

Action Strategies for Improvement in Health Status

Confidence Building of the People

Tribal people have been living under adverse circumstances in hostile terrains developing coping mechanisms for resolving their health and illness problems. For a long time they lived in a time freeze and relied on the magico-religious practices and herbal remedies offered by the *Bhagat*. Their health care concerns have been managed by the benevolent and evil spirits and by white and black magic. Low birth weight babies have, therefore, been preferred for safe delivery instead of risking a woman's life in labour through acceptance of foetal growth interventions. Infant mortality, therefore, would be tolerated in preference to maternal mortality. It has always been customary in all traditional societies to follow the biological cycle of reproduction and allowing the natural cycle of fertility and mortality by marrying at the onset of puberty. People are pragmatic in finding mechanisms of treatment and cure, which are time tested and which are available and affordable in the neighbourhood. Traditional medicine and practitioners continue to provide services to the people. People have to have experience of cure from modern medicine, which would be available and affordable. Tribal people have never sought any facilities apart from what is offered to them by nature and indigenous knowledge. Modern health care facilities and personnel need to reach out to the innocent, tradition bound, tribal people and provide them experience of relief from morbidities and risk situations.

Currently, the health care infrastructure facilities in tribal areas are based on population and geographical area coverage, on the same principle as for other rural areas. The PHCs and sub-centres in tribal areas are designed with less population coverage as compared to other rural areas. In the tribal terrain, with lack of transport and communication facilities, the principle of health institutions and health personnel reaching out to the tribal villages and hamlets, and the patients going to the centres, has to be the time and effort required instead of the distance in kilometres. These institutions have, therefore, to be located within a reachable distance ranging from half an hour by foot for sub-centres and two hours for the PHC. Similarly, the referral centres should not be more than two hours walking distance for the patient and his family.

There is a total lack of mobile treatment teams in the district. At least one such mobile team for each taluka is an urgent need to provide emergency services and experience of health risk management to the people. The services of the specialists such as obstetrician, surgeon, anaesthetist and emergency facilities like blood bank are totally lacking or inadequate in the public sector in Nandurbar district. There has to be a pragmatic tie up with the private sector in hiring their services and facilities by the government when needed. There could be any number of administrative hurdles and bottlenecks in devising the innovative public-private mix in health care. But flexibility in applying administrative regulations to suit the needs of tribals is the key strategy for tribal development.

The bottom-line in dealing with the tribal people, who have experienced exploitation through contact with the outside world of literates, is that they need to get experience of successful treatment management and cure, which would develop their confidence in the government health care system. Tribal society is a close-knit kinship society. In a village, or within a radius of ten to twenty kilometres, people of one tribal ethnic group are all related to each other, either through marriage or through lineage ties. The life experiences are thus shared. Even a *Bhagat* is a close kin of a large number of families. The acceptance and utilization of modern health care facilities require experiences of success.

There are certain special health and disease issues. Women's health is a major issue, which also impacts children's health due to frequent child births, lack of spacing and malnutrition. There are diseases like malaria, TB, leprosy, night blindness and STD. HIV-AIDS has not yet hit the tribal ground. But, with permissive and tolerant sex behaviour within tribal society it could lead to a dangerous scenario in the near future. No doubt there are good schemes like ICDS and maternity benefit scheme, which if implemented efficiently can provide required nutrition to pregnant women and children. It has to be borne in mind that the government schemes cannot continue for unlimited period. The tribal society has to become independent and self-sustaining like the mainstream society. This is possible only through strategies to build the capacity of the local functionaries and people and develop a partnership with the government functionaries in development.

Capacity Building Strategies

At the local level, following functionaries are available in the current system of governance:

1. *Pada* health worker, who could be a female health and development worker in a village and *pada*. She could be addressed as *'Mai'*.
2. ICDS/Anganwadi worker.
3. Traditional birth attendant—*'Dai'*.
4. Traditional health professional—*'Bhagat'*.
5. Gram Panchayat members, particularly women members.
6. Educated young men and women, if any, in the village.

In the public sector there are several functionaries interacting with the tribal people.

1. ANM, MPW.
2. Teachers, particularly from the ashram schools and more particularly the women teachers.
3. Gram Sevak.
4. *Patwari/Talathi*.
5. Forest Guard.
6. Doctors—MBBS, BAMS.
7. Medical interns.

The functionaries at the village level need to be trained and oriented periodically over the feedback sessions. CRHP Jamkhed has been able to upgrade the knowledge and skills of illiterate village level women workers. It has been observed by all action research teams that the TBAs are not being trained properly, although they are conducting majority of the deliveries. Similarly, the Anganwadi worker and her helper have no opportunities to upgrade their skills for personality development of the children. *Bhagat* has good knowledge of medicinal herbs available locally. If he is given proper respect as a health functionary, he could be weaned away from some of the exploitative and superstitious magico-religious practices. PHW has to be a middle-aged woman, who commands respect in the village and not a person in the adolescent age group. Dr. R.S. Arole from CRHP Jamkhed has provided enough proof for the last thirty years of the illiterate village women functioning efficiently as village health worker and as a skilled midwife. BAIF has already started utilizing the indigenous knowledge of *Bhagat* in providing health care to the people. BAMS doctors could have good communication with the *Bhagats* on herbal medicine and can train them in the Ayurvedic principles, which are closely linked with herbal medicine. *Bhagats* could also be trained in the processing of herbal plants. The women Gram Panchayat members could be made aware and be oriented periodically about the health and development issues within their respective Gram Panchayats. They could be trained to monitor and coordinate the activities of village level functionaries with the government functionaries. Due to expansion of education in tribal areas, one comes across occasionally the girls and boys educated beyond seventh or tenth standard in villages. Their resource need to be tapped by further developing their capacities by providing them skills in health care and education. It is very important to educate the community through IEC efforts in health and development issues. These educated boys and girls could be motivated to form Mahila Mandals, youth groups, self-help groups for which they could be remunerated with a very modest activity based honorarium.

Other Action Strategies

Considering the number of *Padas* (Hamlets) and smaller human settlements, the number of revenue villages are far too less and the Gram Panchayats comprising the multiple villages are far too few. As a result, the Gram Panchayat members and particularly the women members are scattered over a wide geographical area making it difficult for them to meet more frequently and to monitor and coordinate the health and development activities. Even if the health committees are formed at the village level, they would not be functional in too much dispersed locations. It would be desirable to have more revenue villages and Gram Panchayats irrespective of the size of population they would cover. Attempts could be made to develop model villages with central settlement patterns to bring home the message of reorganization of very small hamlet settlements into a sizeable, functioning settlement.

Around 46 per cent of land in Nandurbar district is forest land under the regulatory authority of the Forest Department, which functions under the federal authority of Government of India. The environment issues have made the forest laws more stringent and has *de facto* deprived the tribals of their traditional livelihood rights and source of food in the forest. Illegal cultivation of forest land by the tribals, which is construed as encroachment has accentuated the rift between the tribals and the forest department. This needs to be amicably settled permanently between the Central and State Government. There are concepts of joint forest management and social forestry, but the spirit of helping the tribals and to use their indigenous knowledge is often ignored. Forest land is not made available even for construction of Ashram school complexes.

Large-scale seasonal migration to Gujarat has been accepted as an important cause of malnutrition of children and morbidities on account of unsanitary living. The migration of particularly women and children needs to be discouraged by providing work locally to women on the principle of food for work. There are several local works like village and *pada* connectivity and construction of Anganwadi and mini-Anganwadi, where the work could be provided. BAIF through its 'Wadi' project in tribal areas has provided a successful road map to reverse migration by providing livelihood locally and by ensuring the marketing and processing of horticultural products besides helping in the entire process of production by modern methods.

General Recommendations

1. Restructuring of revenue villages and Gram Panchayats to involve more people in democratic participation.

2. Empower Anganwadi and Ashram schools as nodal institutions of development and information of schemes.
3. Gram Panchayats to be handed over some schemes like Maternity benefit scheme and ICDS for implementation.

Livelihood

1. Wadi projects initiated by BAIF be expanded to counteract migration. EGS schemes be made applicable for women for major part of the year.
2. Forest labour could be used for developing medicinal plants, which have a growing internal and export market.
3. Tie up with KVIC for forest produce, honey, handicrafts and hand/ambar charkha production.

Health

1. Health institutions to be located in terms of time required for the people to reach on foot, not in terms of population coverage or distance in kilometres.
2. Local health functionaries like *Dai*, *Bhagat*, Anganwadi worker, *Pada* health worker to get continuous training.
3. Intersectoral coordination at the State, District and Tehsil level under the initiatives of Tribal Development Department.
4. Effective IEC in health by CBOs and NGOs with the help of local functionaries and PRI.
5. Public-Private coordination for health care, particularly the specialist care not available under public health system.
6. NGOs in health and livelihood to be organized for implementing and monitoring development programmes under the leadership of BAIF and CRHP, Jamkhed.

The tribal people in Maharashtra represent the most deprived sections of the population across a range of socio-economic indicators. The concentration of tribal population in particular districts and blocks is reflected in these regions or pockets being categorized as the most backward in terms of human development indicators. For example, Nandurbar district, which is a tribal district in terms of its population composition with about 75 per cent of its rural population being tribal, has been consistently ranked as the lowest ranked district in Maharashtra in terms of the human development index. Nandurbar was carved out as a separate tribal district from Dhule in 1998. However, it may be noted that a discussion on tribal development issues of the region was made sixty years before this in 1938, in the report of D. Symington, ICS, Special Inquiry Officer, who studied the conditions of Bhils and other aboriginal tribes in order to improve their conditions, in the same six tehsils which together now constitute Nandurbar district. He made recommendations about land, rural credit, wages, excise, education, local self-government and public health matters. Some of his observations and recommendations such as the following, continue to be relevant today—"it has hitherto been usually assumed that whatever measures were suitable for the country at large were suitable also for tribal areas...the common law of the land is in many respects highly unsuitable for the tribal areas and produces serious oppression and exploitation...like a child he must be protected from outside interference and victimization and like a child he must be taught how to hold his own. In short, the State's attitude must be paternal" (Government of Bombay, 1938).

It is clear that most of the diseases are water borne or caused by vectors in Nandurbar. Safe drinking water, personal hygiene and sanitation need to be organized. Although, many bore-wells have been installed, the rain water washing down the slopes would be contaminating the water sources. In rural areas where chemical pesticides are being used and where the defecation takes place at high ground, the rainwater creates diarrheal diseases. The TCL is either not used or monitored, the poor quality and expired stock make the effect useless. *Pada* worker scheme for monsoon months is a half-hearted attempt whereby they report emergencies to the PHC. The young *pada*-worker boys and girls cannot command the confidence of people where experience and age is valued. Dr. Arole has shown how the middle aged, properly trained, illiterate women can deliver health care locally. They also know when to refer a case to the hospital.

Tribal Health

Tribal Nandurbar

"Maharashtra has reported progress in all the outcome indicators of health from 2001–2011. The highlights in terms of achievements include a sharp drop in the crude birth rate (CBR), a decline in the fertility rate to below replacement levels, a marginal improvement in the adult sex-ratio with the sex-ratio for the ST well above the state average and improved life expectancy, with a female advantage reported in the same. A significant decrease in the infant mortality rate (IMR) (a drop of 20 points over 2001-2011) is reported with a narrowing of the male-female, rural-urban gap in this indicator. A steady drop in the under-five mortality rate (U5MR), a maternal mortality ratio (MMR) that was half the national average in 2007-2009 are clear indicators of progress, although, there is still a long way to go to achieve the Millennium Development Goals (MDG) for the MMR."

"On the flip side is the low child sex-ratio (for children aged 0–6 years) of 883 in 2011, which could reflect not just male child preference, but also neglect of the female child in terms of the quality of care given. There continue to also exist inter-district, spatial as well as gender and social-group disparities in all these indicators, pointing towards specific interventions that need to be put into place to tackle the same."

"To make the prevailing health scenario in Maharashtra easier to study and understand, it can be arranged under two broad heads, namely, input and outcome indicators. Public spending on health is an important input indicator as it has implications for the availability, provisioning and effectiveness of services provided in this social sector. With less than 2.5 per cent of the state budget allocated to health in 2008–2009, Maharashtra reports low public spending on health. On a per capita basis, at the district level, it is found to be higher for the urban population *vis-à-vis* the rural population. The spread of public health infrastructure and manpower in the state is vast, following a three-tier system and can be considered well above the national average. What needs to be recognized is the presence of a sizeable tribal population spread across 15 districts and the challenges it poses to the outreach of health facilities in the state. Rural hospitals (RHs) have seen a small improvement in population ratios and a lessening in inter-district inequities, which could be a result of the upgrading they have undergone in recent years. Although, there has been an upward trend in the availability of hospitals and beds per lakh population, the latter shows an urban bias. At the district level, many districts

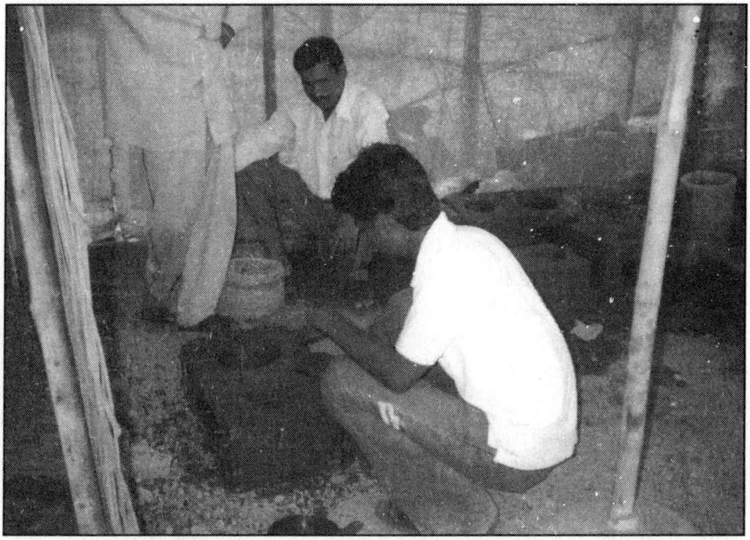

Plate 1: Training to make smokeless

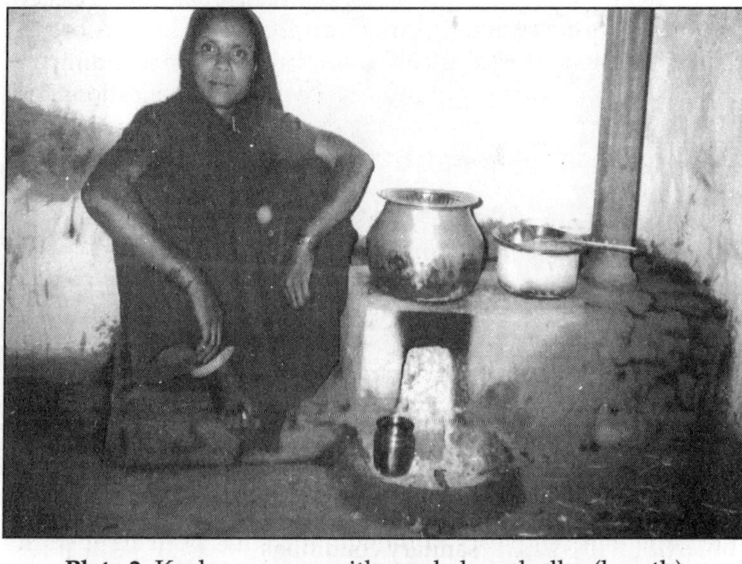

Plate 2: Korku woman with smokeless chulha (hearth) in her kitchen

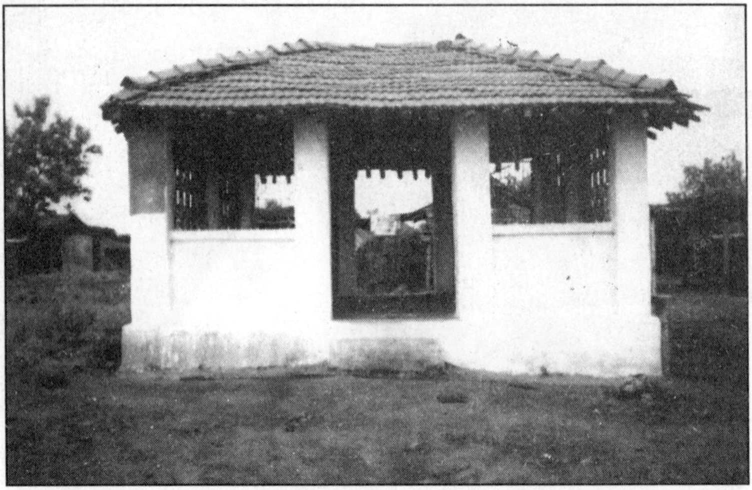

Plate 3: Kolamchavdi – a symbol of ethnic identity

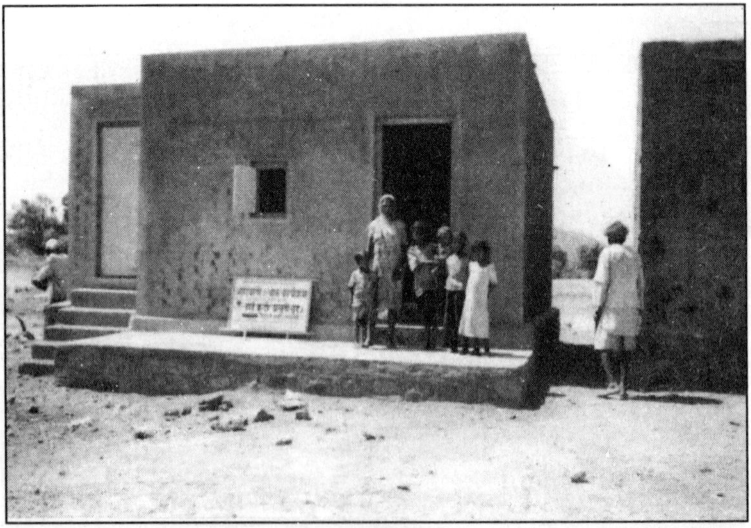

Plate 4: Dai hut (kuti) for safe delivery in the village under sanitary conditions

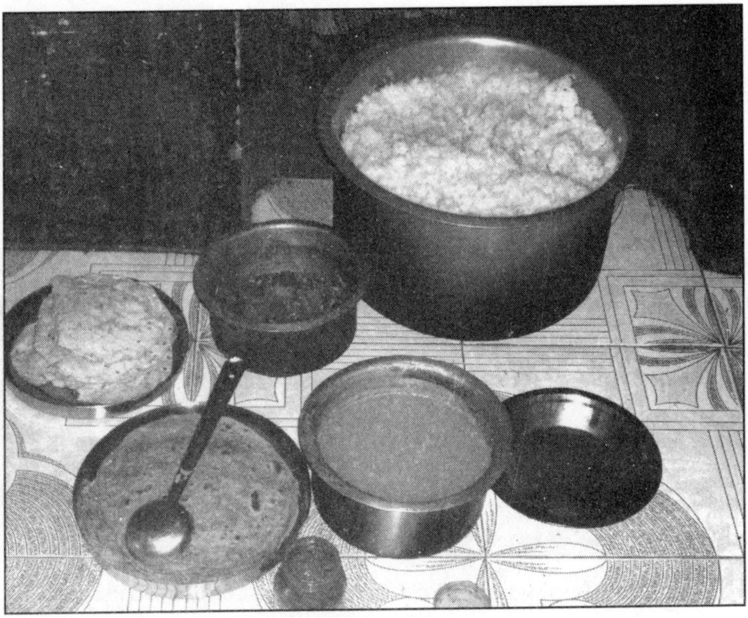

Plate 5: Full meal to a pregnant woman by AUK

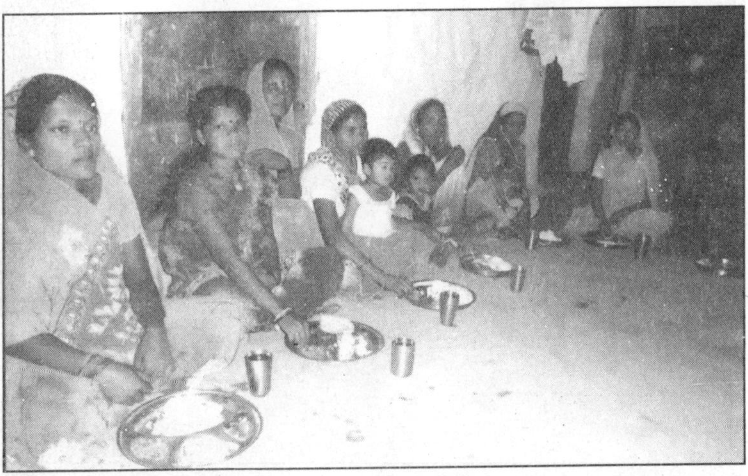

Plate 6: Pregnant women taking meals with kids

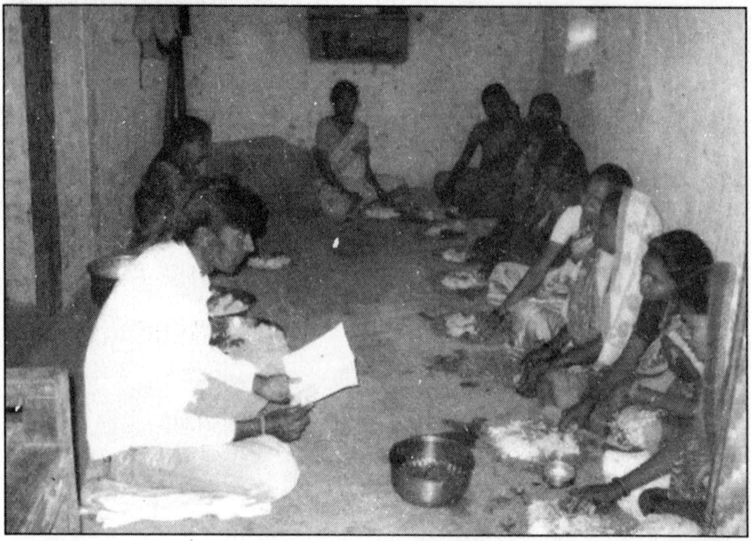

Plate 7: A booklet about pregnancy care being read during meals of pregnant women

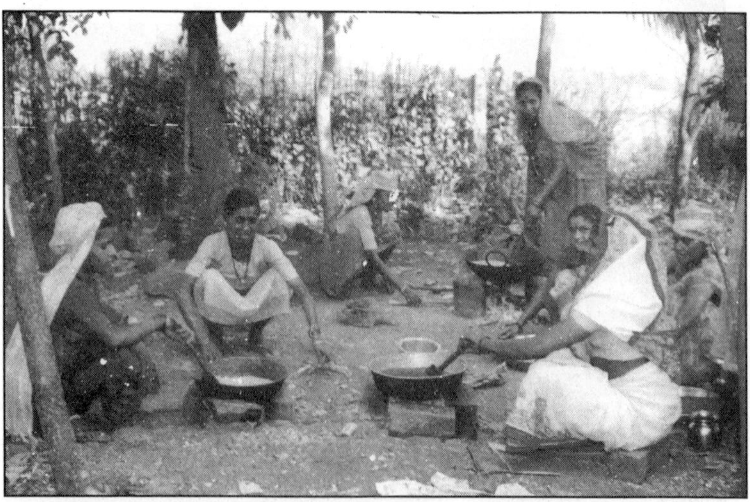

Plate 8: SHG group preparing supplementary food, Sattu for children, pregnant and lactating women

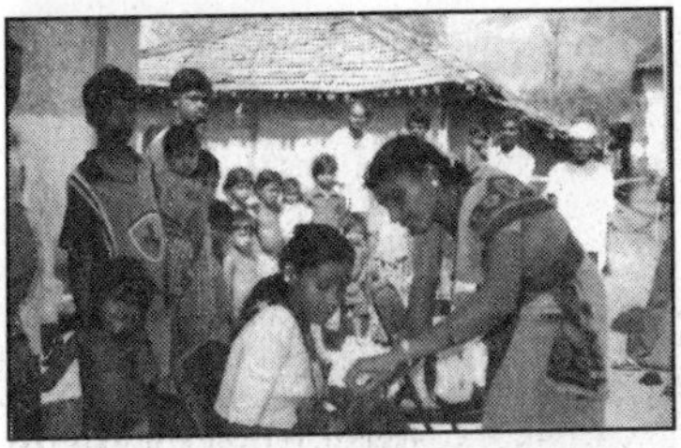

Plate 9: Polio drops given to a baby

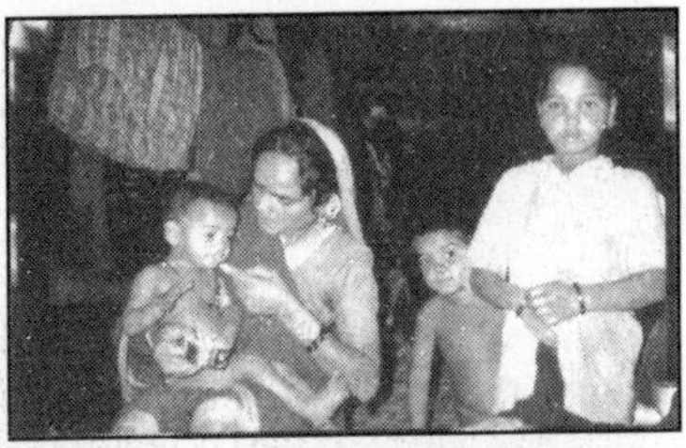

Plate 10: Sattu being fed to a tribal child

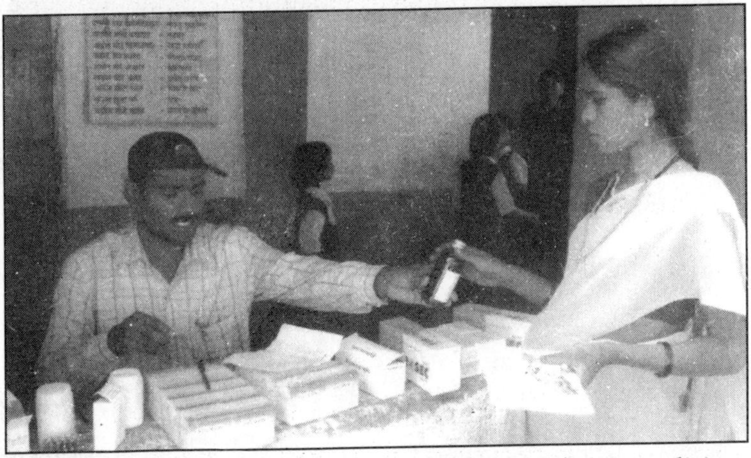

Plate 11: A volunteer dispensing medicine from AUK medicine box in anganwadi

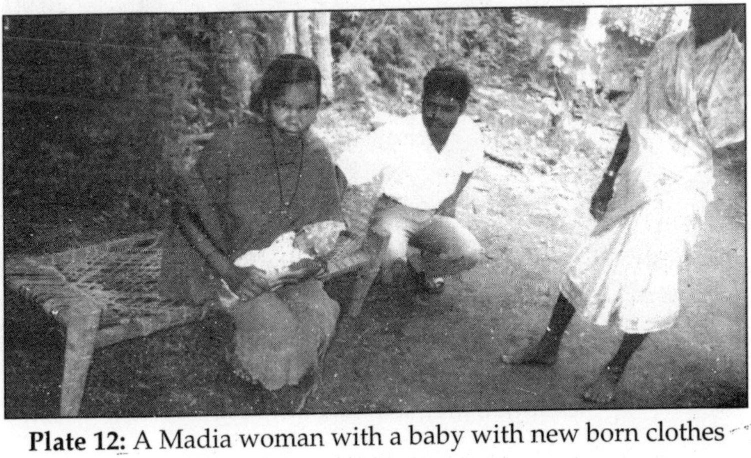

Plate 12: A Madia woman with a baby with new born clothes

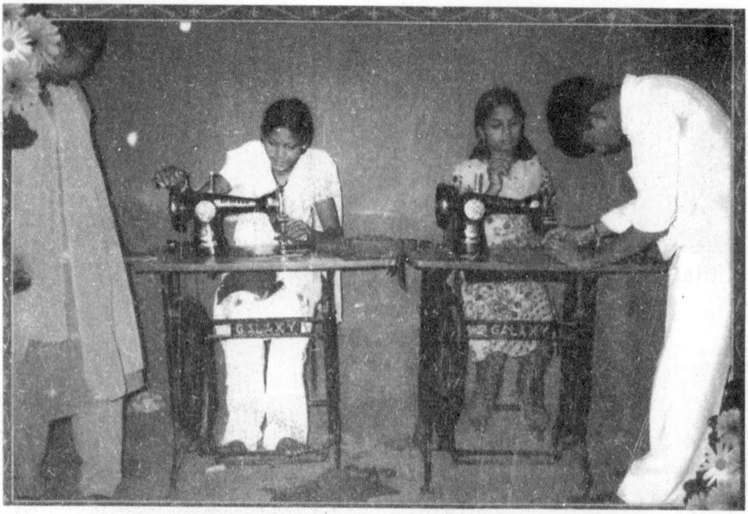

Plate 13: Clothes for new born by tailoring trainees

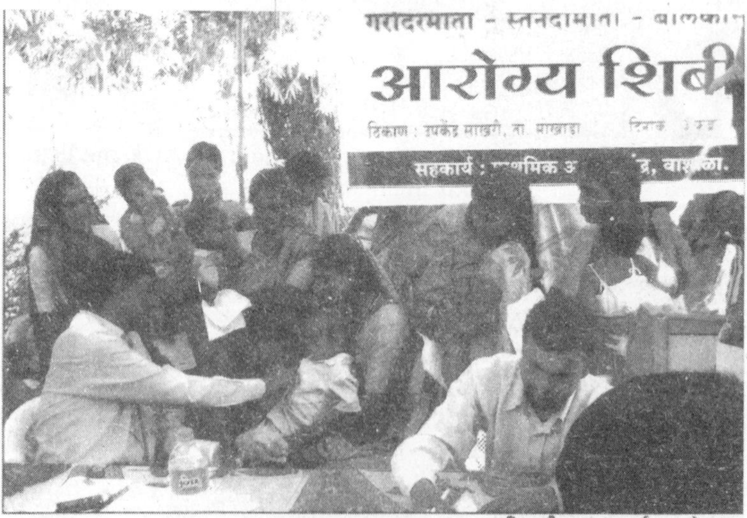

आदिवासी उत्थान कार्यक्रम मोखाडा

Plate 14: Health camp for mothers & children

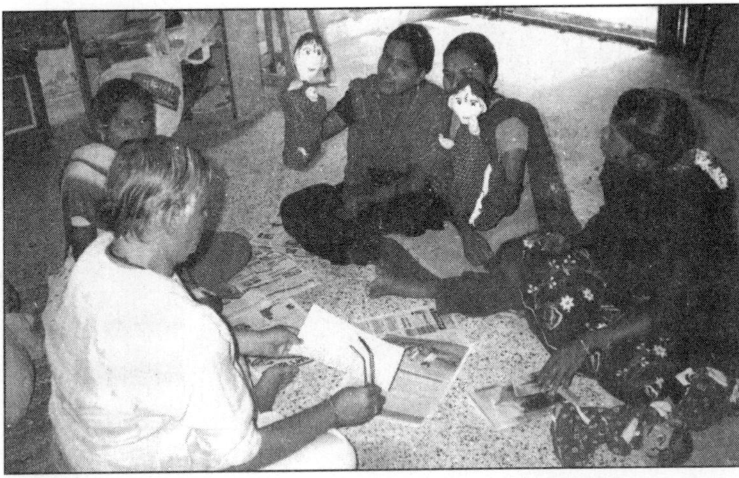

Plate 15: PUPPET making training session

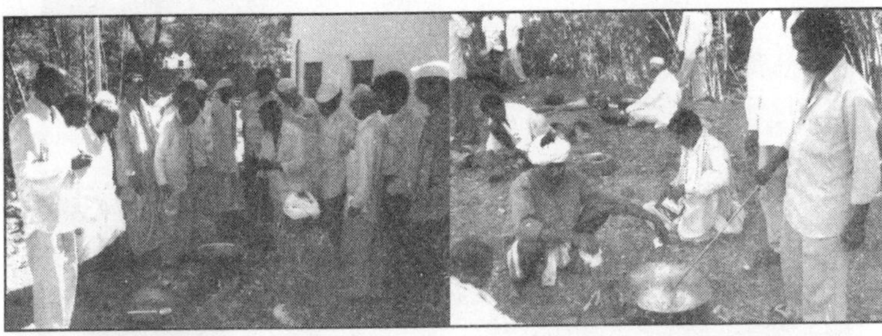

Plate 16: Vaidu training : Making Ayurvedic medicine from herbs

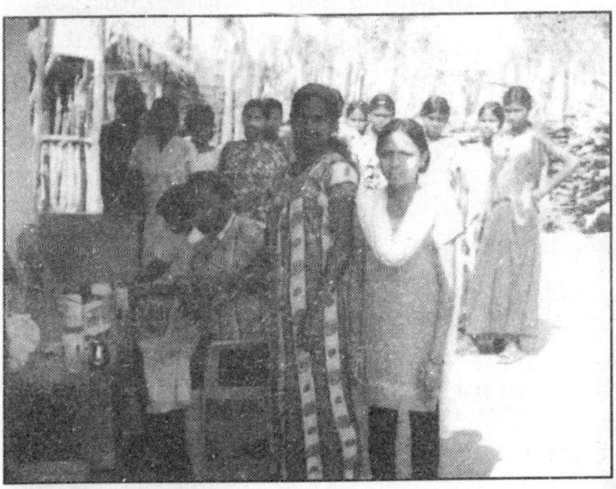

Plate 17: Khelwadi : AUK mini - anganwadi

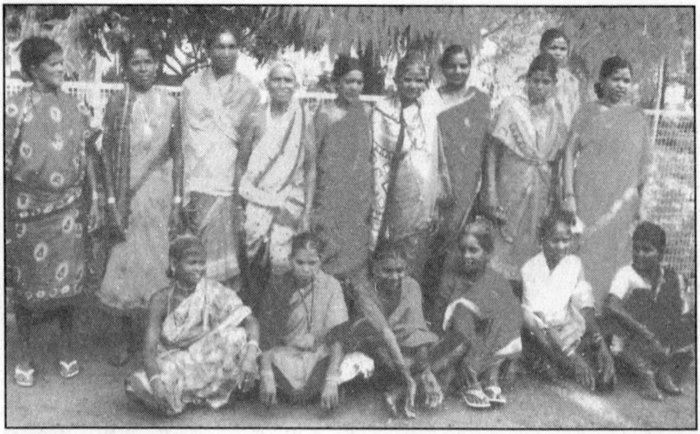

Plate 18: Dais after training session : Etapalli, Gadchiroli

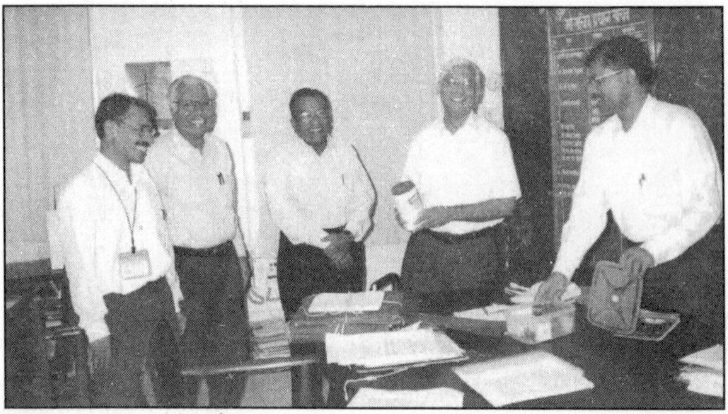

Plate 19: Secretary, TDD, Govt. of Maharashtra appreciating Sattu and medicine box with AUK Directors, Dr. Arole – Prof. Mutatkar

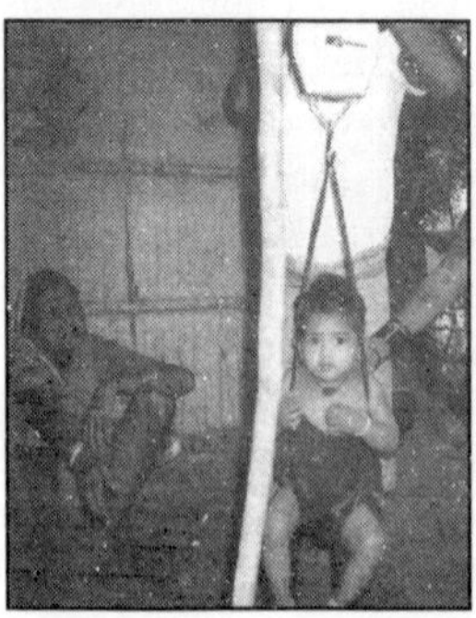

Plate 20: A tribal child being weighed, under grandma's gaze

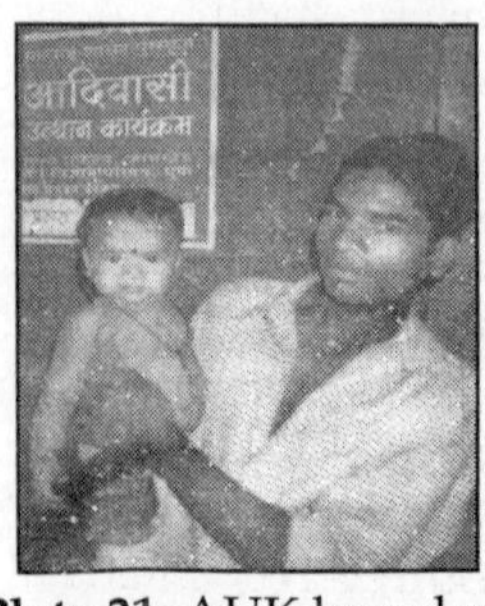

Plate 21: AUK board on volunteer's house

report an increase in population per hospital bed over the last decade, pointing towards the need for improvements on this front."

"Adequate and trained health personnel are essential for the functioning of health infrastructure, and in Maharashtra the numbers of doctors and nurses has been on the rise. Nevertheless, inter-regional variations exist, with urban areas having an advantage in terms of staffing. There is a shortage of auxiliary nurse midwives (ANMs) at the sub-centre level, nurses at the primary health centre (PHC) level and specialists in the Indian Public Health Standards (IPHS) hospitals, with serious consequences for the poor who either have to forgo specialized health care or bear the expenses for availing it. Gadchiroli reports the best doctor-population ratio, but it also has poor utilization of health facilities, which is captured by the very low proportion of institutional deliveries and child immunization rates, demonstrating that mere availability of health facilities and good doctor-population ratios may not necessarily convert to improved utilization rates although they are essential for improving the same."

"Population proportions for inpatient (IP) and outpatient (OP) care are a good reflection of the efficiency of any health care system. In Maharashtra, while there has been an increase in IP and OP cases by around15 percentage points over the period from 1986-87 to 2004, the private sector is found to cater to OP care and hospitalization in larger proportions. Despite such a trend, a large proportion of the poor populace, especially women, access health care from the public sector. There also exists a clear caste disparity with ST households showing very low utilization rates of public health facilities, which could be because of the scattered nature of their habitation and the weak presence of the private sector in tribal-dominated areas. There is thus a pivotal role that the public health sector can play in facilitating inclusion of such excluded social groups into the health-care system in the state."

"While there has been an improvement in the coverage of antenatal care in the state, especially for ST mothers, the third district-level household and facility survey (DLHS-3) reports that only a third of women in the state received full antenatal care during pregnancy. The percentage has improved to 70 per cent in rural area and 61 per cent in urban area in 2011–12 (Government of Maharashtra, 2012). Inter-district disparities are present in the outreach of antenatal care. Women with more years of education, those living in urban areas and those belonging to higher wealth classes were found to access antenatal care in greater proportions. SC and ST women accessed such care from government facilities in larger proportions. One of the highlights of the achievements of the state has been a clear and unambiguous improvement in the proportion of institutional births, an important element for maternal and neonatal survival, seen over the period between the DLHS-1 and DLHS-3 surveys. Combined with it is an increase in the proportion of safe deliveries."

"Overall, while institutional births show an urban bias, the increase in their rates has been higher for rural areas of the state (between DLHS-2 and DLHS-3). What is a matter of concern is the wide inter-district variations in this indicator, with institutional births varying from 93.5 per cent in Mumbai suburban to as low as 24 per cent and 25 per cent in Gadchiroli and Nandurbar respectively, which also report the lowest proportions of safe deliveries. The interventions under the National Rural Health Mission (NRHM) in Maharashtra have had some notable beneficial outcomes, including a marked increase in institutional deliveries to 96 per cent, increase in the per cent of safe deliveries to 98 per cent in 2011-12 (Government of Maharashtra 2012), and OP care, enhanced coverage of the beneficiaries under the Janani Suraksha Yojana (JSY), community mobilization by accredited social health activists (ASHAs), community-based monitoring (CBM) instituted in its first phase and increases in health-care manpower in the state."

"Maharashtra has made progress in tackling under-nutrition for all three measures, indicating improvements in curbing the incidence of child malnutrition, with a considerable reduction in the proportion of underweight children, stunted and wasting children between the second national family health survey (NFHS) and CNSM. The proportion of children suffering from stunting though has not shown a significant decrease and flags a priority area for interventions. Malnutrition is seen to have a larger rural presence, higher prevalence in urban slums and a gender bias. Disaggregated by social groups, the occurrence of malnutrition is found to be higher amongst children belonging to the SC and the ST. NFHS-3 data shows around a third of women have low body mass index or BMI and a little less than half to be anaemic (based on low haemoglobin levels). Women belonging to the lower wealth classes, rural areas and SC and ST groups report low BMI and haemoglobin levels. Maharashtra also reports of high obese or overweight women (higher in urban areas) and a higher proportion of obese men in rural areas."

"Two vital elements for addressing undernutrition are oral rehydration therapy (ORT) and child-feeding practices. In 2007-08 (DLHS-3), close to a fifth of children in Maharashtra suffered from childhood diarrhoea. Awareness about diarrhoea management practices is found to be influenced by a mother's age and education, place of residence, social group and wealth quintile. Maternal illiteracy and belonging to SC households contribute to low proportions of children being breastfed."

"Maharashtra launched the flagship Rajmata Jijau Mother–Child Health and Nutrition Mission (RJMCHNM) in March 2005 with the primary aim of reducing grades III and IV malnutrition in children in the age group of 0–6 years. The RJMCHNM stresses the notion of "the 1,000-day window of opportunity' (–9 to 24 months), during which a significant lifelong difference can be made to the lives of children. With this underlying ideology the second phase of the RJMCHNM was initiated in 2011 with the focus on reductions in under-nutrition amongst children of less than two years of age through a continuum of care. Inclusion of the most vulnerable, youngest, poorest, socially excluded, severely undernourished and difficult-to-reach children is the main aim of the interventions under the RJMCHNM."

"Maharashtra is now positioned such that, although, it has a vast health infrastructure, it needs to be operationalized better so as to be more equitable and inclusive. A multipronged strategy is needed: to tackle regional disparities in the access to and utilization of health care, for effective functioning of referral mechanisms, more efficient utilization of resources, medicine availability and pricing, public-private partnerships and spread of CBM to all districts, deal with the health-care implications of rapid urbanization and last, but not the least, to improve data availability, which could immensely contribute to the formulation of evidence-based interventions for health care. Also, to be more socially equitable, the spread of tribal population across the 15 districts needs to be understood better to facilitate improved provisioning of health care facilities and personnel in these areas. Improvements in the nutrition status of women and children needs increased awareness generation on various fronts, including the benefits of breast-feeding practices, usefulness of colostrums, initiation of complementary foods at the age of six months for infants and usefulness and effectiveness of home based protocols to tackle under-nutrition" (MHDR 2012: Executive Summary : xxxvii-xxxix).

Annexures

Tribal Development in Maharashtra and Odisha: Field Studies

An opportunity was provided to undertake field studies in Maharashtra and Odisha to assess feasibility of horticulture development, supported by NABARD with assistance from German Development Bank, KFW.

The summary of the extensive field feasibility report presented here, represents the studies undertaken by Prof. R.K. Mutatkar, an anthropologist, Dr. A.P. Kulkarni, an economist and Ms. Nancy Gaikwad, a professional social worker and founder of a tribal NGO, during summer of 1996, in Thane and Nasik districts of Maharashtra, and Phulbani, Rayagada and Kalahandi districts of Odisha.

The scientific methodology of rapid assessment was followed, by first running over the area to get a general feel and selecting at least two villages in each taluka for detailed investigation. Detailed family schedules, ten each from the selected villages, were supplemented with interviews of village leaders and women. Group interviews of women were also undertaken. Market surveys were undertaken to judge the present situation and to assess the market forces in order to recommend viable horticulture development programme.

It is believed that traditionally, the tribals have been the collectors of food from the forest, miles away from the market economy. In historical times, caste-Hindu peasantry suffered from drought and famine, but the tribals survived as a result of dependence on the forest food. Now, the depletion of forest and natural resources like soil and water, fodder and fuel, and their exploitation by non-tribals, has resulted in starvation, malnutrition and degradation of the quality of life and loss of nerve. Most affected are the tribal women who face the scarcity of fodder, fuel and drinking water.

This process is sought to be reversed by the Bhartiya Agro-Industries Foundation, Pune (BAIF) and National Institute of Social Work and Social Sciences, Bhuvaneshwar (NISWASS), with the assistance from NABARD under an agreement with a German Development Bank, KFW.

The programme of development envisages what is commonly known as Wadi project of BAIF, whereby the poor tribals are helped to develop horticulture as a means of sustenance. The programme has been successfully implemented by BAIF in tribal areas in Maharashtra and Gujarat.

Maharashtra

Food scarcity leading to migration to urban areas as casual labour is the main problem in the Mokhada taluk in Thane district, and Peth-Surgana taluks in Nasik district. Food lasts in varying degrees for three to nine months which leads to indebtedness. There is plenty of surface water, but there are no watershed development programmes. People are willing to accept modern technology for production of fruits and vegetables, as also take up double crop, depending upon the availability of water. This is visible in Peth taluka where irrigation facilities are available. Scarcity of drinking water in summer is a nightmare to women who were seen lined up at midnight at the village well in parts of Mokhada taluka.

The spread of education in Maharashtra is visible as also the modern amenities like electricity and television. This has led to problem of educated unemployed among the tribal youth who do not want to toil on their lands but aspire for fixed income jobs.

In Mokhada, on the whole, around 20 to 30 per cent tribals are landless and majority of the remaining have less than 5 acres of land under cultivation. Predominant cropping pattern refer to *Nagli* (*Ragi*) 40 per cent, Paddy 30–40 per cent, *Varai* 10 per cent and Lentil, oilseeds and pulses together 10–20 per cent. In Nasik, Paddy is 60 per cent and Nagli or Ragi is 30 per cent.

Encroachment of forest land is very common. There is widespread alcoholism amongst males which is a problem for the women.

Odisha

The striking feature of tribal scene in Phulbani, Rayagada and some parts of Kalahandi is the cohabitation of the Scheduled Tribes and Scheduled Castes in the villages. The traditional hierarchy persists and also gets reflected among those who have embraced Christianity. The ST and SC do not belong to the same Christian order and have separate churches or chapels. The tribals consider themselves as the custodians and trustees of the natural resources such as the forest and the lands, and the SC have to use these at the pleasure of the tribals. However, a symbiotic relationship exists among the two communities. Although landless, the SC are good artisans and make their living on trade, mat weaving, broom making, basketry and carpentry. They do trading for the tribals. SC are relatively better educated and can communicate with the outside world more effectively.

There is more tree cover in Odisha, than in Maharashtra, which is threatened with the shifting cultivation, *Podu*, practiced by the tribals. Unlike Maharashtra, there are no industrial urban areas in the vicinity of tribal areas. Although food security problems are similar, there is no migration to urban areas in Odisha tribal belt under study, but the onslaught is on the forest covered land.

The tree cover on the roadside comprised mango, jackfruit, *sal*, bamboo, occasional cashew, *mahua*, *salap* and *umber*. Within village boundaries and in the backyard of the houses, there is cultivation of mango, jackfruit, papaya, beans, guava and *ber*. Castor and cactus are used as house fence. Turmeric and ginger are the main cash crops in the area.

Podu is practiced on communist principles, each according to the need prescribed by the village council. Destitutes and old widows get their share in the *podu* land and cultivation for their living. The main crops are paddy, maize and occasional *ragi* on flat lands while other crops are raised on *podu* land.

A person with 1 to 3 acres of land gets paddy to last 3-5 months for a family of six members. *Ragi* and millets supplement for another three months which is further supplemented from forest collection of mango, kernel, *mahua* flowers, tubers and green leafy vegetables. Income from sale of pigs, bamboo, tamarind and labour help to tide over the year.

Although drinking water is not a major problem, depletion of forest has led to problem of firewood. Alcoholism among men is being resisted by women by organizing themselves. There is a widespread practice of tattooing of women's faces among the Desia Kondhs on the plains, which is now declining among the adolescents.

Among the Dongaria Kondh in Rayagada district, in Bissam-Cuttack block, the Dongaria Kondh Development Agency has developed horticulture by way of pineapple and banana plantations, as also mango, turmeric and jackfruit. The SC do the trading at Chatikona railway station in the plains, with traders from Raipur in Madhya Pradesh. As a result, *Podu* has distinctly reduced in this area. The fruit processing factory in the plains is, however closed due to political forces. The Kutia Kondh children appear malnourished and afflicted with disorders of the stomach in Belghar hill area.

Expenditure Per Family in Odisha : April 1996

(in Rs.)

Items of Loan	*Family with Land*	*Landless Family*
House Repair (Roof)	3,000–4,000	3,000
Rent : Bullocks for ploughing (per day)	200	—
Vegetables, meat, fish	2,000	1,000 1,500
Edible Oil	250–400	Extracted from Mahua
Clothes	1,200–2,000	800–1,600
Medicine	500–2,000	500
Education (stationery & clothes)	150–400	—
Fuel, Kerosene	250	250
Tobacco	150–200	200–300
Alcohol	700–1,000	200–500
Ceremonies & Festivals	500–1,000	1,000–1,500
Marriage	4,000	4,000
Miscellaneous	800–1,500	900–1,200

Summing up

It is thus clear that one of the ways of developing tribal areas and people is through the method of horticulture development. The people are willing to accept or update the technology which they possess. Along with production, monitoring will have to be done in marketing and by developing the processing industry. Mango is a traditional fruit both in Odisha and Maharashtra. Cashew nut has a potential in Odisha as also improvement in the traditional crop of turmeric. The degradation of tribal life is more marked in Maharashtra due to seasonal migration to the urban areas in construction activities. Odisha tribals still maintain a symbiotic relationship with forest ecology.

Prevalence of Under-Nutrition, by Place of Residence, Sex, Social Group and Wealth Index: Maharashtra

Characteristics	*Height for Age (Percentage)*		*Weight for Height (Percentage)*		*Weight for Age (Percentage)*	
	Stunting (Standard Deviation) (SD < –2)	*Severe Stunting (SD < –3)*	*Wasting (SD < –2)*	*Severe Wasting (SD < –3)*	*Under-weight (SD < –2)*	*Severe Underweight (SD < –3)*
All-India	48.0	23.7	19.8	6.4	42.5	15.8
Maharashtra	46.3	19.1	16.5	5.2	37.0	11.9
Residence						
Rural	49.1	21.0	18.2	5.6	41.6	13.9
Urban	42.2	16.4	14.1	4.6	30.7	9.1
Mumbai (Slum)	47.4	16.1	16.1	4.0	36.1	11.6
Mumbai (Non-Slum)	41.5	15.7	16.4	2.5	25.8	6.9
Gender						
Male	47.3	20.3	17.5	5.2	36.7	12.6
Female	45.1	17.7	15.4	5.2	37.3	11.1
Social Group						
SC	55.2	23.4	20.2	6.6	41.7	13.5
ST	57.8	30.0	18.9	5.6	53.2	21.1
OBC	40.6	14.4	15.7	5.2	33.0	10.0
Others	42.5	16.9	14.6	4.4	32.6	9.6
Wealth Index						
Lowest	63.2	32.9	18.2	5.9	51.8	18.8
Second	55.1	25.1	21.8	6.8	46.6	20.0
Middle	53.6	25.3	19.4	5.3	48.2	13.4
Fourth	45.1	16.4	16.1	5.8	32.4	10.2
Highest	28.9	7.2	10.8	3.3	20.9	4.5

Source: *IIPS and Macro International* (2008), p. 95.

B. TRIBAL NANDURBAR
National Family Health Survey – 4 [2015-16]

Nandurbar, Maharashtra—Key Indicators

Separate data for ST in Nandurbar is not available. However, since about 75 per cent of ST Population is rural, Nandurbar rural data can be surmised as closest to S.T. data for comparison

Indicators NFHS-4 (2015-16)

Population and Household Profile		**Nandurbar Rural**	**Maharashtra Rural**
1.	Population (female) age 6 years and above who ever attended school (%)	51.8	70.3
2.	Population below age 15 years (%)	31.3	25.6
3.	Sex-ratio of the total population (females per 1,000 males)	1,026	967
4.	Sex-ratio at birth for children born in the last five years (females per 1,000 males)	1,050	927
5.	Children under age 5 years whose birth was registered (%)	82.9	94.6
6.	Households with electricity (%)	72.4	90.0
7.	Households with an improved drinking-water source1 (%)	84.2	85.6
8.	Households using improved sanitation facility 2(%)	18.6	44.2
9.	Households using clean fuel for cooking 3(%)	12.0	33.7
10.	Households using iodized salt (%)	98.7	94.4
11.	Households with any usual member covered by a health scheme or health insurance (%)	13.5	13.8
Characteristics of Adults (age 15-49)			
12.	Women who are literate (%)	42.3	74.8
13.	Men who are literate (%)	53.4	91.2
14.	Women with 10 or more years of schooling (%)	21.4	32.6
Marriage and Fertility			
15.	Women age 20-24 years married before age years (%)	24.6	31.5
16.	Men age 25-29 years married before age 21 years (%)	*	17.5
17.	Total fertility rate (children per woman)	–	2.1
18.	Women age 15-19 years who were already mothers or pregnant at the time of the survey (%)	9.4	10.4
Infant and Child Mortality Rates (per 1,000 live births)			
19.	Infant mortality rate (IMR)	–	24
20.	Under-five mortality rate (U5MR)	–	30

(Contd.)

Population and Household Profile		*Nandurbar Rural*	*Maharashtra Rural*
Current Use of Family Planning Methods (Currently married women age 15–49 years)			
21.	Any method4 (%)	55.3	65.5
22.	Any modern method4 (%)	53.4	64.2
23.	Female sterilization (%)	48.7	55.9
24.	Male sterilization (%)	1.4	0.7
25.	IUD/PPIUD (%)	0.2	1.1
26.	Pill (%)	0.7	1.7
27.	Condom (%)	2.2	4.6
Unmet Need for Family Planning (Currently married women age 15–49 years) 5			
28.	Total unmet need (%)	12.3	8.6
29.	Unmet need for spacing (%)	5.1	4.2
Quality of Family Planning Services			
30.	Health worker ever talked to female non-users about family planning (%)	21.7	19.3
31.	Current users ever told about side effects of current method 6 (%)	28.6	32.4
Maternal and Child Health Maternity Care (for last birth in the 5 years before the survey)			
32.	Mothers who had antenatal check-up in the first trimester (%)	53.5	66.8
33.	Mothers who had at least 4 antenatal care visits (%)	52.6	69.4
34.	Mothers whose last birth was protected against neonatal tetanus 7 (%)	80.5	90.7
35.	Mothers who consumed iron folic acid for 100 days or more when they were pregnant (%)	38.5	37.9
36.	Mothers who had full antenatal care (%)	26.5	29.6
37.	Registered pregnancies for which the mother received Mother and Child Protection (MCP) card (%)	73.7	92.7
38.	Mothers who received postnatal care from a doctor/nurse/LHV/ANM/midwife/other health personnel within 2 days of delivery (%)	52.0	75.7
39.	Mothers who received financial assistance under Janani Suraksha Yojana (JSY) for births delivered in an institution (%)	20.2	11.0
40.	Average out of pocket expenditure per delivery in public health facility (Rs.)	15,329	3,653
41.	Children born at home who were taken to a health facility for check-up within 24 hours of birth (%)	5.1	6.9
42.	Children who received a health check after birth from a doctor/nurse/LHV/ANM/ midwife/other health personnel within 2 days of birth (%)	27.3	31.6

Population and Household Profile		Nandurbar Rural	Maharashtra Rural
Delivery Care (for births in the 5 years before the survey)			
43.	Institutional births (%)	52.5	86.7
44.	Institutional births in public facility (%)	41.7	50.9
45.	Home delivery conducted by skilled health personnel (out of total deliveries) (%)	10.4	4.6
46.	Births assisted by a doctor/nurse/LHV/ANM/other health personnel (%)	60.2	88.1
47.	Births delivered by caesarean section (%)	3.4	15.2
48.	Births in a private health facility delivered by caesarean section (%)	(19.9)	27.5
49.	Births in a public health facility delivered by caesarean section (%)	2.9	10.5
Child Immunizations and Vitamin A Supplementation			
50.	Children age 12-23 months fully immunized (BCG, measles, and 3 doses each of polio and DPT) (%)	32.7	56.7
51.	Children age 12-23 months who have received BCG (%)	72.7	89.8
52.	Children age 12-23 months who have received 3 doses of polio vaccine (%)	36.6	69.1
53.	Children age 12-23 months who have received 3 doses of DPT vaccine (%)	47.7	74.8
54.	Children age 12-23 months who have received measles vaccine (%)	68.8	82.9
55.	Children age 12-23 months who have received 3 doses of Hepatitis B vaccine (%)	44.9	63.5
56.	Children age 9-59 months who received a vitamin A dose in last 6 months (%)	71.1	69.2
57.	Children age 12-23 months who received most of the vaccinations in public health facility (%)	93.2	92.3
58.	Children age 12-23 months who received most of the vaccinations in private health facility (%)	6.8	7.6
Treatment of Childhood Diseases (children under age 5 years)			
59.	Prevalence of diarrhoea (reported) in the last 2 weeks preceding the survey (%)	6.1	
60.	Children with diarrhoea in the last 2 weeks who received oral rehydration salts (ORS) (%)	*	58.8
61.	Children with diarrhoea in the last 2 weeks who received zinc (%)	*	11.9
62.	Children with diarrhoea in the last 2 weeks taken to a health facility (%)	*	78.7
63.	Prevalence of symptoms of acute respiratory infection (ARI) in the last 2 weeks preceding the survey (%)	2.6	2.2
64.	Children with fever or symptoms of ARI in the last 2 weeks preceding the survey taken to a health facility (%)	68.9	83.0

(Contd.)

	Population and Household Profile	Nandurbar Rural	Maharashtra Rural
	Child Feeding Practices and Nutritional Status of Children		
65.	Children under age 3 years breastfed within one hour of birth 9 (%)	63.1	59.5
66.	Children under age 6 months exclusively breastfed 10 (%)	*	60.6
67.	Children age 6-8 months receiving solid or semi-solid food and breastmilk 10 (%)	*	38.8
68.	Breastfeeding children age 6-23 months receiving an adequate diet 10, 11 (%)	3.5	4.1
69.	Non-breastfeeding children age 6-23 months receiving an adequate diet10,11 (%)	*	10.0
70.	Total children age 6-23 months receiving an adequate diet10, 11 (%)	2.7	5.0
71.	Children under 5 years who are stunted (height-for-age) 12 (%)	49.7	38.4
72.	Children under 5 years who are wasted (weight-for-height) 12 (%)	40.4	26.1
73.	Children under 5 years who are severely wasted (weight-for-height) 13 (%)	15.2	9.4
74.	Children under 5 years who are underweight (weight-for-age)12 (%)	57.0	40.0
	Nutritional Status of Adults (age 15-49 years)		
75.	Women whose Body Mass Index (BMI) is below normal (BMI < 18.5 kg/m^2) 14 (%)	45.3	30.0
76.	Men whose Body Mass Index (BMI) is below normal (BMI < 18.5 kg/m^2) (%)	39.5	23.7
77.	Women who are overweight or obese (BMI ≥ 25.0 kg/m^2) 14 (%)	7.2	14.6
78.	Men who are overweight or obese (BMI ≥ 25.0 kg/m^2) (%)	3.7	16.4
	Anaemia among Children and Adults 15		
79.	Children age 6-59 months who are anaemic (<11.0 g/dl) (%)	60.8	54.0
80.	Non-pregnant women age 15-49 years who are anaemic (<12.0 g/dl) (%)	61.4	47.7
81.	Pregnant women age 15-49 years who are anaemic (<11.0 g/dl) (%)	(66.2)	49.9
82.	All women age 15-49 years who are anaemic (%)	61.6	47.8
83.	Men age 15-49 years who are anaemic (<13.0 g/dl) (%)	35.4	19.7
	Blood Sugar Level among Adults (age 15-49 years) 16 Women		
84.	Blood sugar level – high (>140 mg/dl) (%)	3.8	4.4
85.	Blood sugar level – very high (>160 mg/dl) (%)	1.0	1.8

Population and Household Profile	Nandurbar Rural	Maharashtra Rural
Men		
86. Blood sugar level – high (>140 mg/dl) (%)	5.3	5.4
87. Blood sugar level – very high (>160 mg/dl) (%)	0.0	2.4
Hypertension among Adults (age 15-49 years)		
Women		
88. Slightly above normal (Systolic 140-159 mm of Hg and/or Diastolic 90-99 mm of Hg) (%)	6.6	6.6
89. Moderately high (Systolic 160-179 mm of Hg and/or Diastolic 100-109 mm of Hg) (%)	0.9	1.4
90. Very high (Systolic ≥180 mm of Hg and/or Diastolic ≥110 mm of Hg) (%)	0.5	0.7
Men		
91. Slightly above normal (Systolic 140-159 mm of Hg and/or Diastolic 90-99 mm of Hg) (%)	12.5	11.0
92. Moderately high (Systolic 160-179 mm of Hg and/or Diastolic 100-109 mm of Hg) (%)	4.1	2.7
93. Very high (Systolic ≥180 mm of Hg and/or Diastolic ≥110 mm of Hg) (%)	0.0	0.8
Women Age 15-49 Years who have ever Undergone Examinations of		
94. Cervix (%)	35.6	44.4
95. Breast (%)	23.5	21.7
96. Oral cavity (%)	14.9	15.3
Available Figures are only for Maharashtra Knowledge of HIV/AIDS among Adults (age 15-49 years)		
97. Women who have comprehensive knowledge 17 of HIV/AIDS (%)	–	22.2
98. Men who have comprehensive knowledge 17 of HIV/AIDS (%)	–	41.3
99. Women who know that consistent condom use can reduce the chances of getting HIV/AIDS (%)	–	61.2
100. Men who know that consistent condom use can reduce the chances of getting HIV/AIDS (%)	–	82.3
Women's Empowerment and Gender Based Violence (age 15-49 years)		
101. Currently married women who usually participate in household decisions (%)	–	89.4
102. Women who worked in the last 12 months who were paid in cash (%)	–	35.5
103. Ever-married women who have ever experienced spousal violence (%)	–	26.2
104. Ever-married women who have experienced violence during any pregnancy (%)	–	3.4

(Contd.)

Population and Household Profile		Nandurbar Rural	Maha-rashtra Rural
105.	Women owning a house and/or land (alone or jointly with others) (%)	–	33.3
106.	Women having a bank or savings account that they themselves use (%)	–	38.7
107.	Women having a mobile phone that they themselves use (%)	–	30.9
108.	Women age 15-24 years who use hygienic methods of protection during their menstrual period 18 (%)	–	55.7
Tobacco Use and Alcohol Consumption among Adults (age 15-49 years)			
109.	Women who use any kind of tobacco (%)	–	7.4
110.	Men who use any kind of tobacco (%)	–	39.3
111.	Women who consume alcohol (%)	–	0.2
112.	Men who consume alcohol (%)	–	18.0
113.	Women who tried to stop smoking or using tobacco in any other form during the past 12 months19 (%)	–	28.9
114.	Men who tried to stop smoking or using tobacco in any other form (during the past 12 months) 19 (%)	–	35.1

Source: *Survey of NFHS*, Done by IIPS, Mumbai.

Appendix 1

District Profile

(I) POPULATION

Nandurbar District Population, Number of Villages and Towns, Area

	Nandurbar District						
	Nawapur	*Nandurbar*	*Taloda*	*Akkalkuwa*	*Dhadgaon*	*Shahada*	*Total*
Population (2001)	238496	293833	128425	177709	135916	334756	1309135
Population (1991)	196550	248363	97931	133880	96912	288909	1062545
% of S.T. population (1991)	85.04	39.28	67.85	81.22	86.13	47.78	62.25
% of Rural Population (1991)	87.8	68.4	77.8	94.2	100	89.2	84.6
% of Urban Population (1991)	12.2	31.6	22.2	5.8	0	10.8	15.4
Number of villages (1991)	155	153	92	186	163	184	934
% of tribal villages (1991)	100	70	100	100	100	94	91
Number of towns (1991)	1	1	1	1	0	1	5
Total area (sq. kms.) (1991)	977	1082	343	868	773	991	5034
% of tribal area	100	56	100	100	100	86	87

Source: (1) Tribal Development Department (TDD), Special Action Plan, Nasik, 2003.
(2) Census of India, 1991.

Sex-Ratio of Scheduled Tribes by Tehsils for Total, Rural and Urban

Sl. No.	Name of Tehsil	No. of females per 1000 males		
		Total	Rural	Urban
1.	Nawapur	1002	1006	902
2.	Nandurbar	1005	1015	902
3.	Talode	1017	1014	1055
4.	Akkalkuwa	1010	1013	–
5.	Akrani	1003	1003	–
6.	Shahada	984	984	990

Source: Census of India, 1991.

(II) VILLAGE AND CONNECTIVITY

Percentage Distribution of Villages by Population Ranges, 1991

Sl. No.	Name of the CD Block	No. of Inhabitated Villages	Percentage of Villages in Each Range					
			Less than 200	200-499	500-1999	2000-4999	5000-9999	10000 and above
1.	Nawapur	150	0.67	13.33	77.34	7.33	1.33	–
2.	Nandurbar	150	4.67	16	68.66	10	0.67	
3.	Taloda	91	10.99	26.37	57.14	4.40	1.10	–
4.	Akkalkuwa	185	13.51	29.73	54.06	2.16	.054	–
5.	Akrani	163	15.34	42.33	39.26	3.07	–	–
6.	Shahada	181	3.87	13.26	63.54	16.02	3.31	–

Source: Census of India, 1991.

The Size of the villages has to be taken into account while demarcating the revenue villages and group Gram Panchayats. Location of educational and health institutions and personnel have to consider the size.

(III) LIVELIHOOD ISSUES

Taluka-Wise Proportion of Forest Area: Nandurbar (2000-01)

Tehsils	% of Forest Area
Akkalkuwa	49.88
Akrani	88.97
Taloda	41.64
Shahada	14.93
Nandurbar	9.76
Nawapur	19.31
Total	**37.41**

Source: Acharya, S., *et al.* (2004), Draft Report, MHDR follow up project.

Appendix 2
Land-Use

Distribution of Villages According to Land-Use

(in hectares)

Sl. No.	*Name C.D. Block*	*No. of Inhabitated Villages*	*Percentage of Cultivable Area to Total Area*	*Percentage of Irrigated Area to Total Cultivable Area*
1.	Nawapur	150	62.25	1.24
2.	Nandurbar	150	77.36	6.49
3.	Talode	91	64.57	8.85
4.	Akkalkuwa	185	42.71	1.36
4.	Akrani	163	75.69	0.62
6.	Shahade	181	77.95	16.73
	District total	1586	64.91	7.79

Source: Census of India, 1991.

Akkalkuwa and Akrani are hilly tracts. There are no watershed projects.

Landless and Landholder Households

Sl. No.	*Particulars*	*Taloda (%)*	*Nandurbar (%)*	*% Total*
1.	Landless families	39191 (56)	42648 (47)	50
2.	Landholder families	30431 (44)	48940 (53)	49
	(a) Irrigated landholders	1774 (06)	2990 (03)	3
	(b) Non-irrigated landholders	27402 (90)	39721 (43)	42
	(c) Both irrigated & Non-irrigated	1255 (04)	6229 (07)	4.6

Total Households = 161210

Total Landholders = 79371

Source: (1) ITDP Taloda at a Glance, TRTI, Pune, 2000.

(2) ITDP Nandurbar at a Glance, TRTI, Pune, 2000.

Many landless families, who have no land as per revenue records, do cultivate forestland, which is considered illegal encroachment.

Landholders Classified by Size or Agricultural Land

Sl. No.	Area in Hectors	Taloda ITDP (%)	Nandurbar ITDP (%)	% Total
1.	Up to 1 hect.	8674 (29)	12258 (25)	26
2.	1-2	13750 (45)	21839 (45)	45
3.	2-3	4082 (13)	7664 (16)	15
4.	3-5	2754 (09)	5270 (11)	10
5.	5-10	1046 (04)	1750 (04)	4
6.	Above 10	125 (00)	159 (00)	0
	Total	**30431 (100)**	**48940 (100)**	**100**

Source: (1) ITDP Taloda at a Glance, TRTI, Pune, 2000.
(2) ITDP Nandurbar at a Glance, TRTI, Pune, 2000.

Season-wise Migration of Families: Taloda & Nandurbar

Sl. No.	Season	Migration Period					
		Upto 2 months		Upto 3 months		Upto 4 months	
		HHs.	Persons	HHs.	Persons	HHs.	Persons
1.	Rainy	816	1952	241	520	317	767
2.	Winter	7600	16124	4287	10332	8205	23302
3.	Summer	8492	18940	4677	11085	8079	20735
	Total	**16908**	**37016**	**9205**	**21937**	**16601**	**44804**

Source: (1) ITDP Taloda at a Glance, TRTI, Pune, 2000.
(2) ITDP Nandurbar at a Glance, TRTI, Pune, 2000.

Major Tribe-wise Number of Migrating Families

Sl. No.	Tribe	No. of Total Families under Survey	No. of Migrated families	Percentage		Percentage of Migrating Families
				Taloda	Nandurbar	
1.	Bhil	114821	20679	12	24	36
2.	Dhanka	6524	1193	16	28	44
3.	Gamit	18990	4335	15	25	40

Source: (1) ITDP Taloda at a Glance, TRTI, Pune, 2000.
(2) ITDP Nandurbar at a Glance, TRTI, Pune, 2000.

About 94 per cent *Bhil* families in Nandurbar and Taloda ITDPs are under BPL. Since Nandurbar ITDP also includes tribal pockets from Dhule district, it is clear that there is no difference in the tribal situation in Nandurbar and Dhule districts for BPL category. Similar is the case with other major tribes, Dhanka and Gamit. Even the Kokna in Nandurbar ITDP, who are better agriculturists among the tribals, have 87 per cent families under BPL. In Taloda ITDP, Kokna numbers are insignificant. There is a significant difference between Taloda and Nandurbar whereby more families migrate from Nandurbar. This is possibly due to proximity to Gujarat where employment opportunities are readily available for Nandurbar tribals in the neighbourhood.

Appendix 3
Health

Water Supply Available as on June 2003

Tehsil	No. Villages under TSP	Drinking Water Facility				
		Tap Water (ZP)	Hand pump	Ele. Pump	Well	Other
Dhadgaon	163	8	624	4	371	71
Akkalkuwa	193	37	590	18	154	211
Taloda	96	54	234	61	37	–
Nawapur	150	143	1054	42	42	–
Nandurbar	107	82	437	65	64	–
Shahada	145	79	311	88	79	–
Total	**854**	**403**	**3250**	**278**	**747**	**282**

Source: Nav Sanjeevan TDD Report, July 2003, Nasik.

Availability of Health Facility in the Village

Facility	Distance Group									
	Taloda ITDP (490 villages)					Nandurbar ITDP (436 villages)				
	0	1-5	6-10	11-15	Above 15	0	1-5	6-10	11-15	Above 15
Primary Health Centre	32	131	146	70	111	31	133	168	62	42
Sub Centre	83	232	97	36	42	101	197	91	25	22
Rural Hospital	10	81	107	96	196	5	40	70	48	273
Government Dispensary	13	72	103	68	234	11	35	47	43	300
Private Dispensary	64	166	110	55	95	73	168	113	38	44

Source: ITDP Taloda and ITDP Nandurbar at a Glance, TRTI, Pune, 2000.

Population-wise, the facilities may not be inadequate, but are non-functional due to distance and the time required to cover distance without public transport. Private overcrowded jeeps are now seen on main roads.

Health Facilities on June 2003

Tehsil	*Rural hospital*	*PHC*	*PHC Sub-centre*	*Mobile Health Unit*	*Primary Health Unit*	*Anganwadi Kendra*	
						Anganwadi	*Mini*
Nandurbar	4	7	37	–	–	175	51
Nawapur	2	9	43	–	–	150	105
Shahada	1	12	59	–	–	221	–
Akkalkuwa	1	9	55	–	3	197	105
Taloda	1	4	25	–	1	142	16
Akrani	1	8	41	–	2	120	120
Total	**10**	**49**	**260**	**–**	**6**	**1005**	**397**

Source: Nav Sanjeevan TDD Report, July 2003, Nasik.

Number of One or More Diseases Occurred during the Year

Disease	*No. of villages where disease found*	
	Taloda	*Nandurbar*
Cholera	113	71
Jaundice	66	64
Dysentery	252	133
Malaria	370	341
Filaria	19	9
Govar (Measles)	100	78
Typhoid	38	11

Source: ITDP Taloda and ITDP Nandurbar at a Glance, TRTI, Pune, 2000.

Child Mortality Chart as on End of June 2003

Tehsil	*Status reported as on 30 June, 2003*				
	Live birth	*0-1 yrs age*	*1-3 yrs*	*3-6 yrs*	*Total*
Nawapur	349	18	3	–	21
Shahada	616	27	7	4	38
Taloda	269	17	5	5	27
Akkalkuwa	507	18	15	9	42
Nandurbar	456	21	4	5	30
Dhadgaon	336	21	4	8	33
Total	**2533**	**122**	**38**	**31**	**191**

Source: Nav Sanjeevan, TDD Report, July 2003, Nasik, Reasons for child mortality need to be studied.

Balvikas Yojana (ICDS) June 2003

Tehsil	*Malnutrition Status reported at June end*				
	Grade I	*Grade II*	*Grade III*	*Grade IV*	*Total*
Nawapur	8786	6065	87	18	14956
Shahada	14126	8238	163	29	22556
Taloda	6223	4214	220	37	10694
Akkalkuwa	12226	9243	259	68	21796
Nandurbar	9796	5283	121	32	15232
Dhadgaon	5419	3755	176	39	9389
Total	**56576**	**36798**	**1026**	**223**	**94623**

Source: Nav Sanjeevan, TDD Report, July 2003, Nasik.

Malnutrition Grade III and IV are a matter of concern.

Supplementary Nutrition Programme: June 2003

Tehsil	*No. of Centres*		*No. of Beneficiaries*					
	Anganwadi	*Mini-anganwadi*	*6 months to 6 yrs*	*Pregnant mothers*	*Lactating mothers*	*Grade III children*	*Grade IV children*	*Total*
Nawapur	150	105	17611	1411	1455	87	18	20582
Shahada	221	–	24771	2022	2027	163	29	29012
Taloda	142	16	14023	1178	1194	220	37	16652
Akkalkuwa	197	105	23701	2076	2014	259	68	28118
Nandurbar	175	51	19767	1545	1715	121	32	23180
Dhadgaon	120	120	20354	1547	1903	176	39	24019
Total	**1005**	**379**	**120227**	**9779**	**10308**	**1026**	**223**	**141563**
Type of diet	Rice *khichdi* and peas curry							

Source: TDD Report: July 2003, Nasik.

Chapter 5

Intervention Programme: Health and Malnutrition

Jointly with ***G.S. Pandit*** and ***Shailesh Dalvi***

Introduction

People living in groups and as communities lead their traditional lives guided by cultural patterns and norms. With basic personality configuration formed due to common child rearing practices within a common cultural framework, people know the tolerance limits of behavioural variations. There are informal and formal mechanisms to set right the deviant behaviour by intervening for correction, to ensure peace and tranquillity in the group or community.

With the advancement of science and technology, and rise of principles of democracy, the benefits of technological advancement have to be shared equally by the citizens of a nation. Knowledgeable people know the road map of getting the benefits of opportunities for their advancement or progress. There are groups and communities who do not have the capacity to use the schemes and opportunities of development. These are branded as backward communities.

Communities in India, usually referred to as caste groups or tribal groups have been categorised as Scheduled Caste, Scheduled Tribe, Other Backward Class and others. Constitutional provisions have been made for SC and ST to offer them reservation in legislatures, in public employment and in educational institutions. Special provisions have been made in respect of tribal communities, i.e. Scheduled Tribes by carving out a separate Tribal Sub-plan and a special administrative mechanism to implement it. However, despite these provisions, tribal regions, as states, districts, talukas or a group of villages are rated lowest on the Human Development Scale. The mortality and morbidity of tribal children, supposedly due to under-nourishment, commonly referred to as malnutrition is alarming.

Background

The national leaders feel embarrassed on global platforms and have expressed child malnutrition among the tribal communities as "National Shame". The higher Judiciary as custodians of human rights enjoined by the Constitution direct the governments to take action and report back to them. The Media keep on reporting the anomalies in the health sector and issues of food security in tribal areas which are taken cognizance of by the Judiciary in *Suo Motu* format, besides taking note of the Public Interest Litigation filed by citizens individually or through an organization.

In response to PILs and Writ petition about malnutrition amongst tribal children, in Mumbai High Court since 1993, it was decided by the Government of Maharashtra to address the issue with the help of NGOs. The initiative was taken by the Ministry of Health and Family Welfare, Government of Maharashtra to involve the NGOs working in tribal areas through Tribal Development Department.

A. CONCEPT AND PROGRAMME DESIGN

The Department of Tribal Development, Government of Maharashtra submitted a Draft Project Proposal about "Improving Mother and Child Health in Tribal Population of Six Districts of Maharashtra," as an NGO-Government of Maharashtra initiative, to Ministry of Health and Family Welfare, Maharashtra, under its Health Sector Development Programme.

Earlier, a meeting on 3rd April, 2003 was convened by the Tribal Development Department, at Mantralaya, Mumbai, with 13 NGOs from various regions of Maharashtra, to discuss the broad issues about the project and the distribution of project areas amongst the NGOs. The project proposal was finalized at a meeting at BAIF on 19th July, 2003 by a committee of Dr. R.S. Arole, Prof. R.K. Mutatkar, Dr. Bhagwat of BAIF and Dr. Dhruv Mankad. Different districts were assigned among the NGOs for implementation. The Maharashtra Association of Anthropological Sciences (MAAS) and Comprehensive Rural Health Project (CRHP) of Jamkhed were jointly given the responsibility for Dhadgaon and Akkalkuwa hilly talukas of Nandurbar District. During 20 – 22 July, Dr. R.S. Arole and Prof. R.K. Mutatkar, accompanied by P.S. Agashe, identified as a coordinator for the project, undertook a tour of Dhadgaon, Akkalkuwa in Nandurbar, to survey the area and meet people for detailed planning (Annexure III).

Probably, in the absence of further development from the Ministry of Health, Principal Secretary, Tribal Development Department invited Dr. Arole and Prof. Mutatkar on 3rd October, 2003 to prepare a fresh proposal for the entire State and requested to take joint responsibility of work. On 3rd November, 2003, Principal Secretary, TDD, Shri Ramesh Kumar visited Jamkhed accompanied by Dr. P.S. Meena, Tribal Commissioner, to explore the possibility of offering a project about malnutrition of tribal children in Maharashtra jointly to CRHP with Dr. Arole and MAAS with me. We all visited a village under CRHP field area where a village meeting was organised. CRHP woman volunteer made a presentation about CRHP work in that village focusing on women and children. Dr. Meena, as a medico, publicly asked her questions about pregnancy care and maternity, including the risk factors. It was a sight to see how confidently and correctly, she answered all the queries. In the evening, while leaving Jamkhed for Mumbai, Principal Secretary asked us to send the protocol of the proposal very quickly and offered, "Let us be partners in development".

Maharashtra Association of Anthropological Sciences, Pune and Comprehensive Rural Health Project, Jamkhed were then jointly offered to be "partners in development" with the TDD, by taking up the responsibility of working in seven districts and nine talukas to address issues of malnutrition of tribal children. In view of the urgency of putting up the formal proposal, at short notice, which was sanctioned quickly as "Adivasi Utthan Karyakram", there was no time to develop and present the programme details for implementation, as a part of the project protocol.

Basic Principles of Programme Design

1. Partnership with the Government which meant utilizing the existing programmes and organizational set up in the public sector by helping to optimize its functioning for measurable outcomes.
2. To function through village-level volunteers/guides as done at CRHP, Jamkhed.
3. Anthropological approach shared by CRHP-MAAS about making interventions of inter-sectoral nature, advocated by "Health for All" strategy of Primary Health Care, known as *Alma Ata* declaration. The components of interventions in the intervention project of AUK have been demarcated as per this approach, although on decreasing priority, after health as the main focus of the project.
4. Activities had to be initiated as Confidence Building activities to solicit people's cooperation and involvement, followed by Capacity Building activities for sustainable development.

The activities documented in the following pages, as Ethnography of Programme Interventions (B) outline the process of implementation of component based interventions. The judiciary and the public required the reduction of malnutrition among tribal children as an indicator of the efficiency of tribal governance by the State Government. Mass Media as one of the pillars of democracy had to recognize the claims by the government.

As understood, the government functions through line

departments, most of which have their own cadres of employees at the district, taluka and village-level. The Tribal Development Department as a single window for all tribal development issues, has no cadre of its own at the block and village-level. It is supposed to function through the cadres of other departments such as Revenue, Rural Development, Mother and Child Health, Education, Agriculture, Public works or Building and Communication Department etc. These departments are funded for their respective works in tribal areas by the Tribal Development Department without having any authority to monitor the activities and schemes undertaken by respective line departments.

Whether the TDD funds from Tribal Sub-Plan (TSP) are meant to be used by the line departments for regular activities as in non-tribal areas, or as top-up funds for tribal development, raise controversies, to analyse the impact failures in tribal development. A case in point could be, as to whether a national highway passing through tribal belt is eligible to appropriate TSP funds for that stretch of road, or the road budget is meant for linking hamlets to main tribal village. Should the Collector's residential bungalow in a newly created tribal district be constructed from TSP funds, in preference to a hospital building? Should it not be constructed from the regular budget of the Buildings and Communication Department?

The AUK project of CRHP-MAAS also had to face the difficulties about coordination of their personnel, with the cadres of the line departments at the grassroots level, without formal authorization and orders by the State, District and Taluka-level supervisors of the respective line departments. It was, therefore, thought more logical and operationally feasible to have a dialogue with the people directly through village/hamlet based AUK volunteers and address their concerns and requirements. Everything was done in consultation with the Tribal Development Department, informally, and through formal channels of joint monitoring committees at the field-level, taluka-level and state-level. The proceedings of these committee meetings have been presented in the chapter on Government-NGO partnership.

Tribal Health Policy Review

A policy review of the Tribal Health Policy of the Government of Maharashtra was being conducted by BAIF Development Research Foundation along with the State Family Welfare Bureau, Pune. This policy review was being undertaken under the Sector Investment Programme (SIP). The SIP was designed to identify and implement Reforms (Administrative, Organization, Technical and Financial) in the Health and Family Welfare Sector. Among other subject areas for policy reviews, the Government of Maharashtra identified its Tribal Health Policy for a review. The general objective was to conduct a review and identify directions to evolve a specific Reproductive and Child Health Programme for Tribal Areas.

Objectives

Specific objectives of the review:

(a) To study the Tribal Health Policy of the Government of Maharashtra.
(b) To study the differences, if any, in the policy across various tribal areas.
(c) To study the specific problems in various tribal areas, and the adequacy of the Policy to address the problems.
(d) To provide suggestions to the Government of Maharashtra on evolving a specific strategy for overall improvement in Tribal Health and specifically on RCH issues.

Salient Results

General

(a) There is no stated Tribal Health Policy of the Government of Maharashtra.
(b) There are a series of GRs, as and when the various Programmes evolved.

(c) A Health Programme for Tribal Areas first evolved in 1974, after the Tribal Sub-plan was drafted.

(d) The Minimum Needs Programme gave an impetus to the health infrastructure development in Tribal Areas.

Organization

(a) The tribal areas/districts have been divided into two categories/groups based on the habitats of PVTG (Katkari, Kolam and Madia Gonds) and others.

(b) There is no separate Bureau for Tribal Health. A Nodal Officer at the DGHS monitors the schemes. There is one officer at the State Family Welfare Bureau for the Nav Sanjeevan Scheme.

(c) The Zilla Parishads implement the schemes at the district level.

(d) Only Amaravati district has an Additional District Health Officer for Tribal Areas. This has been done to comply with the orders of the High Court, due to PILs and Writ Petition about malnutrition in Melghat tribal area in Amravati.

Recommendations

1. The State should have a defined policy to improve the health of Tribal People.
2. The health problems of the Tribals are essentially due to factors outside the control of the health sector. This needs to be highlighted, and necessary coordination with the other Government Departments ensured.
3. Staff should preferably be from the local areas, able to speak the dialects and communicate well with the people. This is especially so with the Paramedical Staff.
4. The experience with the Doctors possessing a Degree in Ayurveda should be evaluated.
5. The families of Staff deputed to tribal areas, may stay in urban areas with Government support, as is practiced by the Armed Forces.

6. There is a need to work closely with the Traditional Healers, and learn from them with a sense of humility.
7. The shortfall in the number of sub-centre buildings should be made up with construction of sub-centres.
8. *Decentralization of the Planning Process*: Presently, the health programmes are planned at the state and implemented in the tribal areas, which therefore, cannot be implemented in a culturally acceptable way to the ethnic tribal groups. This can be addressed if the health problems are studied, identified and a programme planned at the district level, which should be a part of the District Plan.
9. RCH Programme specific for the tribal areas should be evolved.
10. Adolescent health issues need to be addressed and Adolescent Health Programme should be implemented in the Ashram Schools.
11. *Behaviour Change Communication* (BCC): A strategy for behaviour change taking into consideration local cultural practices and beliefs should be worked out at the district and block level to change health related practices of the tribals.
12. *Referral System*: The referral system in the tribal areas needs to be strengthened so that specialist care is available at short distance. Transportation facilities should be made available for patients needing referral services.
13. *Medical Care*: Curative care facilities should be enhanced at the PHC. Mobile units with designated staff and visit schedule should hold clinics in the villages.
14. *Partnership with the Private Sector*: Provision of health care in the tribal areas is a major task and partnership may be explored with the NGOs for effective health service delivery.
15. *Pre-placement Training*: All staff should be briefed about tribal customs and beliefs before posting into tribal areas.

It is possibly in response to this policy review by a prominent NGO, BAIF Research Foundation that the Ministry of Health and Family Welfare of the State Government thought of NGO partnership programme about RCH. However, the TDD owned it by offering "Adivasi Utthan Karyakram" (AUK) jointly to two NGOs, CRHP and MAAS, from the scheme of Nav Sanjeevan Yojana.

CRHP–MAAS AUK Programme: Concept

The State Government had invited a joint proposal from two NGOs, Comprehensive Rural Health Project (CRHP), Jamkhed and the Maharashtra Association of Anthropological Sciences (MAAS), Pune, for intervention in the districts of Thane, Nandurbar, Amravati, Ahmednagar, Gadchiroli, Yavatmal and Raigad in tribal pockets in 9 Tehsils (Talukas), focusing on malnutrition, health and health care as an entry point for comprehensive human development. The proposal presented was titled as "Comprehensive and Sustainable Human Development of the Tribal People of Maharashtra", which has been titled in Marathi as "Adivasi Utthan Karyakram" in the Government order (GR) sanctioning the project for five years. Conceptually, 'Utthan' refers to developing capabilities to solve one's own problems with self-confidence and self-esteem, in the spirit of self-help.

Tribal development refers to comprehensive and sustainable development of tribal people, not the infrastructure development of tribal area. However, generally tribal development refers to area development, i.e. construction of roads and buildings for public facilities like schools, hospitals and offices. In case of urban development, it refers to roads, housing, transport, water and sanitation and does not refer to development of urban people. The same concept cannot be used for tribal development, which should mean human development of tribal people. At best, infrastructure or area development is a tool, as an aid, to achieve human development. Human development has been understood as widening of choices available to people and their capability to access or choose the choices according to one's own liking. The provider-beneficiary relationship is, therefore, not the correct approach of development, and contradicts the principles of democracy as outlined in Lincoln's definition of democracy.

Hypothesis

Development is a process evolving through stages. The hypothesis has been to develop the capabilities of tribal volunteers and other tribal AUK personnel, at the first instance, who are the lay citizens of their respective hamlets and villages. If their capabilities to become self-reliant and self-confident could develop in five years' time in a spirit and action of self-help, it could be surmised that the capabilities of tribal people could also be developed in a reasonable time using the Human Development approach.

Tribal Development

Tribal Development refers to widening of choices and opportunities which are available to the non-tribal caste peasantry in the taluk, district, state and national level, as citizens of nation. There is a difference between the schemes for survival such as *Khavti* or supplementary food in Anganwadi and school, and schemes which would make people self-supporting through their own production or wage-earning. The EGS or MNREGA has to create productive assets or infra-structure such as roads for development, irrigation canals, tanks etc.

In the earlier days of community development initiatives since 1952, while the schools and health centres were started, tribal people did not come forward to take the benefit of these facilities. So, they were branded as superstitious and backward. Even now, it is commonly heard that the Katkari children who were admitted to school left the school. "So, what should we do?" is what the teachers would ask putting the blame on the parents. In case of disease control programmes, people are blamed for not following the regular treatment regimen thereby developing the issues of drug resistance. Are these the answers for the unsolved issues or are these the questions to be addressed, to be resolved? Therein lies the difference between techno-managerial and anthropological approach.

Backwardness can be defined as lacking the capability of accessing the infrastructure of development offered to them, as offered to all citizens of a nation-state, to improve their quality of life. Tribal people are often asked to join the mainstream. What is the mainstream? Is it the culture and life style of caste–Hindu peasantry? Or is it the exploitative social structure of patriarchal and hierarchical caste society whereby there are dowry deaths, female infanticide and molestation of women? Tribal activities frequently ask these questions focusing on exploitative mainstream which poses a threat to tribal identity and self-esteem.

Anthropological Basis of the Programme

The term 'culture' refers to an integrated way of life of a community or society encompassing the economic, social, religious, political, health and aesthetic aspects. The understanding of the issues of tribal malnutrition, therefore, requires the analysis and interventions in health, livelihood and other related sectors. The concept of Tribal Sub-plan and single window Tribal Development Department is based on the principle of integrated culture which requires inter-sectoral coordination between the various departments of the government. AUK offered by the government to focus on malnutrition of tribal children has been designed to initiate activities in other aspects of culture which may have a direct or indirect bearing on the issue of malnutrition.

Culture and Change

Culture refers to the way of life, historically created, which acts as a design and guide for living. Planned change through interventions is expected to bring about social and cultural change. The success and aim of intervention is to perceive change as part of culture, which is reflected in reinterpretation or change in attitudes, behaviour and practices, on a sustainable basis.

Culture is also historically designed as a sustainable entity. The aim, therefore, of any intervention for change has to be designed to be sustainable in a given system. As per Jawaharlal Nehru's philosophy about community development and tribal development, the ultimate aim of such programmes should be human development, and not end in the development of the infrastructure only. Nehru also advocated the single window for Tribal Development and encouraging people to develop according to their own genius (culture). Adivasi Utthan Karyakram (AUK) was designed as per this anthropological hypothesis about cultural and social change. Focusing on health as the first priority, interventions have been tried in six major components such as Education, Livelihood, Community Empowerment, Orientation and Training, and Cultural Identity. Confidence building and Capacity building of the people have been the two major strategies around which the activities were planned.

Symington Report of 1938 about the backward regions in Dhule district, which now constitutes the Nandurbar district, clearly recommends, that the policies of development and their implementation designed for the country should not be replicated in the tribal area. Tribal people need to be helped with hand holding as is done in case of children to become independent.

Following these approaches about inter-sectoral and integrated development, AUK was designed to make interventions in six components of life, although focusing on health and malnutrition. This strategy was accepted by the State Government as mentioned in government order.

Programme Components

Components	*Programmes*
1. Health Maternal and Reproductive Health	Care of pregnant and lactating mothers safe deliveries • Neonatal, infant and child care, care of pre-school children – nutrition, immunization, treatment of simple ailments

(*Contd.*)

Components	*Programmes*
	• Adolescent health education • Water and Sanitation • Personal hygiene
Disease Control and Cure	• Simple symptomatic primary care • Control of common communicable diseases, particularly chronic illness like leprosy, TB or recurrent malaria, gastroenteritis, cholera • Prevention of blindness – nutrition and eye care, cataract and glaucoma
Nutrition and Diet Herbal Care	• Kitchen Garden • Herbal Garden • Nutrition education: for pregnancy, lactation, infant and child care • Healthy locally available diets strengthening local herbal health care and illness care involving traditional health care providers
2. Education Exposure Information	• Strengthening of Anganwadis and primary school education • Improving Ashram Schools and boardings for boys and girls, as demonstration units for nutrition, sex education and personal hygiene; kitchen garden, clean environment and sanitation • Promote vocational education in schools and strengthen ITI training in trades • Provide exposure to information and knowledge • Sensitization of community about superstitions, misbelieves about health and nutrition
3. Livelihood and Income Generation Activities	• Agriculture and farmer • Improved methods of agriculture, horticulture, medicinal plants • Agriculture labour and other labour including women • Livestock development: Collection and processing of minor forest produce, fruits and herbs, sheep, poultry, other animals and birds. • Plant Nurseries • KVIC schemes like Ambar-Charkha and Honey collection and production • EGS: for watershed development, approach roads and local construction
4. Community Development	• Formation of Mahila Mandals and SHGs • Youth clubs and farmer clubs
5. Empowerment	• PRI – strengthening of Gramsabha. Orientation of Gram Panchayat members

(Contd.)

Components	Programmes
	focusing on women members. The information about ITDP and TSP schemes and utilization of the schemes
6. Training and orientation of development functionaries	• ICDS functionaries, Ashram school teachers, Forest functionaries, PRI members and functionaries, TBA and Herbalists, Bhagats will be oriented to health and development information and skills
7. Self-esteem and Cultural Identity	• Promotion of folk arts, music and literature. Use of this media for promoting scientific temper and moral values • Local Kalapathaks to be organized • Local history to be documented

The G.R. about sanctioning the project was issued on 27th February, 2004 to undertake work about malnutrition and mortality of tribal children. The submitted project "Comprehensive and Sustainable Human Development of the Tribal People of Maharashtra" was named in G.R. as "Adivasi Utthan Karyakram (AUK)". The project was to be implemented in nine tribe predominant Tehsils in seven districts of Maharashtra, in selected Gram Panchayat villages. Due to Lok Sabha and State Assembly Elections, the project could actually start the activities only in August 2004. The code of conduct enforced during elections prohibits the government from starting any new activities, by releasing funds, save only for ongoing governance and maintenance. The AUK project was sanctioned for a period of five years. However, due to administrative delays in release of funds, the project was given yearly "no cost" extensions till March 2013. Some of the activities were affected in maintaining regularity. Since the people were kept informed through volunteers, there was no loss of confidence level in interactions with the people.

In the meanwhile, responding to *Suo Motu* writ petition No. 5629/2004, Court Order Dated 8th July, 2004, a meeting of all the Secretaries of all the Government Departments under the Chairmanship of Chief Secretary was convened on 30th August and 9th September, 2004. At this meeting Dr. Abhay Bang made a presentation of his book in Marathi "*Kovali Pangal*" (Falling tender leaves) about tribal children's malnutrition and mortality.

Prof. Mutatkar made a presentation of his report about Health and Education issues in Nandurbar which was prepared for Planning Commission/UNDP. According to Human Development Report of Maharashtra Planning Board 2002, Nandurbar was ranked lowest, i.e. 35th district in HDI ranking. Indira Gandhi Institute of Development Research (IGIDR), a Reserve Bank Institute, had requested Prof. Mutatkar to give a report about strategic planning (Chapter 4B). Third presentation was made by Adv. Sheela Barse who had filed a writ petition No. 2924/1993 at the Nagpur Bench of Mumbai High Court about tribal child mortality in Melghat in Amravati District. Dr. R.S. Arole was also present for the meeting on 30th August.

At the meetings on both the days, the role of PRI was not mentioned even once, during discussions among the Secretaries. The roles and responsibilities of government employees from district to village-level were discussed in detail to address issues of tribal child nutrition.

Operational Strategies

In order to ensure to make it a people's programme with gradual increasing participation and involvement of people, two strategies were designed. Confidence building activities included putting a medicine box of allopathic and Ayurvedic drugs for common ailments in each hamlet with a volunteer, free of charge. Unless people get something concrete which meets with their urgent requirements without any suspicion about extracting or spending cash, which they have to borrow, people's confidence cannot be won which is essential to solicit their active involvement in planning and implementation of programmes.

Capacity building activities included continuing training of volunteers about taking weights of children and charting them on a graph, keeping records of all activities, educating the CBOs and SHGs, monitoring and assisting their activities, dispensing medicine from medicine box etc., in short, to be the change agents with confidence.

Concept of planned change requires interventions in all

aspects of life, since life is an integrated entity. Government functions through line or sector departments. Unless inter-sectoral coordination is successfully implemented, change in the desired direction is not achievable. Some institutions may focus on one aspect such as education, health or livelihood, but they have to link these with other aspects or components. Generally, education is considered as the most important prime mover of development, since it opens choices. Doctors like Dr. R.S. Arole started work in Jamkhed village with curative services, had to extend into preventive care activities, further encompassing the general development with full participation of local peasantry, mostly through marginalised women. To implement the AUK, administrative arrangement had to be designed at the central office level, at each taluka-level and in the villages and hamlets. To cover the entire state, two four wheeler jeeps, Bolero and 9 motor cycles for 9 units were procured as budgeted. The following salaried positions were created.

Sustainable development refers to the process by which the philosophy and direction of development articulated through activities, becoming an aspect or pattern of culture. Culture is a sustainable entity. Culture does get modified in values or hard aspects easily in its process of adaptation, with every generation. Soft aspects of material culture does not easily alter the sustainable aspects of culture expressed through rituals, life cycle, ceremonies and festivals.

Due to technological advancement, soft aspects of culture, that is material and visible aspects of culture, show faster change. Inter-generational perceptions and change are faster. However, harder or value-based aspects of Culture, such as religious issues, life cycle rituals etc. change very slowly. The maternity and child rearing practices and exposure to cultural aspects of life such as kinship, ceremonies and festivals form the Basic Personality of a cultural group with a distinct identity of an ethnic group. The starting of formal education at an early age, such as in Anganwadi, would make an impact on widening of values beyond ethnic group solidarity.

AUK has tried to develop the model of sustainable human development making an entry point for change by addressing the issues of child malnutrition. It becomes necessary to address the mothers, during pregnancy and lactation, the adolescent girls who would become mothers shortly. So, one has to address the formal school education such as the day schools and ashram schools. The issues come up about certain ethnic groups feeling shy or not accessing the free education, issues like drop outs of girls on attaining puberty etc.

Merely giving sermons by way of creating awareness would not be sustainable. People have to experience the results of interventions. Activities planned and executed in consultation with people are sustainable. There is a tendency to assess the effectiveness of such programmes only quantitatively. Qualitative assessment expressed though people's spontaneous expressions are equally important, since it documents the emotional expressions about the process of change and satisfaction.

Administrative Pattern

Government administration whether meant for governance about revenue, law and order or development functions through paid employees. Private sector whether in the service sector or production also functions through employees. The voluntary sector engaged in social service also requires human resources who have to earn their livelihood. Some of the persons engaged in voluntary work have other sources for livelihood, wholly or partly. Voluntary organizations which function through donations and grants have to support their workers wholly or partly from their paltry resources. The most common current term used for voluntary organisations is Non-Governmental organisations (NGO). The NGOs are given programmes for implementation in a government paradigm. Usually, a geographical area is earmarked for undertaking the work as per government pattern for which grants are given. Another term used commonly is outsourcing.

MAAS and CRHP being the voluntary organisations with a paradigm to develop sustainable models, it was necessary to ensure people's involvement in the programme. Minimum employees such as couple of coordinators at Pune to monitor the

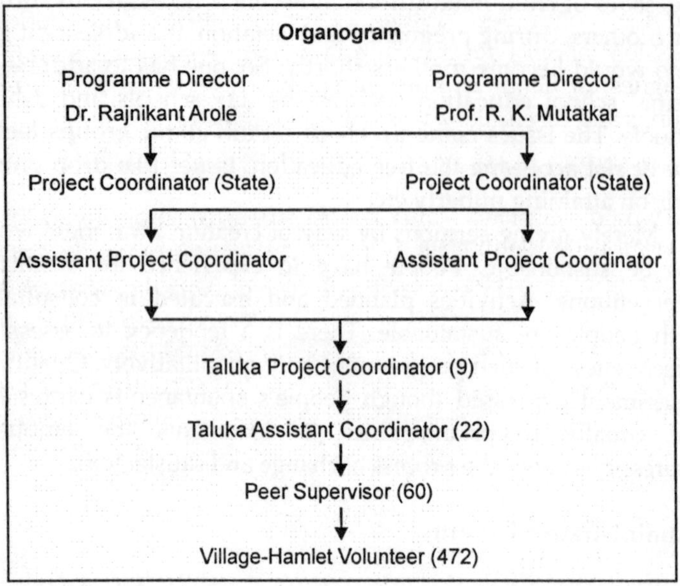

programme in 9 centres all over Maharashtra and one coordinator and one assistant coordinator for each centre were appointed. The taluka coordinator (*Samanwayak*) and their assistants were local persons from the same area. Male and Female tribal volunteers (*Swayamsevak*) from the respective villages/hamlets were appointed. Subsequently, some of them were elevated to function as local peer supervisors (*Margdarshak*) to guide and monitor the work of volunteers.

Pune Central Office

1. State Project Coordinator

He was supposed to be overall incharge of the project, had to do planning and activities for each component of the programme. While on tour, besides meeting the government officials including ATC, he should perform all those functions as done by the Assistant Project Coordinators. He was to monitor the accounts and office audit. His recommendations to TPC even if communicated on phone, should be put in writing and discussed with the colleagues. While in office, he should initiate discussions about field report, training and accounting with the colleagues for about an hour every day. A brief record of such meetings and discussions was to be maintained.

2. *The Assistant Project Coordinators (2)*

They would visit each Taluk centre at least once a month and would meet the volunteers at a training session to get the feed-back. During his presence couple of village meetings were to be organized to be addressed by him personally. Invariably, he should meet the project officer in ITDP office and his colleagues, the BDO and Panchayat Samiti elected representatives such as Sabhapati and Upasabhapati. He should visit the TPC office, look into the files and sign with date. He could put nothing on the file itself, his remarks and recommendations for modifications, if any. His tour reporting format should include all these things in the tabular form usually one of them would cover Eastern and Western Maharashtra every alternate month.

Field Administration

1. Taluk Coordinator: (TPC) (9)

Besides monitoring the activities of the Assistant Coordinator, TPC had to routinely meet BDO and his officials and the project officer of ITDP at least twice a month. He should try to meet the Assistant in the presence of village volunteers and village public. He had to give special attention to Micro-Planning and provide training in micro-planning to the assistants and volunteers. It was necessary to have maps of each hamlet, village and Gram Panchayat to be covered under AUK. All TPC were from some taluka.

2. *Assistant Taluka Coordinator: (9) All Local Tribals*

As a paid employee of AUK, he had to meet every single hamlet very frequently. He had to keep in close touch with the government development officials at the Anganwadi, ZP and Ashram school, Talathi, Gramsevak and Pada Health Worker etc. He had to meet village volunteers in the presence of several villagers and discuss the issues for the villagers to understand that the volunteer was answerable to local community. His reporting format should include village meetings and group meetings and main points of discussion. He should also include his meetings with local government officials and frequency of visits to such institutions as Anganwadi, ZP and Ashram Schools. He was supposed to visit the families of under-weight children and pregnant women in order to monitor, as to the contact and advice provided by the village volunteers.

3. Peer Supervisors (Margdarshak)

Some village volunteers were promoted to these positions to help and monitor AUK work in the neighbourhood villages, besides working in their respective villages.

4. Village /Hamlet (Pada) Volunteers

Selected in the Gram Sabha, village/pada (hamlet) volunteers had to be accountable to the people of the village and would also report about activities and the concerns of the people to the Assistant Coordinator at AUK at Tehsil level. They would visit the tribal families and monitor the Programmes at the local level. They would organize local community to articulate the demands and place it before the government and AUK officials. The reporting format would include number of village or group meetings conducted and the action taken on the programme focusing on maternal and child health.

Selection of AUK Personnel

In August 2004, coordinators and Assistant coordinators at Pune Central Office and at each of the taluka centres were selected after the due process of state-level advertisements in newspapers. Since the basic approach of the programme was to function through community participation and with the availability of residential facilities, the first weak long training was conducted at Jamkhed in the second week of September 2004. Commissioner of Tribal Development Nasik visited the concluding session of the training. After the selection of one coordinator and one assistant coordinator for each field unit in August 2004, training was organized for them during 9-16 September, 2004 at Jamkhed. Hon. Tribal Commissioner visited Jamkhed and provided guidance to the trainees.

Human Resources										
Sl. No.	Tehsils/ Taluka	Tribal Volunteers (Jan. 2005-12)			Tribal Peer Supervisors (Oct. 2005-12)			Local Tribal Assistant Coordinators (Sept. 2004-12)	Local Taluka Project Coordinators (Sept. 2004-12)
		M	F	Total	M	F	Total	M	M
1.	Akole	23	29	52	2	4	6	2	1
2.	Akkalkuwa	34	25	59	7	0	7	2	S.T. 1
3.	Dhadgoan	21	45	66	10	0	10	2	1
4.	Dharani	19	23	42	3	2	5	2	1
5.	Etapalli	20	19	39	6	0	6	3	1
6.	Jawhar	30	27	57	4	3	7	2	1
7.	Mokhada	34	31	65	3	0	3	3	1
8.	Karjat	20	31	51	4	5	9	3	1
9.	Zarijamani	8	33	41	3	4	7	3	1
	Total	**209**	**263**	**472**	**42**	**18**	**60**	**22**	**9**

Grand Total: 563 of which Tribal: 555–M: 274: F: 281 and non-tribals: 8. All workers were from villages, hamlets and local areas.

Monthly honorarium, January 2005 to December 2012. Volunteers: Rs. 250 per month; Peer Supervisor: Rs. 400 per month.

Monthly Honorarium, September 2004 to December 2012. Asstt. Coordinators: Rs. 1500 per month. 9 coordinators got regular salary ranging from Rs. 6000-9000 per month.

During October-November 2004, 25 to 30 male and female volunteers were selected for each field unit in respective Gram Sabha. During 16-29 December, 2004 formal inaugural ceremonies were conducted in all field units with participation of Government officers, elected representatives of the people and the volunteers. An honorarium of Rs. 250 per month was paid to each volunteer since January 2005. During October 2005, some volunteers were promoted as local supervisors.

Training of Coordinators

The training of coordinators at Jamkhed included the knowledge about conceptual basis of Jamkhed model and anthropological basis of holistic, integrated culture which required multiple interventions in various aspects of life to bring about planned change. Issues about selection of volunteers from each taluka centre and villages/hamlets were also discussed. The recording system was also finalised. The trainees visited some villages in Jamkhed area and talked to the people about the process of development, experienced by them.

Soon after, male and female volunteers were selected by convening Gram Sabhas in respective villages. Almost equal number of male and female volunteers were to be selected since it was thought that as livelihood avenues, agricultural sector would have to be empowered with skills and knowledge of scientific farming. Male volunteers were expected to address the livelihood issues, mostly agriculture. Female volunteers were expected to address the issues of pregnancy, safe delivery and child malnutrition. About 50 volunteers were selected to address the population of about 15,000-20,000 in each centre as advised by the Government.

Training Curriculum

What is the meaning of Utthan?

- *Utthan* means standing on ones' own legs with self-respect, self-confidence and self-identity.

What is the goal of Adivasi Utthan Karyakram (AUK)?

- To work towards human development of the tribal people of Maharashtra.
- To develop capacity and confidence to ensure equal opportunities as citizens of one nation.
- To promote self-esteem, cultural identify and national consciousness.

What are the objectives of AUK?

- To achieve optimum health for tribal people, to be active members of the society, to contribute to the production of food and other goods.
- To focus on reduction of child and women mortality and morbility.
- To promote universalization of primary education and vocational training.
- To develop wide range of livelihood opportunities for ensuring food security and nutrition.

What is comprehensive development?

- It refers to development in all sectors of life such as social, economic, political, spiritual, art and aesthetics. These in an integrated pattern form a culture.

What is sustainable development?

- The development that becomes as part of culture and thus perpetuates by itself, without any external monitoring.
- It also means that the psyche of the people or basic personality of the people gets expressed in the attitudes, behaviour and practices about recently acquired knowledge about development.

How can comprehensive and sustainable development be achieved?

- It can be achieved by combined efforts of the Government Development (Tribal) Agencies, Voluntary Organizations (VO), Panchayati Raj Institutions and community based organizations such as Mahila Mandals, Self-Help Groups (SHGs), Youth Clubs and the like.

What is backwardness?

- It refers to lack of capacity and confidence in utilizing and demanding the development opportunities offered by the Government, to the citizens of the nation and particularly to the tribal people.

What is the objective of development?

- To empower and equip the people with information and skills, to utilize and demand development schemes.

What is the role of Voluntary Organizations in human development of tribal people?

- To work in partnership with the Government, to facilitate logistic functioning at the micro-level.
- To develop a do-able model of development addressing all concerns of the local people and by linking it with macro issues and strategies of development.

What is the mechanism with voluntary organizations in working for development?

- *Step* 1: The tribal people in a local settlement like a hamlet have to be informed about development programme.
- *Step* 2: To encourage community to nominate one man and one woman to receive the training with VOs and to monitor partnership programme of VO at their settlement.
- *Step* 3: These community volunteers have to provide a link between the people, VO and the Government Agencies at the local level.
- Government and VO personnel have to train these volunteers and through them, entire local community about development issues, strategies and schemes.

What is human development?

- Human Development (HD) refers to development of common people or the civil society.
- To make alternative choices about development and develop capacity and confidence to achieve them.

Selection of Field Area

As advised by government about the population to be covered in each taluka and as per advice of CEO, Nandurbar Zilla Parishad,

Dr. R.S. Arole and Prof. R.K. Mutatkar selected Gram Panchayats in nine field sites having a population of 15 to 20 thousand each, in consultation with the POs of respective ITDPs, during May and July 2004. Since Gram Panchayat, in effect a group Gram Panchayat, is the financial and administrative statutory body, we were advised to select Gram Panchayats as units of activities. According to PESA, in response to 73rd Constitutional Amendment, even a hamlet could be a functional autonomous unit of development administration. However, PESA has yet to become a functional reality.

Geographical areas, Gram Panchayats, coverage of population, Tribal groups and number of Tribal volunteers

Districts	*Taluka*	*Tribal Population (%)*	*Predominant Tribes*	*Villages*	*Padas, Wadis*	*Gram Panchayats*	*Population*	*Swayam Sevaks Tribal Volunteers (Jan. 2005)*	
								M	*F*
Thane	Jawhar	88	Kokna, Thakar, DhorKoli, Katkari, M. Koli, Warli	19	48	9	19536	30	27
	Mokhada	93		12	75	7	24313	34	31
Nandurbar	Akkalkuwa	81	Bhil, Pawra	11	58	3	16987	34	25
	Dhadgaon	86		31	92	5	25432	21	45
Amaravati	Dharni	75	Korku	19	00	7	16895	19	23
Gadchiroli	Etapalli	81	Madia, Gond, Pardhan	49	20	7	11802	20	19
Yavatmal	Zarijamni	75	Kolam, Gond, Pardhan	23	46	11	14376	8	33
Raigarh	Karjat	25*	Katkari, Thakar	00	67	15	21801	20	31
Ahmadnagar	Akole	46*	M. Koli, Thakar	30	23	14	17306	23	29
Total	**Nine**			**209**	**429**	**80**	**168048**	**209**	**263**

* The tribal people living in exclusive tribal hamlets have 100 per cent tribal population who were selected under the programme.

Source: AUK Report submitted to Govt. of Maharashtra.

Inauguration of Field Units

Inaugural functions were organised at each centre at the hands of local dignitaries such as Zilla Parishad President, MLA, Panchayat Samiti Sabhapati, PO of ITDP etc. with attendance of BDO, teachers and other local functionaries. All the selected volunteers were present as audience. This provided a good back-drop for the volunteers to understand the objectives of AUK activities, to be implemented by them. Common inaugural ceremony was performed for the two centres each in one district, namely for Jawhar and Mokhada in Thane district at Jawhar and for Dhadgaon and Akkalkuwa Centres in Nandurbar district at Dhadgaon. This also provided an opportunity and experience to the taluka coordinators and assistant coordinators to organise public activities with attendance of volunteers. At some places, ladv volunteers spoke boldly using the microphone on the *dias*. The functions also sensitised the local leaders and government officials about AUK project granted by the State Government.

Summary

Briefly, the conceptual framework evolved out of the combination of epidemiological principles of community—public health, and holistic, people-centric anthropological human development approach, goes in line with the primary health care, inter-sectoral coordination approach of "Health for All" strategy advocated by WHO as *Alma Ata* declaration. "Think globally—Act locally," as a slogan validates the emic and micro- approaches of anthropology. When the tribal communities lived in geographic isolation as autonomous entities, not too much disturbed by the river-valley agriculturists, their culture and life style were co-terminus, not in conflict with each other. When the communities became a part of the Nation-State, guided by the Constitution, bestowing special status, using the principle of Equity, the traditional culture was threatened with destabili-sation and identity issues. The culture contact of simple people having cashless, barter, value-in-use economy with the value-in-exchange, market economy at macro, even global level, may lead to their exploitation. Man-Environment (Forest) relationship is threatened, since the natural resources have markets. The natural resources of food used traditionally to satisfy the need and not greed, are denied to tribal communities leading to acute malnutrition, under-nutrition or starvation. Earlier people governed themselves. As the marketable resources or surplus grow, there is organised mechanism of governance controlled by those who have muscle and/or money power. To address the concerns of the people in democratic governance, the people's sector and the government sector have to be bridged. Usually, government system functioning through paid employees cannot act locally at the micro-level. Voluntary organisations can do that.

The government offered an opportunity of addressing issues of tribal child malnutrition, to two voluntary organisations jointly, tacitly approving their respective strengths with a confidence that they could function jointly for the good of the people and could partner with the government system. CRHP-MAAS accepted the challenge to develop a model through a trilogue with the government and the people.

B. ETHNOGRAPHY OF PROGRAMME INTERVENTIONS

Introduction

As mentioned earlier, due to urgency on the part of government to undertake malnutrition related interventions involving the NGOs, probably due to *Suo Motu* injunction from the High Court, there was no focused reflection on the detailed sequence of intervention activities. As anthropologists, we had no experience of planning and implementing schemes for change, and that too with the government as the prime mover in development administration, planted over age-old revenue administration. In case of tribal communities, the regulatory forest administration has been stereotyped as the main hurdle, this image still continuing among the tribal people. It is known that a meek effort was made to resolve this issue by putting together Forests and

Tribal Welfare Departments under a common Minister. However, this arrangement was withdrawn, due to unproductive results, forest superimposing over the tribal section. The CRHP had pioneered community health by capacity building of marginalised women in villages to function as effective health workers which gave rise to CHV, Health Guide and now ASHA, Anganwadi workers, as para-medics. CRHP was in direct communication with the people and not from government funds.

As a result, the intervention activities evolved through communication with the people and with the government system, through informal and formal interactive mechanisms. The anthropological and human development approach to which CRHP-MAAS had wedded put the first priority on winning the confidence of the people through appropriate activities.

Accordingly, the components identified for graded interventions were further classified into those which had an immediate and direct bearing on reducing malnutrition such as supplementary food to children, and to lactating and pregnant women, and full one-time meal during pregnancy. The other components were relating to livelihood issues, education, agriculture-kitchen garden, check dams, new born baby clothes, training of PRI-members, *Dai, Vaidu* etc.

SUMMARY OF INTERVENTION ACTIVITIES

Comprehensive and Sustainable Human Development of Tribal People of Maharashtra

Sponsored by Tribal Development Department—Government of Maharashtra

- **Government Resolution:** To address the issues of health and malnutrition, a partnership has been formed between the Government of Maharashtra and two voluntary organizations, *viz.* Comprehensive Rural Health Project (CRHP) (Founder: Dr. Rajnikant Arole) and Maharashtra Association of Anthropological Sciences (MAAS) (Founder: Prof. R.K. Mutatkar).

- **Duration:** 2004-2013.
- **Geographical Coverage:** The programme covers 7 districts including 9 tribal dominant taluks and prominent tribal groups in the State of Maharashtra. A list of the areas and the tribes covered is given below:
  - **District**: Thane; **Taluka**: Jawhar and Mokhada; **Tribes**: *Warli, Thakar, Kokna, Dhor Koli* and *Katkari.*
  - **District**: Raigad; **Taluka**: Karjat; **Tribes**: *Katkari, Thakar.*
  - **District**: Ahmednagar; **Taluka**: Akole; **Tribes**: *Mahadeo Koli.*
  - **District**: Nandurbar; **Taluka**: Akkalkuwa and Dhadgaon; **Tribes**: *Bhil* and *Pawara.*
  - **District**: Amravati; **Taluka**: Dharni; **Tribes**: *Korku.*
  - **District**: Yavatmal; **Taluka**: Zarijamani; **Tribes**: *Kolam* and *Gond.*
  - **District**: Gadchiroli; **Taluka**: Etapalli; **Tribes**: *Madia Gond.*
- **Population:** Each project unit or Centre included villages and hamlets covering a population of 15,000-20,000 tribal people.

  Unit of Action: Gram Panchayat.

  Number of Centres: 9 centres, covering 250 villages and 2 lakh tribal population.
- **Facilitators:** About 250 Male and 250 Female tribal village/hamlet volunteers selected by the people.

  Guides: 80 tribal guides to guide and monitor the 500 tribal volunteers.

  Project coordinators: 9 project coordinators selected from among the educated locals, one each at the 9 Centres.

  Main Office: Maharashtra Association of Anthropological Sciences (MAAS) Office, Pune.

Findings of the Programme

1. There has been a perceptible change in the malnutrition

rates of the tribal children between the ages of 0-3, due to the interventions of the programme. In comparison to the baseline survey data on weight for age carried out in the year 2005, the percentage of children in the normal weight-range has increased from 31 per cent in 2005 to 39 per cent. The percentage of children in grade III of malnutrition has come down from 9 per cent to 2 per cent, and as for the children in grade IV of malnutrition the percentage has come down from 3 per cent to 0.15 per cent.

The percentage of children in combined grade III and IV of malnutrition has come down from 12 per cent to 2 per cent.

2. The programme's intervention of providing a full nutritious meal to pregnant women from the fourth month of pregnancy onwards has led to various perceptible and positive results. The percentage of low birth weight babies (birth weight < or = 2500 grams) has come down from 39 per cent to 27 per cent. Also the percentage of normal birth weight babies (birth weight > 2500 grams) has increased from 61 per cent to 73 per cent.

   In the common Indian population the percentage of Low birth weight babies is 30 per cent, whereas in the tribal population where the programme's intervention of providing a full nutritious meal to the pregnant tribal woman has been implemented, the percentage of low birth weight children is only 20 per cent. The birth weight of the children born to the mothers benefitting from this intervention is 2.76 kilograms on an average. Through this we can conclude that providing a full nutritious meal to pregnant women leads to the birth of children with normal birth weight.

3. **Human Resource Development:** The 500 tribal volunteers and the 80 tribal guides were given training twice a month. 500 *Dai* in the programme areas were trained by elderly and experienced *Dais* working at Jamkhed for CRHP. Other than that around 2500 tribals

were trained in various fields. These include 350 *Vaidus,* 250 Gram Panchayat members, 150 puppeteers, 200 bamboo artifact makers, 300 girls for tailoring training etc.

Many of these trained tribals have now been appointed as ASHAs, Anganwadi Workers, members of Gram Panchayats and Secretaries etc. The volunteers were paid Rs. 200-250 per month, while the guides were paid Rs. 400 per month.

- *Structure and Function of the Programme*: The volunteers selected by the locals and the educated youth of the villages carried out the baseline survey in 2005. Though the main aim of the programme was to address health and malnourishment, since all aspects of culture are inter-related, hence, the programme planned for intervention in other components of life such as education (Ashramshala, Anganwadi), livelihood, community development, training and cultural identity etc.

  Confidence and capacity building of the tribal people has been the strategy of the program. Some of the activities of the programme are listed below:
- Providing medicine-boxes to the volunteers in the villages, so that medicines are made available to the villagers easily and free of cost. In many places the medicines made by the local herbalists trained during the programme has also been in these medicine-boxes.
- Kitchen gardens have been a cultural component of the tribal society. Hence free seeds of 12 types of nutritious vegetables were distributed among the tribal families having pregnant women or malnourished children and they were also distributed among the tribal volunteers. In many of the 'Ashramshalas' drumsticks, 'Amla', custard-apple, papayas, lemon etc. were planted in the school nurseries.

- *Jhabla-topda-duppate* (cotton wrappers) were provided to new-born to provide protection from cold and prevent respiratory infections. This led to an increase in birth registrations. The garments provided were sewn by the young girls who were given training in tailoring during the programme.
- Good quality weighing machines were provided to all the tribal volunteers in order to take and maintain accurate weight data of infants, children and pregnant women.
- The villages in which the demand for services of the *Dais* was very high, in such villages *Dai-Kutis* were constructed in order to provide a hygienic and convenient place for carrying out deliveries.
- In order to fulfil the nutrition requirements of children in the age group of six months to three years, nutrition supplement made of wheat flour and flour of dried gram was given. This supplement is called as *Sattu* and it was prepared by the local Self-Help Groups. *Sattu* fortified with *Shatavari, Jyesthmadh, Ashvagandha, Pimpli* and other Ayurvedic medicines were given to pregnant and lactating women.
- Fourth month of pregnancy onwards, the pregnant women were given a full nutritious meal daily. The arrangement and preparation of the meals was done by the tribal volunteers and these meals were given to the pregnant women at the volunteer's home. This activity led to an increase in ANC registration and also the children born to these women had an increased birth weight.
- To improve the condition of the 'Ashramshalas', the following activities were undertaken by the programme:
  - Providing solar lamps.

- Arrangement of good quality drinking water.
- Building of toilets and bathrooms, especially for the girls.
- Coaching for tenth standard students (SSC examinations).
- Computer repair and training.
- Development of kitchen garden and nursery.
- 'Khelwadis' established in villages and hamlets with no 'Anganwadis'.

- **Other Activities**
  - Arrangement of Health camps.
  - Building check dams.
  - *Chaupal/Chawdi* repair.
  - Building soak pits.
  - Training of Gram Panchayat members.
  - Training for puppet shows.
  - Building raised platforms for seedlings.
  - Training for making smokeless *Chulhas*.
  - Training for Biogas development.

- **Government-voluntary organization partnership**: A joint coordination committee for monitoring was formed at the Taluk, District, State and Mantralaya level. This committee included members from the Government, the two voluntary organizations running the *Adivasi Utthan Karyakram* and people's representatives. This presents a good example of Government-Voluntary Organization-People's partnership.
- The programme resulted in the development of a model for tribal development. The programme sets an example of how tribal development can be achieved through Government and People's partnership without increasing the expenditure of the current Government system. The programme also aims at demonstrating that sustainable development is not achievable without Human Development.

Activities directly related to under-nutrition and child mortality

Sl. No.	*Activity*
Health	
1.	One square meal per day to pregnant women after registration of pregnancy with ANM of Primary Health Centre. Food was cooked in ANM volunteers kitchen and method of spot feeding was adopted for quality results. After meals, spot feeding of iron tablets from ANM was done. Discussion about pregnancy care, lactating mother's care and new born care was done during after meals.
2.	Herbal medicine fortified *sattu* to lactating women after delivery and up to period of six months. Three kilogram of herb fortified *sattu* per month per lactating women.
3.	*Sattu* to children of age group 6 months to three years, as weaning food to introduce concept of weaning at proper age. One kg *sattu* per child per month for age group six months to one year. Two kg *sattu* per child per month for age group one year to three years. *Sattu* prepared by SHGs.
4.	(*Jhabale-topade-dupate*) wrapping cloth for protection of hypothermia in newborn babies.
5.	Medicine—Ayurvedic and allopathic for treatment of common ailments.
6.	Kitchen garden to improve quality of diet by use of vegetables for provision of vitamins and micronutrients.
7.	Health camps with focus on pregnant women, lactating women and children up to age of six years. General health check-up and treatment follow up in critical cases was taken by project with help of government health facilities.
8.	*Dai* hut for safe delivery of women in the village and rest for three days. *Dai* hut was constructed in a village of trained *dai*. *Dai* hut was also utilized by ANM for health check-up and immunization of pregnant women.

(*Contd.*)

Sl. No.	*Activity*
9.	Coordination with anganwadi in weighing of children and improving anganwadi enrolment.
10.	Adolescent health check-up and education mostly done with focus on Ashram school. The girls who were anaemic were referred to Primary Health Centre for further follow-up action.
11.	*Dai* training was given to local tribal dais. Training was for five days every year and was given by master trainer *dais* from Comprehensive Rural Health Project Jamkhed.
Education	
12.	*Khelwadi*: Children from some tribal hamlets were not getting acess to Anganwadi due to their location at a distance in caste-peasantry village (and also social distance). To provide pre-primary education and supplementary food, Khelwadi (mini-anganwadi) were introduced in tribal hamlets with focus on PVTG, viz., Katkari, Kolam.
13.	*Libraries in Anganwadi*: twenty anganwadis from each field unit were provided with books.
14.	*Health check-up of out of school adolescent girls*: The percentage of out of school adolescent girls is quite high, in Ettapali, Dharni, Jawhar, Mokhada, and Akole.
15.	*Ideal Ashram School*: Extra coaching classes for SSC students, drinking water facility, Kitchen garden, Biogas plant, Compound and Painting of ashram school, strings for drying clothes and other activities like sports.
16.	Activities like repair of bathrooms, latrines, buckets, solar lamps and botanical garden in Jawhar and Mokhada, particularly in girls ashram schools.
17.	Medicine box in Ashram School, for common ailments. Two bathroom scales were given to each ashram school in field areas of Akole, Jawhar, Mokhada.

(*Contd.*)

Sl. No.	*Activity*
Livelihood	
18.	Check dams built by local community in Dhadgaon and Akkalkuwa tehsil of Nandurbar. Check dams were built with gunny bags filled with stones (supplied by AUK).
19.	*ARTI training*: 145 tribal youths from nine field areas were in Appropriate Rural Technologies Institute, Phaltan, Maharashtra, such as smokeless *chulha*, bio gas, vermi-composting, nursery.
20.	Fish rearing was done in field areas of Jawhar, Mokhada, Dhadgaon, Akkalkuwa by self-help groups. In Ettapali, fish rearing was done by families in their own ponds. Half of the fish thus produced was distributed free of cost to families of pregnant, lactating women and malnourished children. Fish seed supplied by AUK.
21.	Bamboo training was given to tribal youths from Dhadgaon and Akkalkuwa. Total 184 youth were trained in bamboo art.
Community Development	
22.	Panchayat Raj training was given to all elected members from eight field units except at Ettapalli due to volatile political (Naxal) situation there. About 344 members were trained.
23.	SHGs were trained about *sattu* preparation. Some SHGs from Jawhar and Mokhada were trained in processing of herbal medicine.
Training and Orientation	
24.	*Swayamsevak training*: Tribal village volunteers selected by community were given training and orientation on various aspects of health and development and continuing monthly training. Every quarter, there was residential training of three to five days for peer

(Contd.)

Sl. No.	*Activity*
	supervisors, taluka and state-level coordinators.
25.	*Vaidu training*: Local tribal *vaidus*/herbalists were trained at local level in processing of herbs to medicine. These medicines were purchased from them and included in Ayurvedic medicine box in each hamlet. State level workshops of same type were organized first at Pune. At State level workshops, 53 *vaidus* were trained and 296 at field level.
26.	*Puppet show training*: 150 tribal youths were trained in Puppet making and play by an organization "The Puppet" at Karjat. The trained youths gave performances in their areas on health and development issues.
27.	**Cultural Identity** Kalapathak, Musical instruments distribution, Ghotul and Chavadi repair.

Note: Unless specific source-reference is given, all data is generated from field activities.

Preparatory Phase

There was no idea of implementing parallel interventions since the programme was to be undertaken in partnership with the government with institutions like anganwadi meant for children under six, pregnant, lactating women and adolescent girls. However, it was realized that the Anganwadi Sevika was too much busy and occupied with filling about 18 registers for monitoring by the higher authorities. We understood that AWW had no instructions from her superiors to formally coordinate with us. We also realized that the people were not bringing their children to anganwadi for regular weight check up as they had no knowledge of its significance as an index of health. They had qualitative indicators like a child not playing, or not eating properly or looking weak etc. We also observed that our own lady volunteers and their children were visibly malnourished.

Since AUK was a project focusing on malnutrition, the first concern had been to decide about the indicator of malnutrition. Epidemiologically, the first issue would be to assess the prevalence of the problem, according to geographical region, ethnic group, age and gender. Anganwadi in the public sector was already responsible for weighing the children and maintaining a growth chart for every child. It was, however, observed that the children were not brought to anganwadi by the parents. There was too much pressure on AWW to keep all the records and not report to higher ups of those who were in grade 3 and 4 for fear of being held responsible for their malnutrition. At one point of time, the Chief Minister of Maharashtra sent a letter to every AWW assuring that the correct picture about children's grades be reported and that she would not be held responsible for poor health of children.

At some centres, there was a good coordination among the AUK volunteers and AWW. However, there were no instructions from ICDS to share the data with AUK.

It was, therefore, decided to purchase the weighing scales for the new born, for children up to 6 years and for taking weights of pregnant women periodically.

The programme had to start with health component having direct bearing on malnutrition. Malnutrition or malnourishment is a term which commonly refers to undernourishment, probably due to the vernacular expression as *Kuposhan* with English equivalent term as malnourishment. Malnourishment among children is measured according to three anthropometric indices of nutritional status.

Stunting: Measure inadequate height-for-age; Wasting: Measure inadequate weight-for-height; Underweight: Measure inadequate weight-for-age. In the Anganwadi, weight for age is recorded on a graph and a child is graded as normal or in grade 1, 2, 3 or 4. Grade 3 and 4 are ranked as acute malnourished which would require hospital intervention, including hospitalisation or special nourishment centre.

Confidence Building Visible Activities

One of the first programme was about weighing new born and children up to 6 years, and pregnant women. Three types of weighing machines, one for the new born, spring balance for children and bathroom scale for pregnant women were purchased. About 1400 weighing machines were supplied to the volunteers besides the 445 available in the Anganwadis. Volunteers were trained to take the weights and chart them as per Anganwadi pattern. Another major activity has been to provide a medicinal kit box for common ailments with allopathic and Ayurvedic medicines kept with every volunteer. The medicine was available all the time free of charge. Simultaneously, the *Vaidus* were given training to prepare Ayurvedic drugs from the herbal plants available in the neighbourhood forest. Taking into account the cultural practice of kitchen gardens, seeds of about 12 kinds of vegetables and some fruits were provided free of cost to the volunteers and to the families where malnourished children were identified. In order to prevent respiratory infections, new born children were provided with two sets of traditional baby cloths, culturally called, *Jhabale, Topade* and *Dupate.* First time, the clothes were stitched by Tata Gruhani Udyog at Pune, a woman's non-profit, in-house subsidiary of TELCO. Afterwards, training in tailoring was given to adolescent girls in tribal area and were provided with tailoring machines under the government scheme. The *Dais* were trained every year by the senior trainers from Jamkhed about pregnancy and birthing practices. In order to ensure sanitary conditions for delivery, *Dai* huts were constructed in the villages where *Dais* were in great demand. All these activities were initiated in the year 2005 immediately after the Base Line Survey.

Weighing Children

There are various ways of measuring the degree of malnutrition among children, most commonly termed as stunting (Height-for-age), wasting (Weight-for-height) and underweight (Weight-for-age). However, Dr. Arole had recommended weight-for-age, since we were dealing with the weights of thousands of tribal children across the state, coordinating with anganwadi. In the public sector, weighing machines are supplied to anganwadis. However, due to lack of awareness about the quantitative measurement of weight as an indicator of child health, children were not taken to anganwadi for recording weights.

One of the first issues when AUK started functioning in the field with the nominations of male and female volunteers by the respective village/hamlet Gram Sabhas, was to train than to measure weights. Realising that children needed to be weighed at their respective homes, volunteers were provided with three types of scales (a) Baby scale for new born to 6 months; (b) spring balance for children 6 months to 3 years; (c) Bathroom scale or floor scale basically to weigh pregnant women. In an average-size village or hamlet, 4 or 5 births took place in a year. Accordingly the baby scale and bathroom scales were purchased for 2-3 hamlets together and kept with a volunteer who was easily accessible.

A new born baby had to be weighted within 24 hours of birth. If a scale was not functioning properly, it was replaced immediately and the old one was repaired at Pune. The volunteers were trained to use the scale by putting the scale at a place where the pointer remained at zero indicator before weighing. Weights had to be recorded immediately in a register which was supplied. In case of a volunteer being totally illiterate, weights were recorded by a literate member of volunteer's family or by a neighbour.

Co-ordination was established with anganwadi. AUK figures were shared with anganwadi worker to update her record and register. All children were weighed during 25th to 28th of the month in every home by the volunteers.

Dr. Nagapure, a retired Assistant Director of health with the State Government had joined us as one of the state-level coordinators. I was with him in a village when we carried a spring balance to an open verandah of a house and hung it appropriately. Several women from various ethnic tribal groups came with their children for weighting. The discussion was initiated about the reasons for variable weights among the children with same age. It included such issues as the food taken during pregnancy, iron tablets, and lactation and diet of children, weaning food etc. It was quite revealing to all the women present there that the weights of children from Kokna and Mahadeo Koli who were land owners were normal, while those among Warli, Katkari, Dhor-Koli who were either marginal farmers or farmless labour, their children weighed less than normal.

This message of relationship of weight as an indicator of measuring degree of malnutrition was disseminated by volunteers as an alert information. Volunteers were trained to plot the weights on anganwadi pattern of graph.

Over a period of time, people understood the relationship of weights with degree of malnutrition and the need to feed the children properly. As a result ready-to-eat *Sattu* became popular and was meticulously fed to children as directed.

Response

"It is to understand why weights of children go up or down, that weights have to be recorded periodically."

"People know what food to be taken. Pregnant woman also understands this. However, due to poverty, it is not possible to follow this" (Laxman Mukane, Karkari, Jawhar).

Medicine Kit

Traditionally, Man has been getting or collecting his food and medicine from the natural environment around his habitat. Tribal communities in the collection stage knew the difference between food and herbal medicine as also the value or quality of food as medicine. Processing of food and herbs has been minimal. With domestication of fire, food processing developed into recipes. Herbs were mostly eaten in raw form after breaking or beating it to become chewable or possible to swallow it.

While the rulers exploited forest as wealth and the regulatory forest department was established, the traditional use of forest resources as food and medicine got restricted, due to depletion of forest.

With Community Development Programme initiated in India as a transformation programme of rural development in 1952, health centres were designed to be established as health care delivery centres. It took quite some time to establish such centres in tribal areas due to weak infrastructure of connectivity and buildings to house such centres. The formally trained medical manpower was also not available in requisite numbers. Even now, these problems of physical inaccessibility exist and several posts of doctors trained in modern medicine remain vacant, which are now filled by medical graduates in Ayurveda. Health care or illness care is based on Allopathic system. So, there is a mismatch between the doctors in position, mostly trained in Ayurveda, without requisite supply of Ayurvedic drugs. Health centres function as per government rules and regulations whereby the availability of doctors in the OPD is for limited duration. The tribal patients have to walk or reach the health centres or sub-centres, which may not be possible during stipulated hours of OPD. If the free medicines were denied at these centre due to short supply, the people had to go to nearby towns to purchase from pharmacy shops in the nearby town.

Private medical facilities are usually not available around tribal villages, except at Taluka or District headquarters and would not be financially affordable to the tribals.

Accessing the services of traditional *vaidu* in the village or in the neighbourhood remains the only choice. However, for some communicable disease conditions, modern medicine may appear or function more effectively in short time, showing the reduction in symptoms of illness to make it possible to attend to usual work schedule.

To tide over these difficulties and to win over the confidence of the people, it was decided to keep a medicine box with every volunteer for treatment of common ailments. The medicine was to be given free of any charge. These medicine kits were also supplied to Ashram Schools.

The boxes included following medicines—

Allopathic Medicine Kit

Furazolidin
Paracetamol
Septran
Sodamint
Vitamin B-Complex
Gentian Violet
Tr. Iodine
Band-aid
Eye ointment (applicaps)

Ayurvedic Medicine Kit

Mahanarayan Tail
Kuda Ghanvati
Shatavari Vati
Sitopaladi Vati
Krumighna Vati
Cough Tablet

Volunteers were trained to give medicine, and dosage, as per symptoms and age group of the patients. The peer supervisors, assistant coordinators who were also tribals were residents of the same area and could monitor the activities. Drug supply was immediately replenished. There used to be training sessions every month for the volunteers about the activities of AUK. They would also report the activities undertaken by them. The honorarium was also paid to them on this day. The volunteers were trained to maintain a record of dispensing of medicine in a register with the name of patient, age, gender, symptoms and medicine given.

Ayurvedic medicines were first purchased from two sources. At Pune, a social service oriented senior *Vaidya* produces medicines for his patients and also sells it from his outlet. He holds training sessions for making Ayurvedic medicines for common ailments, traditionally used as kitchen medicine. He has written several booklets about pregnancy care, geriatric care etc. with a price ranging from Re 1 to Rs. 3 per copy. He was happy to supply us medicine at 20 per cent discount of the usual price. Zandu Pharmaceutical Works, Mumbai also gave us Ayurvedic medicines at reduced rates under their corporate social responsibility scheme (CSR).

Subsequently, *vaidus* were trained to process herbs into medicine as done in pharmacies or by Ayurvedic physicians and were purchased as buy back by AUK. A series of training workshops were conducted at Pune and in the respective field centres.

Beneficiary of Medicine Supply 2005-2012

Year	Akole	Akkalkuwa	Dhadgaon	Dharni	Etapalli	Jawhar	Karjat	Mokhada	Zarijamni	Total
2005	4500	5700	7400	3000	2800	3200	3500	4000	3000	37100
2006	10000	10000	9000	10640	5358	6385	7338	6987	4343	70051
2007	16479	7000	10000	11950	6104	8431	13975	5845	6836	86620
2008	16420	8949	12942	10561	6532	9120	9685	6582	6952	87773
2009	15345	7853	10313	10241	5885	6721	8322	6314	6448	77442
2010	14200	8431	11221	10442	6321	8251	7544	6826	6822	80058
2011	13185	8300	9351	10900	5412	8435	8355	5419	5424	74781
2012	15123	7135	10824	10403	6400	7300	7835	5356	6221	76597
Total	**105252**	**63368**	**81051**	**78137**	**44812**	**57843**	**66554**	**47329**	**46046**	**590422**

Source: AUK Report submitted to Government of Maharashtra.

Responses

"There is no ANM centre in our village, nor private doctor, we are deep in a forest village. In case of fever, vomiting, diarrhoea, we go to AUK volunteer any time of the day or night. We do not have to go to Etapalli. So, our expenditure is saved without loss of wages." Village Launji, District Gadchiroli.

"As a volunteer, my stature has gone up in the village since I give medicine to the people. I am getting the status of a doctor which makes me self-confident and proud." C.K. Durva, Todsa.

"After delivery, I had adequate lactation for about 10 days. Due to reduced lactation afterwards, I gave cow milk and sheep milk to the baby. I had home remedies, consulted local medicine priest, and a doctor with no effect. AUK volunteer gave me *Shatavari Kalpa*. After a week, I had adequate lactation to feed my baby. Baby's health is normal." Village Parsalgondi.

"My son's birth weight was 2300 gm. There was no problem about adequacy of breast milk but had no improvement. The volunteer gave *Mahanarayan* oil for massage of the baby. After three weeks, the baby was shining and had weight gain." Launji.

Keeping medicine kit with the AUK volunteers was one of the first confidence building activities of AUK in 2005 and remained the most popular. In the initial phase, there were two Assistant State Coordinators at Pune who were retired medical officers from the Government of Maharashtra, one with MBBS degree and another BAMS. They organised and monitored this programme at all stages from purchase to delivery, to use and replenishment, in consultation with Dr. Arole.

Kitchen Garden

Kitchen Garden to grow vegetables, irrigated by kitchen waste water has been a part of tribal culture among the communities. However, only few vegetables were grown. The programme of giving seeds of about 11 types of vegetables, i.e. cow peas, bitter gourd, ladies fingers, cluster bean, bottle gourd, papaya, green chilli, brinjal, tomato and spinach free of cost was started in 2005. This was meant to provide vitamins and other micro-nutrients to pregnant, lactating women and children. Tribal communities have been collecting green leafy vegetables during rainy season from the fields and forest. First the seeds were given to families with pregnant and lactating women and in the families of malnourished children. Later, it was extended to giving free seeds to all the volunteers.

Seeds were purchased from established seed merchants and were dispatched from Pune in April every year. The vegetables were available from kitchen garden in August-September. The vegetables from kitchen garden were also exchanged among the families. The pregnant women several times carried vegetables from their kitchen garden to the volunteers' kitchen when meal programme for pregnant women was introduced.

Seeds were also provided for kitchen gardens in Ashram

School. People got the message of significance of vegetables in their diet for better health.

Response

"We got good seeds which gives better yield as compared to our seeds."

"Some tribal farmers planted seeds in their agricultural field."

"In Akkalkuwa, irrigation from AUK assisted check dams was used for growing vegetables."

Beneficiary of Kitchen Garden Seeds 2005-2012

Year	Akole	Akkalkuwa	Dhadgaon	Dharni	Etapalli	Jawhar	Karjat	Mokhada	Zarijamni	Total
2005	513	700	700	350	358	807	454	266	216	4364
2006	1047	1713	1593	628	1125	1680	2500	507	1012	11805
2007	350	988	1200	442	356	367	627	920	238	5488
2008	289	479	1109	366	533	705	209	297	664	4651
2009	1129	486	660	220	299	501	127	318	241	3981
2010	557	520	686	444	285	524	148	614	245	4023
2011	575	535	544	432	231	565	144	670	250	3946
2012	580	490	473	189	192	530	144	526	280	3404
Total	**5040**	**5911**	**6965**	**3071**	**3379**	**5679**	**4353**	**4118**	**3146**	**41662**

Source: AUK Report submitted to Government of Maharashtra.

New Born Baby Clothes

Neo-natal mortality has been a significant problem in tribal belts. A new born baby has to get warm environment. Although culturally, babies are wrapped in a piece of cloth and kept close to mothers' breast, there have been interior areas in Gadchiroli among the Madia Gonds where no clothing was available. Men always wore only *'langoti'* and women hardly wrapping their thighs (above knees) with a piece of cloth and remaining top-less. During severe winter, open fire inside a kitchen or in the courtyard provided warmth, which sometimes led to burns.

Even among the non-tribal peasantry villages or urban areas, new clothes were not traditionally presented or made for the new born. Old sarees were used as baby wrapping. Usually, the naming ceremony or 12th day was celebrated with new wrappings, and small clothes. It was believed that the chances of neo-natal mortality kept on receding with passing of days, 5th and 6th day after birth being considered crucial, supposedly visited by the spirits to decide the life destiny of the baby. These days were celebrated with rituals by the kin and neighbourhood. The woman who had delivered a baby was considered ritually impure till the naming ceremony on 12th day, thereby also protecting her from outside contact since she was isolated as much as possible, and not visited except by *dai* or close female elders who observed cleanliness by way of bath.

The AUK project, in order to prevent mortality due to hypothermia decided to present a set of new clothes, a uni-sex frock, cap to cover head and wrapping to cover whole body, within 48 hours of birth. This was linked with weighing the new born and registering the birth in Gram Panchayat. This was one of the first programmes undertaken in the year 2005 in August. The first lot was stitched by TELCO women's group at Pune, at cost. Later, training sessions for stitching were organized for tribal women and adolescent girls in each centre. New born baby clothes were stitched by them. Wherever available, government schemes at district level were used for getting tailoring machines for the trained women, which also became a source of livelihood for them.

Before initiating this programme by AUK, at some places, ANM used to advise baby to be protected in a thermocol box during rainy season and winter. It was further decided to give two sets of baby clothes to new born to wash them regularly.

Beneficiary: New born baby clothes: 2005-2012

Year	*Akole*	*Akkalkuwa*	*Dhadgaon*	*Dharni*	*Etapalli*	*Jawhar*	*Karjat*	*Mokhada*	*Zarijamni*	*Total*
2005	50	40	40	50	50	50	55	72	50	457
2006	235	315	650	319	201	215	87	293	164	2479
2007	249	335	841	382	239	345	70	407	201	3069
2008	252	461	631	372	244	402	132	401	170	2705
2009	267	229	404	225	111	274	55	528	91	2184
2010	244	250	485	210	123	350	100	400	80	2242
2011	96	404	472	234	155	310	100	400	80	2251
2012	280	353	502	240	145	280	80	435	90	2405
Total	**1673**	**2387**	**4025**	**2032**	**1268**	**2226**	**679**	**2936**	**926**	**17792**

Source: AUK Report submitted to Government of Maharashtra.

Tailoring

Some of the tribal girls who have been educated up to 9th-10th standard have had no avenues of gainful work except working as labour in the fields. There has been a scheme of getting a sewing machine from ITDP provided some formal training in tailoring had been done. AUK started the training in tailoring in Etapalli, Zari-zamni and Jawhar. Six months training was initiated free of cost. Some sewing machines were purchased, some were hired on monthly rental basis. A room on rent for training was also hired. A training teacher was appointed on an honorarium basis ranging from 150-1800 per month. The girls learned to stitch women's clothes such as blouses, *salwar-kameej*, gowns etc. The baby clothes which were supplied to new born by AUK were also stitched by these trained girls.

In Etapalli, 43 girls, in Zari-zamni 33 girls and in Jawhar 60 girls received training in tailoring. Subsequently, about 70 girls received sewing machines from ITDP. Some of them were hired by ready-made garment industry in the nearby towns while some of them purchased machines on their own.

Response

Niroja, 12th pass have two brothers and a sister. I had my education staying in a hostel at Etapalli. Back home, I had work in the house, in the field and as farm labour. Since AUK stared a tailoring class in my village, I contacted AUK volunteer and joined the class. During six months, I can stitch baby clothes, *salwar-kameej*, petticoat, Gown and Blouses. I charge 80 Rs. for *salwar-kameej*, Rs. 30 for blouse, and Rs. 20 for baby clothes of AUK. I also own a tailoring machine of my own given by ITDP. Now, villagers know me as tailorbai. I am helping my family living, two-three marriage proposals have been offered. I am thankful to AUK for making me self-reliant." Village Yemli, Etapalli,

"Earlier we were using old clothes. Now, these new clothes protect the baby from getting unwell."

"Weighing the new born, registration of birth and baby

clothes gave a message to people that the programme was sincere about baby and child care."

Dai Training

In the living world, perpetuation of ones' own species is a matter of prime concern. In the animal world, birthing is an instinctive and natural process, unaided by peers or elders. Among the human beings also, birthing is a natural process. Human baby remains biologically dependant for a long period, until the baby becomes a child as a biped, capable of searching food or other things in the kitchen, in the house. A foetus is precious since it continues the family and kin-group. There is no family without a baby-child, own or adopted. Husband-wife are a couple, not a family. As a result, loss of foetus due to miscarriage or during birthing process is regretted. The woman has to bear another pregnancy, mostly soon after such wasteful episodes, which is a drain on her health and which compromises her other economic functions.

Internationally, midwife or Traditional Birth Attendant (TBA) or *Dai* in India is a universal health functionary, assisting the birthing process. In caste-Hindu peasant society, *Dai* has become a caste with hereditary occupation. In tribal communities, in the absence of division of labour, any woman could function as *Dai*. *Dai* not only conducts birthing process but is available for oil massage of mother and baby varying from 5 days to 15 days in different ethnic tribal groups. During this period, she also washes clothes of the new mother. This has traditionally been a common practice among the caste-peasant rural or in urban families at all socio-economic levels.

In order to reduce neo-natal mortality, *Dai* training has become a formal programme in public health. Dr. R.S. Arole, Co-programme Director of AUK is credited with the pioneering effort, with success, to create good trainers from among the rural women who were socially marginalised. This has been the Jamkhed Model. These experienced women, now old, were available for *Dai* training in the AUK Centres.

It is interesting to find documentation of birthing practices of the indigenous people of America, the American Indians.

"The Indian practices associated with child birth have been called more rational than those of Europeans of an earlier period. ....Dr. George Engelmann, whose study of labor among primitive peoples was first published in 1883, regarded the obstetrical method of primitive tribes as more reasonable than those used among civilized peoples. He described massage and manipulation techniques used in various tribes for the expulsion of the foetus and after birth which were in his own time just beginning to be adopted in white medicine" (Virgil J. Vogel, 1970: 232).

"Delivery takes place while the woman is squatting, or on her knees, or on hands and knees or elbows, or lying down; frequently she holds on to an attendant, or to a sash, rope, strap, or stick which is fastened somewhere for the purpose. ..... The assistance given by a midwife or female relative consisted, 'mainly of pressure or kneading with the hands or with a bandage about the abdomen, the object of which is to give direct aid in the expulsion of the child" (Virgil J. Vogel, 1970: 234-235).

Every year, during March-April, residential training was imparted to *Dais* at each centre by the trainer *Dais* from Jamkhed, accompanied by a senior supervisor, Smt. Ratna Kamble and a gynaecologist Dr. Mrs. Kalpana Mutatkar from AUK. Besides *dais,* other women or AUK volunteers who volunteered for such training were also included for training session. Dummy delivery models were used for training.

Major Components of *Dai* Training

(A) *Pregnancy*

1. Identification or confirmation of pregnancy.
2. Registration of Pregnancy with ANM and her services.
3. Special food during pregnancy and its frequency.
4. Immunisation schedule such as T.T. injection.
5. Risk factors and their recognition/identification.
6. Weight gain during pregnancy and its process.
7. Home remedies during pregnancy for common ailments.
8. Things to be avoided during pregnancy.
9. Management of risk factors and referrals.

10. Management of transverse abnormal position in uterus, Twins.

(B) Delivery

1. Care to be taken by *Dai* for safe delivery.
2. Identifying safe and at risk delivery to decide about referral services.
3. What is still birth?
4. How to clean new born baby? What if the baby becomes blue/black?
5. Examination of new born.
6. How to ensure normal respiration of new born?
7. Care of new born baby and low birth weight baby.

(C) Care of infants (0-1 year)

1. Bath of the baby—when to start bathing?
   Necessary everyday? When to be avoided?
2. What about pre-bath oil massage?
3. Breast milk? When to start? How long breast feeding? What about weaning ?
4. Immunisation schedule. What vaccines?
5. Care to prevent from pneumonia.
6. What should be weaning food? How much?
7. How to prevent diarrhoea? Home Remedies.
   When to refer to dispensary?
8. Care of low birth weight baby. Risks.
9. Care about measles and chicken pox.

(D) Care of Lactating Mother

1. Benefits of breast-feeding within half an hour of birth.
2. Care of breasts.
3. Food of lactating mother and quantity.
4. Food after delivery. Other nutritious supplements?
5. How to improve lactation? Traditional or herbal tonics?

(E) Care of Children (1-3 years)

1. What general care?
2. What is malnourishment? Causes?

3. Child morbidity. Common ailments, like fever, diarrhoea, cough-cold, pneumonia, measles, chicken pox.
4. What preventive care?
5. Management of malnourished child. Home remedies besides cleanliness and clean potable water.

Response

"I had no knowledge about delivery. As an AUK volunteer, I attended training sessions. In my village, there was a case of complicated pregnancy with a woman in labor. This was a care of transverse position which needed hospitalisation. However, I tried soft massage on the stomach which resulted in normal delivery. So far, I conducted three deliveries." Village Markal, Etapalli.

A Bhil woman in Akkalkuwa who had undergone *Dai* training conducted 25 deliveries and narrated her experiences in Bhilli dialect on public platform. She replied to the questions posed in Bhilli dialect by the Minister of State for Tribal Development, a Bhil himself, who was a Chief Guest at an AUK programme at Pune.

As a result of *Dai* training programme for three years, it was decided to construct *Dai* huts in selected villages in AUK centres.

Health Care Practices about Mother and Child Health

Sl. No.	*Delivery Practices and Care*	*Maharashtra Tribes*
1.	*Dai's* help	5-15 days.
2.	For easy Delivery	Decoction of black pepper and cumin. Put root of Calotropis plant (Rui) on scalp.
3.	After Delivery	Massage by coconut oil or mahua seed oil.
4.	For Lactation	Asparagus (*Satavar*) roots, Paste (*Chattany*) made up of Earthworm, Ginger, Garlic, Black Pepper. Rice with Sesame chutney. Prawn curry fortified with earthworm extract. *Ladoo* made up of common cress (*Ahaliv*)
5.	Breast-Feeding	½ hr. after birth
6.	Weaning Food	After six months, (*Dal*) Soup of pulses, thin porridge of *ragi*.
7.	Massage of Baby	Mahua oil, *Til* oil, Coconut oil.
8.	Recovery after Delivery	*Fenugreek* (*Methi*) *Ladoo*, Dry fruit *Ladoo and Ladoo* made up of Common Cress (*Ahaliv*)

Source: Author's Field Survey.

Dai-hut—Institutional Delivery

As evident from the baseline survey, most of the deliveries in tribal areas we conducted in the respective houses. With the mobility of other members of the family, with cattle, sheep, fowl in the house, it would be difficult to maintain sanitary conditions required for delivery. Sri Shivaji Dudhwadkar, then ATC of Thane suggested the utility of *Dai*-hut for institutional delivery at the village-level, particularly in the inaccessible areas, away from PHC or Sub-centre, without private or public transport.

Some *Dais* who had also undergone training were in demand by families to perform home delivery. A clean place in the hamlet was selected in consultation with the villagers for construction of *Dai*-hut. It could be easily accessed by the hamlets and villages in the neighbourhood.

In *Dai*-hut, a big utensil for heating water for bath, a kerosene stove, small utensils for making tea and porridge were supplied. A bucket, soap, utensil for storing clean drinking water, an iron bed with mattress, plastic covers for bed etc. were provided. Five packages of delivery kit including gloves were kept in the hut. Food during delivery was supplied by the village volunteer. A baby scale and an adult scale, a small table clock/watch, a calendar and baby clothes for new born baby were also kept in the hut. Mother's other small children had access to *dai*-hut to meet the mother. The hut was also used for ANM to examine the pregnant women from the neighbourhood on a pre-determined specific day.

Margaret Mead, an eminent anthropologist has given her opinion on the basis of international experiences in a book prepared for UNESCO in 1955.

"This author gives the favourable and unfavourable aspects of maternal care here as follows: the woman feels secure through the authority of the family medicine man who is a personal friend and who supervises the pregnancy. Her muscles are active, she eats little. Her genital tract has not been handled during pregnancy, so the danger of infection is reduced. She is used to pain. Her friends are with her during delivery. Against this, the author sets the fact that no one present knows how to deal with complications and unusual presentations, that there is no fresh air in the delivery-room and that hygienic measures are lacking, thus exposing the infant to infection". [*Ref*: *Cultural Patterns and Technical Change: Cross-cultural Studies of Technical Change* (ed.) Margaret Mead, p. 211].

A Tribal Atlas for Maharashtra TISS, Mumbai

Percentage of Deliveries* Conducted in Health Institutions among Total and Scheduled Tribe Population in Maharashtra and TSP Districts, 2002-04 & 2007-08

TSP Districts	*2002-2004*		*2007-2008*	
	Total	*ST*	*Total*	*ST*
Maharashtra	**57.9**	**28.7**	**63.5**	**34.0**
Nandurbar	28.4	9.2	25.3	13.6
Gadchiroli	20.4	14.2	23.3	12.5
Dhule	38.1	8.6	50.5	26.9
Nasik	47.2	17.8	63.9	40.2
Yavatmal	53.2	33.3	53.6	34.8
Chandrapur	41.4	25.9	54.7	34.7
Gondiya	36.7	28.9	53.8	47.0
Jalgaon	51.6	31.3	53.4	25.5
Amravati	56.7	12.3	63.2	22.2
Thane	68.6	27.6	72.4	52.2
Raigarh	63.5	32.2	68.9	46.2
Nagpur	73.2	58.2	81.9	72.7
Nanded	39.4	19.9	56.3	45.0
Ahmadnagar	65.7	33.2	80.4	58.1
Pune	79.4	56.4	83.1	61.5

Reference: *For women age 15-49 years, Asked for the last two live/still birth born in last three years Reference period: Deliveries of women who has their last two live/ still birth since 01-01-2004 (DLHS-3) and live/still births during three years preceding the survey (DLHS-2).

Source: DLHS-2 (2002-04 & DLHS-3 (2007-08).

This data about institutional deliveries amongst ST clearly brings out the importance of *Dai*-hut as an alternative institution readily accessible.

There are two issues (1) Institutional Delivery for cleanliness, safety and availability of referral services. (2) In tribal terrain and due to difficulties at home, tribal women do not go to PHC (Primary Health Centre) for delivery. The Primary Health Centre, also are not properly equipped in terms of personnel and referral services. Almost all the deliveries continue to be done in their respective homes, with the help of the local *Dai*. However, house may be small, crowded and not as clean as desirable. We, therefore, proposed to construct *Dai* huts in our project area for which the following guidelines were followed:

1. An experienced and trained *Dai* who was in demand by the people in the radius of five kms, should be identified.
2. The community could make land available for *Dai*-hut over which, community would have common ownership rights.
3. The construction could be made in the style in which the local houses are made.
4. The construction could be done by the villagers on the same basis as they made their houses. In no case could the contractor make the construction. The expenditure could be borne by AUK. In these efforts, *Dai* could be consulted and village meeting could be held for discussion and decision.
5. *Dai*-huts could have a bed, mattress, sheets (Bed sheets cloths), mackintosh. There would be place for bath with the facility of drainage, or soak pit. Allopathic and Ayurvedic drugs be placed in *Dai*-hut. There must be a kitchen corner in the hut or outside the hut for heating water and making food for new mother and her other children up to the age of 3 years, if they visited her.
6. We had to plan the utilization of *Dai*-hut when not in use. Preferably, the place was used for health check-up of women and adolescent girls. It could also be used by ANM during her visit. In no case *Dai*-hut should be used for storing or dumping any material. For assistance to *Dai* conducting labour and for up-keep of *Dai*-hut, amount needed to be standardized.

In Jawhar field area, in three *dai*-huts, 37 deliveries were conducted in nine months in 2008, the most prominent being 19 in the village Kayari, habited by very poor tribal group, Dhor-koli. The weights of new born babies varied from 2.5 to 3 kg. Two babies were born with weight 2 kg and 2.2 kg. Ten *dai*-huts were constructed in nine field areas of AUK.

Health Camps

Health camps serve dual purpose in tribal areas. Besides providing multiple medical facilities with expert doctors at one place, it also has social potential. Patients coming from one village/hamlet could share transport charges and families could interact with each other. No fee was charged from patients. In Jawhar, couple of general health camps were organised which created problems of large numbers. We restricted health camps to pregnant women and children. Couple of exclusive eye camps were organised where spectacles were also distributed free of charge.

The AUK volunteers proved very useful since they accompanied the patients to camp site and back to the respective villages. Volunteers could also get to know about the care they needed to take of the needy from their villages/hamlets.

More health camps were organised at Jawhar, Mokhada and Zari-zamni. Due to nearness to towns like Nasik and Yavatmal, the NGOs like Indian Medical Association and doctors from other voluntary organisations and charitable hospitals also participated in health camps. Otherwise, the PHC, and Rural Hospital doctors were always available for health camps. AUK met with the expenditure of medicines, travel and honorarium to doctors and food charges. At several places the expenditure of transport for patients accompanying volunteers was also met by AUK.

Health Camps for Pregnant women and New born 2005-2012

Year	Akole	Akkalkuwa	Dhadgaon	Dharni	Etapalli	Jawhar	Karjat	Mokhada	Zarijamni	Total
2005	105	–	330	–	–	–	400	–	–	835
2006	–	292	200	208	69	830	456	386	586	3027
2007	–	–	–	–	278	476	35	400	130	1319

(Contd.)

Year	Akole	Akkalkuwa	Dhadgaon	Dharni	Etapalli	Jawhar	Karjat	Mokhada	Zarijamni	Total
2008	750	–	–	–	–	872	60	200	547	2429
2009	100	300	–	–	–	300	–	368	423	1491
2010	–	–	–	269	–	264	–	455	688	1676
2011	100	50	–	–	–	452	–	512	369	1483
2012	–	–	–	–	–	–	–	–	–	–
Total	**1055**	**642**	**530**	**477**	**347**	**3194**	**951**	**2321**	**2743**	**12260**

Source: AUK Report submitted to Government of Maharashtra.

Interventions Directly Impacting Malnutrition

At least for the couple of decades, malnutrition of tribal children in India has been at the centre-stage of political and judicial review, as reported in the media. As discussed earlier, it is treated as a seasonal epidemic to be addressed by feeding programmes by the government and the NGOs. However, the vicious cycle of low birth weight baby, growing into an anaemic adolescent girl to marry and beget children at an early age and the survivors suffering from food security throughout life, due to livelihood issues, resulting in migration is a complete circle. The government does have supplementary food and mid-day meal programme, but caught into administrative and financial delays, it continues to function through contractors who have a capacity to absorb the delays, unlike the NGOs and CBOs like SHGs.

Anthropological understanding based on tribal field experience about the "cashless economy" till the wage labour for migrants or such schemes as EGS (MNREGA) started with cash payments, cautions about the exploitation of tribal people, with linkage to market forces. We had no inclination to start a parallel system of providing supplementary food or a meal to pregnant women. However, the sustainable and replicable model had to be developed for reduction of malnutrition. It was not enough to weigh the children, pronounce grades of malnourishment and direct them to anganwadi, without any follow-up activity from our side, to find solution.

Supplementary Food *(Sattu)*

Coming from Gwalior, I had the experience of consuming *Sattu* which was made at home for children. *Sattu* was made of baked wheat and Bengal gram in equal proportion. It is used as ready to eat supplementary food for children and even for adults. It can be taken in different forms such as with water and sugar/ jaggery, with milk, with curd or butter milk, and with oil, red chilly powder, salt and *jeera*. *Sattu* is the most common ready-to-eat supplementary food for children and adults in North India. It was common for the villagers travelling by passenger trains to carry *sattu* and a *katori* (bowl) for mixing with water. *Sattu* has been seen being purchased in a liquid form in a glass outside New Delhi Railway Station by hand cart pullers, from ladies selling it under the bridge.

Accidently, I came to know that a reputed food production company at Pune was manufacturing the *Sattu* and was available in the market. We approached the owners and told them about our issues of tribal malnutrition. They readily accepted to supply us in whatever quantity required, at concessional price. Accordingly, we purchased *Sattu* worth Rs. 16 lakh, by single payment, and transported it to the centres all over Maharashtra. It was given a brand name of Sakas fortified medicinal food. The packing was of 1 kg. plastic container with a bowl (*katori*) and a spoon for 20 gm. measurement. This was meant to be given to infants and children in the age group of 6 months – 3 years. Pregnant women were given 3 kg. of *Sattu* per month. At a later date, lactating women were also given *Sattu* fortified with Ayurvedic lactogens such as *Shatavari*, *Jeshthamadh*, *Ashwaganda* and *Pimpli*.

Sattu was purchased only once from the manufacturer. Initially, the production was not given to SHGs for fear of stomach ache and digestion problems, lest the grain and pulses were not baked properly. The response of the people also had to be assessed. Afterwards, the tribal volunteers were trained to prepare *Sattu* at home or through Self-Help Groups (SHGs). The SHGs were provided with big utensils such as *Kadhai* for baking the wheat and Bengal gram. Grinding was done at the flourmill available in the area. In Akkalkuwa, women prepared *Sattu* at the household level, on the stone grinding wheel, available in every house.

The wheat was purchased from the PDS Ration Shops using the family cards issued under BPL scheme with subsidized rates. Bengal gram was purchased directly from the farmers or from the market. Wheat purchased on Antyoday Card was Rs. 2 per kg. which we purchased at Rs. 4 per kg. and gave it back to SHG. As a result, the cost of *Sattu* came down very drastically since wheat in the open market was Rs. 13 per kg. There have been minor variations in the content of cereals and pulses in the making of *Sattu* in different field sites. In some places *Ragi* has been used in addition to wheat while at some other places, rice, soybeen and green-gram has been used. This programme has resulted in the weight gain of children and that of the pregnant women. Lactating women had improved lactation as a result of fortified *Sattu*.

The programme was monitored by the village volunteer, peer supervisor and assistant coordinator, at the family level. Volunteer used to visit each house for measurement of weight in the last week of every month. *Sattu* was supplied to families twice a month in polythene bags which people transferred to the container bottle supplied first time when it was purchased from a production company at Pune. *Sattu* was being propagated as medicinal supplementary food, to avoid its sharing in the family. This ready-to-eat supplement could be taken in different forms to suit the taste. *Sattu* could also be kneaded like wheat flour, to bake it on *Tawa* on open fire, with or without seasoning of oil, commonly known in Maharashtra as *thalipeeth*, similar to a north Indian *paratha*.

Response

"With *Sattu*, there is definite weight gain of children. *Sattu* is given in good quantity. As a result, children started looking bright and healthy". "Women got empowered. They formed groups to prepare *sattu*. They realised that they could produce and distribute as is done in government system. The awareness about health dawned on them. Self-Help Groups producing *Sattu* gave us income of our own. People have now realised that if the weight goes down, something could be prepared at household level from the available grain in the house, such as rice, ragi and pulses." "I gave to my children porridge made with baked rice and Bengal gram or ground nut and jaggery for weight gain."

A news item about ready-to-eat food supplement as accredited by UN bodies, should motivate all of us to document the traditional home made supplements. These could be popularised instead of getting something from the market on a large scale, with a risk of financial scams.

Fortified, Ready-to-use Food can Cure Malnutrition

"New evidence highlights that about three-quarters of children with severe malnutrition, those who have a good appetite and no medical complications can be treated at home with highly fortified, ready-to-use therapeutic foods (RUTFs), which are palatable, soft and crushable nutrient- and energy-rich foods that can be eaten by children over the age of six months without adding water, and thus reducing the risk of bacterial infection. RUTFs provide the nutrients required to treat a severely malnourished child at home, without refrigeration, and even where hygiene conditions are not perfect, the World Health Organisation (WHO), the World Food Programme (WFP), the United Nations Standing Committee on Nutrition (SCN) and UNICEF said in a joint statement" (Statesman News Service, New Delhi, June 9, 2007).

"Sufficient evidence exists to show that the best window of opportunity to prevent chronic undernutrition in children, including *adivasi* children, is the period from conception to the first two years of life. The damage caused in this period is largely irreversible. Unfortunately, the child feeding and care practices, particularly after the child turns six months of age, are abysmally poor. A 2013 UNICEF study in rural areas of the top eleven tribal populated states shows that the proportion of chronically undernourished *adivasi* children increased with increasing age – one-fourth in the age group 0-5 months, which doubled in 6-11 months period and at 18 months, 75 per cent *adivasi* children were already chronically undernourished. With only 2 per cent *adivasi* children between 6 and 11 months fed complementary foods in recommended quality and frequency, such levels of undernutrition should not trigger surprise. But the fact that this is considered the norm should cause outrage!"

"The study also revealed that if the mother herself was chronically stunted, the likelihood that the child being chronically undernourished increased twofold. The reasons for high maternal undernutrition in *adivasis* were obvious—68 per cent mothers under 20 years and 48 per cent mothers overall were themselves undernourished, inter-pregnancy intervals were narrow and birth orders ranged from 1-12. We need to remember three things—first, 50 per cent of the growth failure that accrues by two years of age actually occurs in the womb; second, foetal stunting is largely because of problems in the first trimester and pre-pregnancy; and third, pre-pregnancy weight and weight gain during pregnancy have independent and additive effects on foetal stunting. This compounds the problem for India since the focus of nutrition interventions for Indian children have largely been interventions after birth. Clearly, we are missing the critical time period in which stunting takes place" (*Journal 'Seminar—The Malnourished Tribal'*, No. 661, September 2014, p. 45, "Mind the gap" by Biraj Swain and Vani Sethi).

Reduction of Child Malnutrition

	Dec. 2005 Baseline Survey	*Dec. 2006*	*Dec. 2007*	*Dec. 2008*	*Mar. 2009*	*Dec. 2010*	*Dec. 2011*	*Dec. 2012*
N	2791	4391	3481	3697	4421	4168	4081	3974
%	31.5	35.7	31.7	33.88	38.32	39.97	42.8	47.24
I	2813	4548	4273	4177	4182	3685	3061	2612
%	31.8	37	38.9	38.2	36.25	35.34	32.9	31.05
II	2212	2865	2780	2846	2679	2403	2109	1604
%	25	23.3	25.3	26	23.22	23.04	22.11	19.07
III	777	427	394	191	238	144	261	192
%	8.8	3.5	3.6	1.7	2.06	1.38	2.74	2.3
IV	264	74	58	15	17	28	27	31
%	3	0.6	0.5	0.1	0.15	0.27	0.28	0.37
%	100	100	100	100	100	100	100	100
III & IV	1041	501	452	206	255	172	288	223
%	11.8	4.1	4.1	1.9	2.21	1.65	3.02	2.7
TOTAL	**8857**	**12305**	**10986**	**10926**	**11537**	**10428**	**9539**	**8413**

Source: AUK Report submitted to Government of Maharashtra.

In respect of data based on weight for age, 30 per cent of child population of 0-5 years age group was covered by baseline survey investigators in December 2005. As per GR issued by the State Government, AUK was to end by March 2009. Was given yearly no cost extension up to March 2013 due to default in release of grants.

Data based on weight for age conducted by volunteers for total child population of 0-3 years age group. Grade III and IV has reduced from 11.08 per cent in baseline survey to 2.7 per cent by December 2012 as a result of AUK intervention.

Summary

Baseline: December 2005, First end point, Dec 2008 if the AUK was to end by March 2009. Second end point, December 2012 since AUK extended up to March 2013.

Reduction of Child Malnutrition: Tribe-wise

	Baseline Survey: Dec. 2005			Volunteers Data Dec. 2008		
Tribes	Gr.: Normal-1	Gr. 2	Gr. 3-4	Gr.: Normal-1	Gr. 2	Gr. 3-4
	2005			2008		
Kokna	61.1	28.5	10.4	73.9	25.7	0.4
Katkari	59.9	28.9	11.1	68.1	28.2	3.7
Thakar	52.5	30.4	17.1	68.7	29.2	2.2
Warli	57.7	28.8	13.5	65.9	32.7	1.4
Dhor Koli	62.6	25.5	11.9	71.8	27.9	0.3
M. Koli	65.1	23.5	11.4	69.5	29.9	0.7
Bhil	65.2	25.1	9.7	76.7	21	2.3
Pavra	63.9	19.3	16.9	76.6	19.7	2.6
Kolam	67.7	22	10.3	68.9	31.1	0
Gond	71.1	19.4	9.5	73.1	26.9	0
Korku	70.8	19.8	9.4	74.8	22.2	3
Madia	60.1	25.3	14.6	73.2	23.7	3.1

Tribe-wise Nutrition Grade: December-2005

Grades	*Bhil*	*Pavra*	*Dhor-Koli*	*Mahadev Koli*	*Korku*	*Madiya*	*Kolam*	*Gond*	*Thakar*	*Warli*	*Kokna*	*Katkari*
Normal	500	107	105	420	501	250	108	75	188	160	156	206
%	30.94	42.97	33.87	32.41	42.03	27.23	30.86	37.3	25	28.5	26.3	27
Grade1	554	52	89	424	343	302	129	68	207	164	207	252

(Contd.)

%	34.3	20.9	28.7	32.7	28.8	32.9	36.9	33.8	27.5	29.2	34.8	33
Grade2	405	48	79	304	236	232	77	39	229	162	169	221
%	25.1	19.3	25.5	23.5	19.8	25.3	22	19.4	30.4	28.8	28.5	28.9
Grade3	120	26	28	115	77	97	30	13	101	55	45	68
%	7.4	10.4	9	8.9	6.5	10.6	8.6	6.5	13.4	9.8	7.6	8.9
Grade4	37	16	9	33	35	37	6	6	28	21	17	17
%	2.3	6.4	2.9	2.5	2.9	4	1.7	3	3.7	3.7	2.9	2.2
Total	**1616**	**249**	**310**	**1296**	**1192**	**918**	**350**	**201**	**753**	**562**	**594**	**764**
Tribe-wise Nutrition Grade: December-2008												
Grades	*Bhil*	*Pavra*	*Dhor-Koli*	*Mahadev Koli*	*Korku*	*Madiya*	*Kolam*	*Gond*	*Thakar*	*Warli*	*Kokna*	*Katkari*
Normal	1311	182	125	84	249	167	94	81	282	180	187	95
%	40.66	39.39	33.88	28.19	37.61	26.05	28.92	34.03	29	27.8	33.4	31.6
Grade1	1163	172	140	123	246	302	130	93	386	247	227	110
%	36.1	37.2	37.9	41.3	37.2	47.1	40	39.1	39.7	38.1	40.5	36.5
Grade2	677	91	103	89	147	152	101	64	284	212	144	85
%	21	19.7	27.9	29.9	22.2	23.7	31.1	26.9	29.2	32.7	25.7	28.2
Grade3	68	12	1	2	18	19	0	0	20	9	2	11
%	2.1	2.6	0.3	0.7	2.7	3	0	0	2.1	1.4	0.4	3.7
Grade4	5	0	0	0	2	1	0	0	1	0	0	0
%	0.2	0	0	0	0.3	0.2	0	0	0.1	0	0	0
Total	**3224**	**462**	**369**	**298**	**662**	**641**	**325**	**238**	**973**	**648**	**560**	**301**

Source: AUK Report submitted to Government of Maharashtra.

Meal to Pregnant Women

"Under-nutrition in children is influenced not only by food and child-feeding practices in the first two years after birth, but also by maternal nutrition before and during pregnancy, narrow inter-pregnancy intervals, gender inequity, household poverty, and other such issues. This makes it clear that any meaningful solution must follow a holistic approach addressing issues related to nutrition, health, family planning, water and sanitation, poverty alleviation and women empowerment simultaneously, and the concerned ministries should join hands to plan and implement effective inter-sectoral interventions and not leave the responsibility to only one or two ministries. The Ministry of Tribal Affairs (MoTA) being the nodal ministry for tribals can convene various Ministries for policy, planning and programme coordination for tribals to ensure that basic nutrition, health and sanitation and development reaches them". (*Journal 'Seminar—The Malnourished Tribal'* No. 661, September 2014, p. 13, "The Problem" by Vani Sethi).

It is usually remarked that the problem of child malnutrition is rooted in the malnourished mother. It is alleged that the tribal women not only do not take any special care during pregnancy, but deliberately eat less for fear of birthing problems in case of large foetus. The statistics about tribal maternal mortality are not projected in national surveys. The general observation of non-tribal functionaries in tribal area is that maternal deaths are very less, although neo-natal and infant deaths are very high. We observe that not only tribal people appear stunted but also their cattle.

To address the issue of low birth weight babies, it was decided to provide at least one meal during pregnancy. It is believed that traditionally tribal pregnant women did not "eat more for two" to ensure smooth and safe delivery and avoid maternal mortality. A woman during pregnancy did not get any rest from her daily schedule of household chores and work in the field or forest. As we know, most of the tribal families are nuclear families and not joint families.

The programme was initiated in August 2008, but had to be discontinued after an year due to funding crunch from the government. After the initial survey of pregnant women in each hamlet, it was decided to cook the meal in the house of the female volunteer. Time of meal was decided in consultation with the pregnant women. No take home meal was permissible. All pregnant women in a hamlet would eat together. A pregnant woman on visit to the hamlet from other village was also invited for a meal. Cooking utensils were managed by the volunteer. Eating plates were sometimes brought by the women from their respective homes. Menu for the week was scheduled which included *chapati*/Millet *Bhakar*, Rice, *Dal*, Curry and seasonal vegetables. Once a week, egg or fish or other non-vegetarian item was included. Occasionally, pregnant women brought vegetables from their kitchen garden. A woman had to first register her pregnancy with the Anganwadi with the knowledge of ANM who was supposed to provide ANC services. Iron tablet given by ANM was taken during meal time. The woman volunteer was not given any additional remuneration for cooking but she with her small children were permitted to partake the meal. Shopping of provisions was done by the lady volunteer at the village shop, if available, otherwise at the weekly market. No vouchers or accounts were demanded, as evidence of expenditure. Several times, the pregnant women helped the volunteer in cooking or in cleaning of utensils. Every week, weight was taken of pregnant women by the volunteer with weighing scale already provided to her. During meal, there was discussion about pregnancy and child care. Sometimes, the local supervisor (*Margdarshak*) or Assistant coordinator would read a booklet about pregnancy care prepared by AUK. If fuel wood was not readily available from the forest, it was purchased from the market.

Meal was supplied usually from the fourth month of pregnancy until delivery. The birth weights of babies born to these women increased, i.e. those with more than 2.5 kg were 2167 (73.0%) out of available field records of 2964 babies born to these women. Food was a big attraction, inasmuch as some women who missed their menses reported for meal programme claiming pregnancy. However, nobody was welcome without registration with ANM Anganwadi.

Impact of meal intervention on birth weights (All Nine Centres) January to December 2008

Period	*Available Birth Wt.*	*No.&%*	*Birth weight groups in kg*				
Jan. to Aug. 2008 (Before) Intervention	1892		**1.5 – 1.9**	**2.0 – 2.4**	**2.5**	**2.6 – 2.9**	**3+**
		No.	28	227	484	649	504
		%	1.48	12	25.58	34.3	26.64
Sept. to Dec. (After) Intervention	1173	No.	20	107	195	520	331
		%	1.71	9.12	16.62	44.33	28.22

Source: AUK Report submitted to Government of Maharashtra.

Pregnant Women's Spontaneous Reactions from different Centres

"We are getting full meal from AUK. Ours is a large family. We women used to get food whatever was residual being the last to eat in the family; we had no special treatment in the family due to pregnancy."

"Earlier we were getting only rice and green from the wild or porridge. Expensive pulses were out of reach. Earlier we used to feel weak, now with full meal, we feel energetic."

"Everyday, our weight was recorded. We also received ANMs black tablet (Iron) during meal. We received information about government schemes. A booklet about pregnancy and maternity was also read during meals."

"We now listen to the volunteers carefully and follow it."

Baseline Survey

Usually, the projects start with baseline survey. The purpose of baseline survey as explained to the people usually refers to benefits that the post-survey activities would accrue to the people. However, it is the experience of several people that the promises of activities to be undertaken after base line survey are never implemented. It is very important that people's confidence has to be won, if we want people to participate in the activities and turn it into their sustainable programme. It was, therefore, decided to start some primary activities to gain the confidence of the people. The Base Line Survey was undertaken during December 2005 covering about 30,000 tribal families in nine field sites giving due importance to all the ethnic tribal groups. In anthropological studies, sampling is not done. The entire population is covered from the selected area. Baseline survey provides an opportunity to have first hand contact with the families and neighbourhood families who hover around the family house where the information is being sought. Dialogue with the people is very important for involving them in the activities. Sometimes, there is a discussion as to why some information is being sought. Particularly, the school going children want to know the process, although, they may not ask questions. When the surveyors are local youth, the surveyors as also the families get information and knowledge which potentially develops their capacities.

The analysis of the data is, therefore, two-fold, taluka-wise and as per ethnic tribal groups. It is to be understood that ST is a general administrative category and not a cultural or social and economic category. It is, therefore, necessary to collect and analyse data as per each ethnic tribal group, since there are wide socio-economic and cultural disparities amongst them.

The survey was undertaken by local educated youth and the volunteers after due training and pilot testing. Supervision and monitoring was provided by the coordinators from Pune and some faculty members from the University of Pune.

Summary Findings

Baseline Survey for Adivasi Utthan Karyakram was conducted during the period November 2005–January 2006. The main findings are as follows:

Population

Survey covered 28,608 tribal families from 7 districts and 9 talukas and population of 1,48,427 individuals.

Average family size was (5.2). *Bhils* had highest family size of (5.8) while Kolams had lowest—only 4 individuals per family.

Sex-ratio for total population was 957 females per thousand males. Pawra (1030) and Kolam (1012) communities had highest sex-ratio while Korku from Dharni taluka had sex-ratio of 911.

Marriage

About (74%) females and (80%) males had married before the legal age of 18 and 21 years respectively. More than (40%) males and females from Madia, Gond and Kolam tribal groups had married after the legal age of marriage. All these groups belong to Vidarbha region.

About (48%) individuals got married within a radius of 10 kilometres indicating small social sphere.

Education

Total literacy rate for all talukas was (42.5%). Literacy rate among males and females was (50%) and (35%) respectively. Korkus from Amravati district had highest total (62%), male (70%) and female (53%) literacy rate. Mahadev Koli tribe from Akole taluka also showed similar trend. PTG community Katkari had lowest literacy rates—less than (31%) for males less than (16%) for females and total rate of (24%).

Only (4%) individuals had passed matriculation while another (1%) had education up to graduation level. Bhils from

Satpuda region had highest number of graduates and post-graduates. (60%) children in the age group of 6–14 years were attending the school at the time of survey. Bhil and Katkari tribal groups had highest number of out of school children (60%), in this age group.

Occupation

Individuals (76%) above the age of 10 years were engaged in main occupation of agriculture. Nearly (84%) Katkari individuals reported labour work as main occupation.

Labour work formed subsidiary occupation for about (83%) individuals.

Maternal Health

About (25%) Kolam and Katkari women remained pregnant at the age less than 20 years. *Bhil* tribal group had (25%) pregnant mothers with age greater than 30 years. (74%) pregnant mothers had registered with PHC. Highest registration was reported by Korku (88%) while Katkari mothers had lowest registration rate (61%).

Eligible pregnant mothers (91%) were examined by the ANM. (87%) mothers received TT injection while same number of pregnant women consumed iron tablets. (54%) pregnant women and (52%) lactating mothers received *Matrutva Anudaan*. Less than (15%) pregnant mothers from Kolam and Katkari community received *Matrutva Anudaan*. Similar trend was also observed for lactating mothers. In (94%) cases delivery was conducted at home. Most of the deliveries (93%), were conducted by *Dais* in villages.

Child Health (0-5 Years)

Immunization coverage for Polio and DPT vaccines showed gradual decline from first dose to third. Akole taluka along with talukas from Vidarbha region had high coverage for child immunization. Akkalkuwa and Dhadgaon taluks reported low coverage (less than 60%) for all the vaccines.

About (32% each) children belonged to Normal and Grade I categories. Another (25%) children had Grade II. Nearly (9%)

children belonged to Grade III while another (3%) children belonged to Grade IV. The proportion of Grade III and IV children was comparatively high for the tribal groups—Thakar and Madia.

Comparison with WHO standards showed that Weight-for-Height and BMI-for-Age indicators are slightly lower than the WHO standards. However, Height-for-Age and Weight-for-Age indicators, there is considerable difference between the study population and WHO standards.

Child Deaths

There were 348 child deaths (0-6 years) in the surveyed population. *Bhils* from Satpuda region reported highest child deaths. Among the three PVTG communities Katkaris had highest child deaths. Out of the total deaths (31%) were neonatal deaths and children (35%) died at the age of 1 month to one year. Thus there were 66 per cent infant deaths.

Diarrhoea/Gastro (20%), Fever (19%), Sudden Death (15%), Malnutrition/Low Birth Weight (7%) and Pneumonia (6%) were the main causes of child deaths.

Morbidity

During the rainy season June–September 2005 there were (12%) cases of morbidity.

Tribal group Korku (17%) reported highest morbidity while *Bhils* (8%) had lowest morbidity.

Fever, cough and cold, diarrhoea and gastro were the main causes of morbidity.

Patients utilized private health care services (52%) than government facilities (35%).

About 34 per cent Madia patients went to '*Pujari*' (Shaman) for the treatment. Use of home remedy was negligible.

On an average patients spent Rs. 516 on the treatment. In Akole taluka treatment was costly, Mahadev Koli patients spent Rs. 900 per illness episode. Madia patients on average spent Rs. 178 only for the treatment.

Korku and Madia tribal groups reported highest number of malaria cases.

Disability

There were 1993 cases of disability. Totally deaf (21%) and totally blind (20%) were the major forms of disability.

House

Tribal families (11%) had benefited from the government housing scheme. Katkari (22%) families, benefited from the scheme. About (11%) families lived in houses with thatched roof.

Only 16 per cent household had electricity and only half of them possessed electricity with meter connection.

Only 10 per cent families had constructed latrines and out of them only 28 per cent were used for the purpose.

Agriculture

There were 31 per cent landless families. The two PTG communities – Katkari (88%) and Kolam (55%) had maximum number of landless families. Among the land holder families, Kolam families possessed average land of 8 acres while Katkari families from Karjat had average land of 3.7 acres only. Only (8%) tribal families had irrigated land. About 10 per cent families borrowed land for cultivation. There were (9%) tribal families who cultivated forest land. About 39 per cent Madia families cultivated forest land while forest land cultivation by tribal groups—Pawra and Korku was negligible (less than 1%). More than 85 per cent families from *Bhil, Pawra, Korku* and *Kolam* communities purchased seeds from the market and used fertilizers. *Gond, Pardhan* and *Kolam* communities reported highest average for fertilizer use—more than 350 kg. per family while for Warlis from Jawhar taluk fertilizer use was minimal—44 kg. per family. On average fertilizer use for all communities was 142 kg. per family.

Livestock

Tribal families reared she-goats, fowls, cows and bulls. Madia families from Gadchiroli district had highest livestock.

In total 8450 (30%) families owned milk animals, out of these families only 1467 (17%) families extracted milk. Most of the milk was consumed at home. More than (50%) Mahadev Koli families sold milk in the market.

Food Security

About 63 per cent families reported that food grain produced in farms was not sufficient for family for whole year. About 4 per cent families consumed *'Ambil'* and same number consumed roots and tubers to overcome food shortage. Most of the famiiies belonged to Warli, Thakar and Kokna tribal groups. Tribal families (74%) possessed ration cards. Tribal groups—*Warli, Kokna, Thakar, Mahadev Koli* and *Dhor Koli* had more than 80 per cent families with ration cards while *Bhils* and *Pawra* communities had less than 65 per cent ration cards. For PTG community Kolam, 85 per cent families had *Antyodaya* ration cards. 4695 families didn't lifted ration quota, 66 per cent families were compelled to do so due to the non-availability of money/purchasing power.

In total 34 per cent families received Khavati loan during the recall period of three years.

More than 40 per cent families from *Warli, Dhor Koli, Pawra, Kolam* and *Korku* communities received loan under the scheme. Only 5 per cent Madia families were benefited. Only 6 per cent families made partial repayment while another 5 per cent families repaid loan totally.

Migration

Nearly 9.4 per cent individuals from the surveyed population migrated seasonally for earning livelihood. Katkari tribal group had 23 per cent individuals who migrated for livelihood. While only 1 per cent individuals from PVTG Kolam migrated. Among the migrants 76 per cent were males and 24 per cent females.

Highest migration took place in the months of October and November, i.e. after the *Kharif* season. Migrants from *Bhil* and *Katkari* communities on an average worked for 120 days, while migrants from Madia community worked for 22 days only. On an average migrants worked for 60 days.

Daily-wage rate varied from taluk to taluk, migrants from *Dhor Koli, Warli* and *Kokna* who went to metropolitan area of Mumbai and nearby urban area earned on average more than

Rs. 75 per day. Katkari migrants who worked on brick kilns earned average daily wages of Rs. 52. On average migrants earned Rs. 61 per day.

Bhil migrants from Satpuda region who worked for longer duration earned average income of Rs. 6100. Migrants from Madia community had lowest average income of Rs. 1318. Average income for migrants from all taluks was Rs. 3238.

Loans and Advances

Nearly 40 per cent families took loan for agriculture and 14 per cent for health care. 94 per cent families from Kolam community had taken loan for agriculture. About 42 per cent families had taken loan for the period 7-12 months.

Money lender (33%), Relatives (18%), Friends (16%) and Shopkeepers (14%) were the main sources for loan. 79 per cent Kolam families took loan from the money lender.

Loan amount ranged from minimum of Rs. 100 to maximum of Rs. 2,00,000. On average each family took loan of Rs. 5076. Families from Gond community on average took loan of Rs. 8500 Families from *Dhor Koli* community took average loan of Rs. 1100.

Annual rate of interest varied from zero interest to more than 60 per cent. Kolams from Zarijamani taluka had to pay interest rate of 50 per cent irrespective of loan amount or period. 5 per cent families took advances from their employers. About 28 per cent Katkari families took advances.

Work on Government Schemes

Individuals from 37 per cent families worked on government schemes for short duration, i.e. 5-15 days. 65 per cent families from tribal groups *Warli, Dhor Koli* and *Kokna* worked on such schemes while only (10%) *Kolam* families got opportunity for work.

On average families earned 121 kg. of food grain and cash income of Rs. 855.

Benefits of Government Schemes

About 61 per cent families received benefit of at least one scheme during the recall period of three years. Tribal communities—*Kolam* (86%) and *Korku* (77%) families reported benefits while only (41%) *Mahadev Koli* families received benefits during the period of three years.

Beneficiaries of the schemes—Janashree Insurance, Grain Bank, Well for Irrigation, Diesel Engine, Farm Pond, Goatry, Milk animals; Vocational training and Loan for Self-employment were negligible. Land development and horticulture schemes by Agriculture department benefited tribal communities from Jawhar and Mokhada taluks only.

Food Security: Food grain adequacy and tribes (% of population)

Tribes	*Adequate*	*Not adequate*	*No ration card*	*Have ration card*	*APL*	*BPL*	*Antyodaya Card*
Kokna	**46.5**	53.5	13.3	86..7	10.9	60.1	15.8
Katkari	**6.2**	**93.8**	**23.7**	**76.3**	**0.9**	**11.7**	**63.7**
Thakar	33.7	66.3	15.8	84.2	7.6	60.3	16.4
Warli	35.3	64.7	12.1	87.9	2.7	59.5	25.7
Dhor Koli	25.0	**75.0**	18.3	81.7	5.9	55.0	20.9
M. Koli	29.0	71.0	16.8	83.2	16.4	59.3	7.5
Bhil	**62.8**	37.2	**46.5**	53.5	1.9	44.3	7.3
Pawra	59.2	40.8	38.5	61.5	3.1	52.1	6.3
Kolam	24.7	**75.3**	12.6	87.4	0.9	1.4	**85.2**
Pardhan	21.3	78.7	31.4	68.6	9.2	6.3	53.1
Gond	35.7	64.3	32.1	67.9	7.3	9.7	50.9
Korku	18.9	**81.1**	24.1	75.9	2.2	30.5	43.2
Madia	41.5	58.5	31.0	69.0	7.1	16.8	45.2
Other	30.4	69.6	24.6	75.4	4.3	39.1	31.9
Average	**37.2**	**62.8**	**25.9**	**74.1**	**6.1**	**41.2**	**26.8**

Source: AUK Report submitted to Government of Maharashtra.

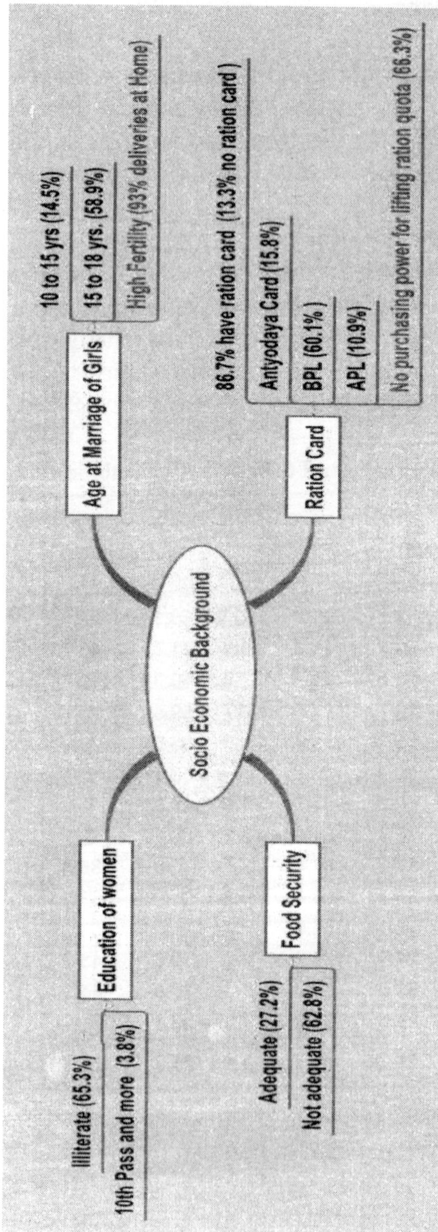
Socio Economic Background
Education of women
Illiterate (65.3%)
10th Pass and more (3.8%)
Age at Marriage of Girls
10 to 15 yrs (14.5%)
15 to 18 yrs. (58.9%)
High Fertility (93% deliveries at Home)
Food Security
Adequate (27.2%)
Not adequate (62.8%)
Ration Card
86.7% have ration card (13.3% no ration card)
Antyodaya Card (15.8%)
BPL (60.1%)
APL (10.9%)
No purchasing power for lifting ration quota (66.3%)

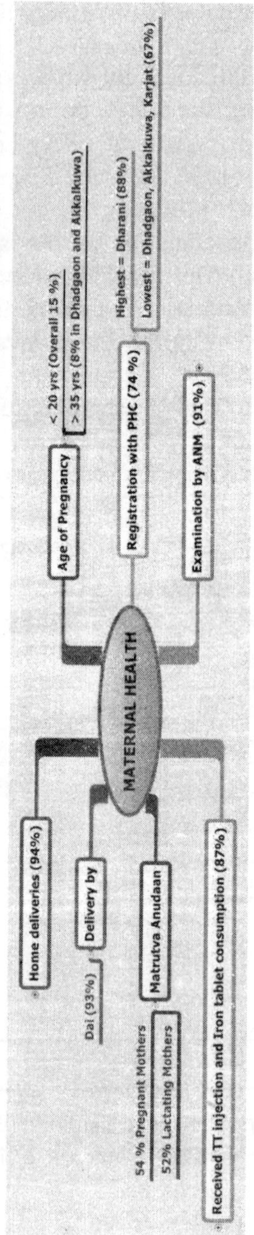
MATERNAL HEALTH
Age of Pregnancy
< 20 yrs (Overall 15 %)
> 35 yrs (8% in Dhadgaon and Akkalkuwa)
Registration with PHC (74 %)
Highest = Dharani (88%)
Lowest = Dhadgaon, Akkalkuwa, Karjat (67%)
Examination by ANM (91%)
Home deliveries (94%)
Delivery by
Dai (93%)
Matrutva Anudaan
54 % Pregnant Mothers
52% Lactating Mothers
Received TT injection and Iron tablet consumption (87%)

Education of Women and Tribes (% Women)

Tribes	*Illiterate*	*Std. 1-3*	*Std. 4-6*	*Std. 7-9*	*Std. 10 +*
Kokna	55.9	11.2	13.0	14.3	5.5
Katkari	83.5	8.2	5.6	2.4	0.3
Thakar	69.7	13.1	10.5	6.1	0.6
Warli	69.2	10.5	10.9	8.0	1.4
Dhor Koli	75.5	8.6	8.2	6.6	1.2
M. Koli	50.3	12.9	14.6	14.4	7.7
Bhil	78.7	8.1	5.9	3.5	3.7
Pawra	74.3	11.1	7.5	3.8	3.4
Kolam	58.1	18.0	15.9	6.4	1.7
Pardhan	37.1	10.7	16.5	21.7	14.0
Gond	51.5	14.4	14.5	13.2	6.3
Korku	46.6	21.1	17.2	11.1	4.1
Madia Gond	77.0	9.6	6.6	4.9	1.9
Other	50.8	13.4	13.9	16.0	5.9
Average	**65.3**	**12.0**	**10.8**	**8.2**	**3.8**

Source: AUK Report submitted to Government of Maharashtra.

Nourishment Centre

A pilot project for emergency feeding programme for children in Grade 3 and 4 according to Anganwadi scale was initiated in Jawhar at the instance of Thane district authorities during 2007-08. The same afterwards was adopted by the government as Child Development Centre (CDC) and later as Village Child Development Centre (VCDC).

At a meeting in October 2007 at Panchayat Samiti, Jawhar, attended by DHO, BDO, ICDS, PHC doctors from four PHCs, BAIF and AUK Jawhar centres, DHO invited AUK and BAIF to undertake emergency feeding centre for children under Grade 3 and 4 malnutrition scale.

"The ICDS system is also singularly unable to identify, let alone address, malnutrition. As Supreme Court Commissioners, we find that in most States with significant tribal populations, the ICDS system is unable to identify more than 1 per cent of malnourished children, whereas NFHS-3 surveys suggest the numbers to be around 17 to 20 per cent in these states."

"There needs to be a more robust system for early detection and treatment of malnutrition as it sets in among young tribal children. Not only does this require that all ICDS centres, even small and remote ones, are well equipped with weighing machines, but also training and monitoring of workers. Nutrition tracking needs to become a community based activity, involving organized groups of mothers. Community based treatment of malnutrition, with locally produced therapeutic calorie dense food, needs to kick in universally after a child is identified as malnourished. All primary health centres in tribal areas need to be urgently upgraded to include nutrition rehabilitation centres, to save lives of severely malnourished children, especially those with infections which—because of their poor nutritional condition—are potentially life-threatening". (*Journal 'Seminar'—'The Malnourished Tribal'* Journal No. 661, September 2014, p. 51, 'Unequal destinies' by Harsh Mander).

The concept was to admit a batch of 20 children, under Grades 3 and 4 for 20 days at the Centre with their parents under the supervision of a doctor. Children would be provided with nourishing food and tonics and weights regularly recorded. Food was to be provided to parents also and a compensation of Rs. 40 per day against loss of wages. Some toys for children were also available.

Besides breakfast in the morning and snacks at 4 p.m. lunch and dinner was provided to everybody. A spoonful of cooking coconut oil was fed to every child in the morning. Fresh milk was not available for children. Breakfast usually included wheat porridge and boiled egg. Soup of pulses, *khichdi*-mix of rice and pulses, banana, boiled potato were other items for meals spread over a weekly menu.

In the first batch of 20 children, there were children from 16 hamlets and villages, represented by ethnic tribal groups, Thakar, Katkari, Dhor-koli, Warli between the age group of 1 year 3 month to 4 year 5 months. All admitted were from Grade 3 except one in Grade 4. In the first batch 6 children improved to Grade 2. Remaining children were again readmitted for second batch whereupon 9 children improved to Grade 2. Later on, the batches were admitted under respective PHCs. These PHCs were designated as Child Development Centre (CDC), later converted to Village Child Development Centre (VCDC).

Thus, a pilot experiment implemented with the assistance of AUK became a government programme.

Plant Nursery

Although, livelihood was not the main focus of AUK, some pilot initiatives were undertaken by way of combining livelihood and nutrition. One such effort has been developing nurseries for selling plants. At Phaltan (District Satara) there has been an Institute of Appropriate Technology developed by a well-known Botanist, Dr. Anand Karve, son of famous anthropologist Prof. Irawati Karve. From amongst the coordinators and peer supervisors, about 50, who volunteered for such training were sent to Phaltan by AUK. One of the training modules has been about nursery.

In Akkalkuwa in Nandurbar district, at Bardi-Rautpada, nursery of drumstick, papaya, hadga, nimb etc. was prepared. A forest tree Mokha whose leaves are popular with the tribals for making vegetables was also grown in nursery.

Besides getting micro-nutrients from vegetables, those who developed nurseries also got some additional income. Further, they learnt to prepare nurseries by making special field for the proper growth of plants.

Plants Grown in Bardi, Rautpada (Akkalkuwa) Nursery

Sl. No.	*Plants*	*Numbers*
1.	Drumstick	1400
2.	Sesbania (Hadga)	3560
3.	Papaya	3200
4.	Nimb	100
5.	*Schrebera swietenioides* (Mokha)	40
	Total	**8300**

Source: AUK Report submitted to Government of Maharashtra.

Fish Nursery—Etapalli

Gadchiroli district was constituted as a distinct district on 26th August, 1982 by dividing Chandrapur district (earlier Chanda, until 1964). The district has 76 per cent forest cover.

District capital Gadchiroli was a village when the district was formed. Etapalli taluk is inhabited by Madia Gonds who have been given the status of PVTG. Madia traditionally have been the collectors of food from the abundant forest in which they live. Paddy is the main cereal crop supplemented with kitchen garden and collections form roots, tubers and small game and fish from rivers.

When we had our first field trip of the anthropology students from Pune University during December 1963-January 1964 in Laheri village, ahead of Bhamragad, we could experience absence of cash economy. No tribal could count currency beyond Rs. 20, very few of them could count up to Rs. 100 in terms of 2, 3, 4, or 5 twenties. There are several stories about how the tribals were exploited since they were not familiar with paper currency. In case of hunting expedition by all the villagers in the forest, a pregnant woman was given two shares while dividing the game equally to all the villagers. There has been a tradition of pond irrigation extending widely going into Chhattisgarh with family ponds in Bengal, where fish were reared, like kitchen garden vegetables.

The influx of (East) Bangali refugees particularly after the Bangla Desh war in 1971, added a new dimension to the fish in the pond phenomena. The Bangalis hired the ponds of Madia for fish rearing for a sum of Rs. 1000-2000 per year and pocketed all the profits. Madia had to purchase fish reared in their own ponds. Similar exploitative phenomena is rampant among the PVTG Kolams in Yavatmal district where the farmers from Andhra hire the tribal fields for 'Mirchi', red chilli production and the tribals work on their own fields as labour.

AUK decided to train Madia in pond fish rearing as a livelihood and food security issue. It was, therefore, decided to follow the pattern of kitchen garden seeds, by purchasing and distributing fish-seed to the families with pregnant and lactating women, families with malnourished children and later to AUK volunteers.

Fish seed is put in the pond (*Bodi*) generally in June-July after a good monsoon whereby the ponds are filled with enough water for fish rearing. Fish seed was distributed to about 240 families in the presence of Sarpanch, village head, Patil, *vaidu* and Anganwadi worker. The volunteers were trained to monitor fish rearing in the pond, to ensure that the ponds did not overflow in the nearby fields. After about couple of months, fish having attained the weight of 300-400 gms were to be harvested for meals. ITDP personnel visited these ponds to see fish-rearing. Fish rearing programme was also initiated on a small scale in Jawhar, Mokhada village ponds.

Anganwadi

It appears that the concept of Anganwadi evolved out of the experimentation with Balwadi developed in India out of the concept of Kinder Garden School which was initiated by Smt. Tarabai Modak based in Kosbad, near Bordi on the sea coast in Thane (now Palghar) district. Smt. Tarabai Modak and Smt. Anutai Wagh had pioneered pre-school Balwadi in the Bordi area on west coast at Kosbad to attract tribal children to school education. Experiments such as meadow school, in the open, under a tree, by river-side, were successfully conducted. Balwadi became a government programme which later was turned into Anganwadi.

The disciples of Mahatma Gandhi like Sri B.G. Kher who was 'Prime Minister' of Bombay in 1935 and later first Chief Minister of bilingual Bombay State after Independence with colleagues like Acharya Bhise Guruji, usually referred to as Sarvodaya workers, were crusaders for education in tribal areas. Simultaneously, they also initiated Forest Labourers' Co-operative Societies to function as autonomous bodies instead of being subordinate to Forest Department. Smt. Tarabai Modak and her junior colleague Smt. Anutai Wagh were trying to get tribal children to schools. Since they had no liking for sitting in a school, since they were used to playing in the natural environment of trees and streams and rivers, innovations were tried to have informal education under the trees giving examples from nature to teach them arithmetic or science or language.

The main question haunting the child educationists was, how to attract tribal children to school. This developed into concept of Balwadi which further evolved into a wider frame of anganwadi as a centre of playful education, nutrition and later adding services to pregnant, lactating women, and adolescent girls.

Anganwadi is a universal national programme providing pre-school education and supplementary food to children up to 6 years Anganwadi also provides supplementary food to pregnant and lactating mothers and to adolescent girls.

Initially, it was decided by AUK to address the issues of child malnutrition in chose collaboration with anganwadi. However, it was found that the attendance in anganwadi was limited to children in the age group of 3-6 years while the malnourishment was targeting children up to 2 years So, the regular weight check was also not possible. Anganwadi had only one spring balance for weight of children. If it was out of order, it could take several months through red tape administration to get it repaired or replaced.

These observations and experiences led to redesigning the AUK programme. Further, anganwadi is not owned by any vertical line department of the State Government. Programme is largely owned by Central Government financially. Earlier, anganwadi employees, i.e. teacher and attendant were given honorarium, not salary as an employee. While other state-level line departments are headed by the Secretary, anganwadi is headed by the Commissioner at the State level. Anganwadi is under pressure not to report acute malnutrition to higher authorities or to media.

Reflecting on all these issues, AUK functioned through male and female volunteers, for weighing the children in their homes every month, and providing ready-to-eat and ready-to-make pre-cooked. *Sattu* in their homes.

At an informal level, close coordination with anganwadi was maintained. She was allowed to copy our weight charts for her reporting. Every attempt was made to see that anganwadi staff did not feel threatened by AUK programme working among the same population which was statutorily her responsibility.

Model Anganwadi

There is a booklet of the government for guidance to anganwadi. It was decided that AUK could try to follow the manual in letter and spirit in respect of some anganwadis under AUK centres' jurisdiction, to project some anganwadi as role model to others. The idea was to make anganwadi a part of the village to be culturally and socially owned by the community.

Anganwadi has to be a health centre for children, pregnant and lactating women, a recreation and play school for children up to 6 years and information centre for the village. During discussion with Anganwadi workers, supervisors and project officer of ITDP, they said that they were criticized and targeted, if there was neo-natal or child mortality or malnutrition, despite supplementary food to pregnant and lactating women and children. "However, nobody understands our problems, nobody appreciates our work".

Some anganwadis were selected in Mokhada taluka, Dharni and Etapalli centres of AUK to develop as models following the anganwadi manual.

Sakhari village at a distance of 4 km. from Mokhada is 2 km. for the road situated on a hillock. One had to walk 1 km. to reach the village. Of the two rooms, windows were broken as also the floor of stone slabs. Rooms were stacked with cupboards, medicine boxes and toys. There was no place for the children to sit or play in the open. Without water supply, toilet was not being used. About 10-12 children attended anganwadi. Supplementary food was being cooked in the village and given in the homes of pregnant and lactating mothers as take home food. The taluka coordinator of AUK went to anganwadi at 9 a.m. everyday and visited the houses with anganwadi helper to persuade parents to send children to anganwadi. In about a month's time, attendance rose to 35 children. Behind anganwadi was open space of Zilla Parishad school which was made available for playing in the open. Behind kitchen room, kitchen garden was developed for growing vegetables. Building was repaired including the floor and windows. Building was painted in bright colours.

Every fortnight, children's nails and hair were cut. In fact, AUK, had supplied large number of nail cutters to the centres like weighing scales. Assistant coordinator of AUK, every Tuesday, Thursday and Saturday visited anganwadi to tell stories about animals and about national leaders to children. They would mimic the voices of animals and their behaviour, which was quite entertaining. He also helped anganwadi worker in weighing children every month and recording the weights of pregnant and lactating women. Villagers, AUK volunteers, pregnant-lactating women, adolescent girls and ANM are invited to anganwadi every month. ANM is doing immunisation work every month. As supplementary food, Porridge, *Khichdi*, *Shira*, *Upma* are given.

Sanitary block was repaired. A 200 litre capacity syntax tank was installed and plumbing undertaken for a tap. Sarpanch of Gram Panchayat arranged to supply water in bullock cart.

As a result, anganwadi became functional on all days, even during absence of anganwadi worker. AUK volunteer, ASHA worker and helper took the responsibility of running the anganwadi all the days. Food was cooked and consumed in anganwadi instead of in the village. AUK meal programme for pregnant women was also administered at anganwadi instead of in volunteers' house elsewhere. The Sarpanch visited anganwadi regularly for monitoring.

At Tingrya village anganwadi, in Dharni AUK centre, a coordination committee of Up-Sarpanch, anganwadi worker, police patil, AUK volunteer and taluka coordinator was formed for planning, monitoring and implementation. 41 children in anganwadi were provided with two sets of uniforms and identity cards. Parents provided shoes. Plays, games and songs were taught in Korku dialect, not in Marathi. Uniforms were kept in the school and were washed regularly. About 100 booklets were kept for reading and were circulated.

Two groups of adolescent girls were formed, with membership respectively of 16 and 12 girls in each group. Pregnant women registered in anganwadi were provided one full meal in the house of AUK lady volunteer everyday in the evening as decided by them. The meal consisted of rice, pulses, wheat or millet *roti,* fruit and green vegetables, maintaining the variety of pulses and vegetables. A lady animator was appointed by AUK at the anganwadi to teach Korku songs and games and monitor personal hygiene of children. She was paid an honorarium of Rs. 400 per month for four hours attendance during 10.00 a.m.—2.00 p.m.

A similar programme was implemented at Manger village anganwadi in Etapalli district. A committee of Anganwadi worker who belonged to Oraon tribal community, her husband, AUK volunteer, taluka coordinator was formed to prepare an action plan. Children were given uniforms which were kept and washed at anganwadi, twice a week, by *anganwadi sevika.* Pregnant women took AUK meals in the house of lady volunteer as in other places, after registering the name at anganwadi. A water filter was supplied by AUK for potable drinking water, since the one supplied by ITDP was not functioning and required considerable amount for repairs.

If coordination committees are formed with participation of Gram Panchayat, anganwadi could function properly with good attendance. In general, the participation of adolescent girls in anganwadi is very poor. Even the attendance of children up to age of 3 years is unsatisfactory. The community has to be motivated to use and monitor the anganwadi facilities.

As per Culture and Personality theories, a child's Basic Personality is formed by the age of 6 years. Thus if a child spends few hours in anganwadi in his village peer group, exposed to culture system though stories, songs and dances, his basic personality and capacity to widen his horizon, world view and choice will broaden. With nutritious supplementary food, diversified on week days, would have a positive impact on their physical and mental health.

Khelwadi

Anganwadi which is universal in tribal areas in Maharashtra meant for children up to 6 years, also caters to the supplementary food requirements of pregnant, lactating mothers and adolescent girls. However, there are certain pockets whereby tribal communities are located in hamlets of the villages inhabited by Caste-Hindu peasantry.

Invariably, the anganwadis are distance-wise and socially not accessible to the tribal children. One of the issues before the higher judiciary related to inadequacy of anganwadis as one of the causes of tribal child malnutrition. The State Government took a plea that the Central Government had to release the funds as per funding pattern for anganwadi. Although the judiciary directed the Central Government to release funds to open more anganwadis to cover tribal hamlets, AUK could assess that it would take lengthy administrative procedures to implement these directives.

It was, therefore, decided to start the anganwadis in tribal hamlets as AUK activity, in concurrence with the State Government. However, we were advised not to name it as Anganwadi since AUK funds were State Government funds and the state had put the plea of providing additional funds for starting new anganwadis. Through mutual consultation, it was decided to call these centres as Khelwadi, since Balwadi had earlier preceded Anganwadi.

The pattern of anganwadi with food supplementation, playful education, personal cleanliness and hygiene was followed from AUK funds. A local lady was appointed in each Khelwadi and was given some honorarium. In majority Khelwadi, uniforms were given to children. The lady helper would cook supplementary snacks and food, at her residence and bring it to Khelwadi. The actual play-school for three hours was held at a common meeting place of the hamlet or in the house of the helper.

Majority of Khelwadi were started in Karjat taluka of Raigad district, not far from Mumbai. Majority of hamlets belonged to Katkari PVTG group who habitually migrated for work. Some were opened in Yavatmal District and couple of them in Gadchiroli district. Totally 21 Khelwadi were started under four AUK centres in four districts/talukas. All shopping of provisions was made by tribal Khelwadi teacher and helper from local shops or weekly markets.

Subsequently, all the Khelwadi were co-opted by the State Government as mini-anganwadi and the staff was absorbed in anganwadi cadre.

Khelwadi (Mini-anganwadi) started under AUK: Karjat Taluka, Raigad District

Village/ Hamlet	*Population*	*No. of Children*	*Lactating Women*	*Pregnant Women*	*Adolescent Girls*	*6 m-3 Years Children*	*3-6 Years Children*
Chinchwadi	200	18	4	—	12	10	8
Mohpada	200	21	2	4	7	15	6
Damsewadi	150	24	4	2	10	12	12
Jambhulwadi	170	37	4	3	9	23	14
Lakhachiwadi	160	34	1	1	8	4	30
Pulachiwadi	155	32	7	1	12	17	15
Mugpe	150	22	3	—	11	12	10
Ambewadi	170	12	—	1	4	8	4
Vame	160	22	2	1	5	10	12
Total	**1515**	**222**	**27**	**13**	**78**	**111**	**111**

Source: AUK Report submitted to Government of Maharashtra.

Tribe-wise Mini-anganwadi (Khelwadi)

Tribe/Hamlet		*Children*	*Pregnant Women*	*Lactating Women*
Katkarivadya	6	149	17	7
Mahadevkoli	2	45	6	6
Thakarwadi	1	18	4	—
Total	**9**	**212**	**27**	**13**

Source: AUK Report submitted to Government of Maharashtra.

Ashram School

Education as an instrument of social and cultural change is an accepted fact. A tribal child may not have the congenial social and economic environment in the family for education. Residential schools have been instituted with the basic idea to treat an Ashram school as a Nodal Agency of development and subsequent change. Ashram school has yet to have agriculture land to train the children in scientific production. It could also incorporate various trades and skills necessary for earning livelihood. The Ashram school need to be strengthened to play such a role. Ashram school is not just an educational institution for curriculum based certificate granting institution, but refers to a school for living and personality development.

The first Provincial Government during British Raj was formed in 1935 for Bombay Presidency with Sri B.G. Kher as the 'Prime Minister'. After Independence also, he was the first Chief Minister of bilingual Bombay State, constituting the present Maharashtra and Gujarat. He held the education portfolio. He had appointed the Symington Committee in 1938 about indebtedness and backwardness in tribal areas in Khandesh which has become the present Nandurbar district.

A Committee under the Chairmanship of Sri D.N. Wandrekar was appointed to recommend about educational issues. The Committee recommended that Ashram School as a residential school for personality development of children and skill development for settled agriculture was the solution to propagate education among the tribal people. Sri B.G. Kher, Acharya Bhise, Janardan Valvi, and such other disciples of

Gandhiji who were called *sarvodaya* workers were trying to introduce education as an agency of change in tribal areas. They started some schools which were opposed by landlords who were exploiting tribals as cheap and bonded labour. Smt Godavari Parulekar, a Communist activist organised the Warli on west coast against this labour exploitation, commonly referred as "Warli Revolt."

Ashram School became a Government Programme after Independence. Currently there are about 1000 Ashram schools in Maharashtra, 50 per cent of which were established and administered by voluntary organisations with substantial government aid. In the geographical area allotted to AUK by State Government for model development activities, there have been 40 Ashram Schools, including the exclusive girls' ashram schools. Some of the older schools had an extensive land area. However, the children had to go to river for bath since the availability of water in ashram school premises was scarce. Being residential school, food was supplied to children. All such facilities as dining space, water and space for cleaning eating plates etc., supply of electricity for study at night had bottlenecks. The medical facilities to cope up with sickness were lacking. Although improving Ashram Schools was not one of the approved programmes under AUK, the emphasis being on addressing malnutrition issues, it was decided to do networking with Ashram school. Children educated at these schools have become the participants in governance and have contributed to tribal work force in the mainstream, as technical professionals, as doctors, engineers, elected representatives of people etc. Ashram school having a campus and students-teachers at one place, it is easier to address them to further develop their knowledge, skills, world view and aspirations.

Model Ashram School

The AUK coordinator from Dharni in Amravati district took initiative in developing Government ashram school at Bijudhawdi near Dharani as an ideal institution. The PHC and branch of Bank of Maharashtra are also located in the village.

The school had classes up to 10th standard. There have been issues about tribal dialect Korku of the Korku tribals, since the medium of instruction at the school has been Marathi. There have been communication issues between the teachers and students. The performance at the SSC Board examination has been poor. Due to shortage of potable drinking water, which was frequently purchased, there have been illness episodes. Prevalence of malaria has been high due to menace of mosquitoes with grassland on the open fields on the campus.

Normally, vegetable supply is done by contractors on a weekly basis which precludes fresh vegetables in the meal. AUK with the help of students and teachers developed vegetable garden in the open spaces and arranging irrigation by digging drainage line to supply waste water.

Medicine kit boxes were supplied by AUK to ashram school. There were five computers in the school which were not in use. They were repaired and brought in use. AUK provided computer training to teachers and 104 boys and 85 girl students.

The performance of students at SSC examination was 48 per cent in the year 2007. The students were weak in English, Marathi and Mathematics at the 10th standard. Their mother tongue was Korku and language of communication was Hindi. There are Korku across the State border in Madhya Pradesh. In consultation with Headmaster and ITDP project officer, coaching was provided to the students which improved the performance to 88 per cent in the year 2008.

There was an issue about disposal of leftover food in the kitchen and in the plates of students as also the week-old rotting vegetables supplied by the contractor. AUK volunteers from each of the nine centres in a batch of 20 each, were sent for training in appropriate technology to a voluntary institution at Phaltan, district Satara. They learnt about bio-gas being made from such left-over food and vegetables. Technicians from the institution were invited to install the bio-gas unit at the ashram school.

There have been two bore-wells in school compound of which one was usually out of order. Water from one of the bore-well is not potable for drinking. Water borrowed from an agricultural field in the neighbourhood was stored in a syntax tank which had only one tap. This was insufficient and inconvenient for all to drink water and clean their eating plates, which further dirtied the surrounding for breeding mosquitoes. AUK supplied with another syntax tank and installed 10 water taps with drainage facility.

The girls' hostel on the campus had bath rooms of which the flooring and doors were broken. The same were repaired by AUK providing clean bathroom with privacy. Even new buckets were supplied.

The school walls were painted afresh on which messages from great men and saint-poets as also proverbs were written. Hangers in the rooms and strings were supplied for clothes. Circular platforms around the trunk of big trees were constructed for informal discussions and chatting. The ground was levelled to make it fit for sports activities. Sports material was supplied by AUK.

Such facilities as were lacking were supplied in the ashram schools in other centres of AUK. At one school in Jawhar, solar panels were installed while at another girls school, solar lamps were distributed for study. Bathrooms at the girls' ashram school were repaired to ensure sanitary conditions, personal hygiene and privacy. Kitchen gardens, nursery of vegetable and medicinal plants and medicine boxes were the common facilities supplied by AUK. In Jawhar and Akole ashram school, training about making sanitary napkins was given to girl students.

Actually, the basic issue boils down to, as to why the Tribal Development Department could not provide these basic facilities from their own budgets. We were told that the Department which supplies budgets to line departments made requests to these departments like Public work or Health etc. but failed to get these done in reasonable time despite several reminders. The TDD had no formal authority to monitor the functioning of line departments in the tribal areas, despite the funding being provided by TDD.

It seems, Ashram Schools have again fallen in disrepute. Some tribal students are being supported in English Medium Schools where they are socially ridiculed. Ashram Schools managed by voluntary sector complain about irregular funding from the government while the government sources point out irregularities in such ashram schools. The good concept of Ashram School need to be operationalised and monitored by an autonomous organisation, to avoid lack of coordination between TDD and Education Department.

Ashram School: Vision

On the ground, Anganwadi and Ashram Schools are the nodal institutions for children and women. The tribal persons who are in positions of leadership and employment are all the products of Ashram School. Historically, created Ashram schools were not meant to be schools as per the definition of Education Department. Ashram School was supposed to have more than 10 acres of land to educate tribal children about agriculture to orient them to the psyche of peasantry, which has been the mainstream society. Without residential school, it was not possible for the parents to allow children to be away from the families to wean them away from traditional task of food collection in preference to food production. However, the discussion about Ashram School has always revolved around quality of food and high cost, as compared to other educational schools. Even Anganwadi has been reduced to a centre for supplementary food programme for the age group above 3 years while malnutrition is an issue up to 2 years of age. The management issues or the contractor system is tarnishing the two important institutions which can play a nodal role in tribal development focusing on women and children. Such micro-issues as number of bathrooms or number of buckets for adolescent girls in an ashram school or a hostel to address the issues of menstrual hygiene are not addressed in a macro-design of administration. We have experienced, SHGs could manage nutrition issues if they were provided with assured funds when needed for cooking utensils or grains. SHGs do not have corpus funds or borrowing capacity unless they become sub-ordinate to contractors. How long should tribal children use a classroom as a hostel dormitory?

We need good micro-level village based studies of Anganwadi and Ashram school as an exercise in participatory research. PVTG and some other ethnic groups who are not formally branded as PVTG need special attention due to migration. Katkari are the most marginalized among the ST in Maharashtra. They are a classical example of "Ascribed Deprivation" as studied by Dr. Rohit Mutatkar from TISS. Several times we recommended separate Ashram School for Katkari since they are ridiculed by teachers and peers from better off ethnic tribal groups like Mahadeo Koli and Kokna, in the regular Ashram Schools. As a result, Katkari do not go to Ashram School or dropout soon.

AUK could change the face of Biju Dhawdi Ashram school in Dharni block in Amrawati district by small interventions for improving the school grades by special coaching within the school.

Volunteer Training

In the beginning of AUK, after the selection of volunteers, some centres organised awareness tour of the volunteers for exposure of other NGOs' work among tribals, especially in the area of health care. A tour was organised to visit Shodhgram (SEARCH) in Gadchiroli district, a Health NGO of Dr. Abhay and Dr. Rani Bang. Similarly, a tour of Dr. Satish Gogulwar's project about traditional medicine in Kurkheda was also organised. Volunteers at Wardha visited Sevagram Ashram of Gandhiji and Pawnar Ashram of Vinobaji besides visiting Magan Sangrahalaya and Centre for Science for villages established by Sri Davendra Kumar, former Secretary of Gandhi Smarak Nidhi.

The formal training and feedback sessions of the volunteers were organised every month either at taluka AUK office or at a place equidistant to volunteers. Honorarium of Rs. 250 per month, per volunteer was also paid to them on this day. Local travel was reimbursed. Food was served during training. Resource persons for training included besides coordinators and experts from Pune, the BDO, PHC doctors, ANM, CDPO, PO and trained village volunteers from Jamkhed. Method included group discussions, use of booklets, participatory enactment of plays, use of puppets etc. Subjects for training:

1. Use of weighing scales and charting the grades
2. Baseline survey methods
3. Pregnancy and home remedies
4. Child morbidity, mortality and malnutrition
5. Supplementary food to children at home
6. Meal programme to pregnant women
7. Health camps
8. Supplementary food to lactating women
9. Drainage and soak pits
10. Government schemes of tribal development
11. Networking with Anganwadi
12. Kitchen garden seeds
13. Medicine box: Distribution and record keeping
14. Self-Help Groups and participation
15. Use of AUK calendar and diary, for planning and documentation
16. Presentation of monthly reports.

Trained Volunteers in Action

Since the weighing scales to weigh new born and children, were given to all volunteers, weights of children up to 3 years were taken at the residence of the child. The communication about relationship of weight, nutrition and diet, for increasing the weight, about the risk factors, and need of referral to SC or PHC was a natural process. Networking with anganwadi and ANM was useful. Anganwadi worker who was burdened with multiple record registers could update her weight register of children. Activities about kitchen garden, baby clothes to new born, dispensing medicine at all hours to fellow villagers, were performed at family level. At the village-level, participation in village meetings, helping to get requisite validity or birth certificates for admission to ashram school, accessing referral health services when needed, were the activities of the volunteers, sometimes performed alone or with assistance of supervisor, guide (*margdarshak*). Specially designed AUK calendar as an educative manual, helped to record neo-natal death, pregnant, lactating women, malnourished children, special events in a village for the whole month.

Peer-Supervisor-cum-Guide (*Margdarshak*)

From amongst the alert and articulate volunteers, one of them to supervise and guide the volunteers of 5-8 hamlets was promoted and given additional responsibilities. All these guides met at AUK Taluka office once a week to exchange notes and discuss issues with Taluka coordinator. He would also meet PHC doctor, other government functionaries and Ashram School teachers to inquire about the well-being and difficulties of students from the area.

Special training and 4 day orientation workshops of these guides were organised at Pune during February 2008 and again during August 2009 to do micro-planning for the hamlets under their jurisdiction, including budgeting. Another major programme has been one time meal to pregnant women which was to be organised and monitored properly. Accordingly, activity road maps were prepared for their respective hamlets.

Couple of training workshops were also organised for assistant coordinators, once at Pune and during November 2008 at Velhe, a taluka capital town in Pune district. Taluka coordinators were the main pillars of AUK. The performance of all activities as per objectives depended on their management skills and capacity, to involve the community and volunteers in the work. He also had to function like a PRO, keeping in touch with the revenue, rural development and tribal development government functionaries on one hand and elected representatives of the people at all levels. After the first training workshop at Jamkhed in September 2004, residential workshop for four days during April 2005 was held at a Christian Seminary Convention Centre at Pune, who allowed their facilities to be used by voluntary organisations at concessional rates. During this workshop, issues like baseline survey, government system about tribal development, feedback of 9 centres' work, documentation, conducting group discussions and FGDs in the community, and planning for the next quarter were undertaken. It was decided to have quarterly meeting-*cum*-workshops at one of the AUK centres to get a feel of the work in the whole State. In these meetings, field visits were planned including Gram Sabha, discussion with ITDP functionaries to organise activity planning for the next quarter. Couple of times, Additional Tribal Commissioner (ATC) of Tribal Development, incharge of the region attended the workshop and provided guidance. At Rajur, the taluka coordinators had discussion with the Hon. Minister of Tribal Development at his residence.

Response

(1) "As a village volunteer, first training was given about malnutrition. I also received guidance about health, women's common ailments, home remedies. After village survey about pregnant, lactating women and under three children, I started taking weights of children in their homes. After monthly training, started giving medicinal tablets to about 20-25 persons everyday on common ailments. There was remarkable improvement due to medicine box. Pregnant women and families with malnourished children were given seeds of vegetables for kitchen garden like Black eyed beans/cow peas (*Chawali*), Bitter gourd (*Karli*), Ladies fingers (*Bhendi*), Cluster bean (*Gavar*), Bottle gourd (*Doodhi bhopla*), Spinach (*Palak*), Papaya (*Papai*), Green Chilli (*Mirchi*), Brinjal (*Vangi*), Tomato etc.

Due to clothes for new born, child deaths got reduced. Due to supplementary ready-to-eat *sattu*, there was weight gain amongst children. Self-Help Groups of women who prepared *sattu* benefited economically. In coordination with anganwadi worker, ANM and Pada worker, we could weigh children, do immunisation and examine pregnant women (ANC). Due to monthly training, I could get information about Ayurvedic medicines, Ayurvedic herbs and about various aspects of health. Due to full meal to pregnant women, babies with 3 kg. and more were born. I am happy that as AUK volunteer, I could be of help to villagers." Ashok Pocham, Alenga-Tal. Etapalli, District Gadchiroli.

(2) "Because of AUK, I have reached this position. There was lot of malnutrition in my village. There were several children in Grade 3 and 4. After training, we started taking weights of children. We could understand that malnourished children cannot learn, their mind and intellect becomes weak. Due to meals to pregnant women, they got weight gain and birth weight of new born improved. Lactating women were given fortified *Sattu* and *Ragi laddoo*. We prepared all these things in our self-help group. We got livelihood in village itself."

"Earlier, we spent all our lives in our house, looking after household and children. Due to AUK, we could travel, go out to Pune, to taluka and district places. I have been selected as ASHA. Now, I can speak boldly in Gram Sabha, in public meetings over the microphone." Laxmibai Bhangre, Akola District Ahmednagar.

(3) "Government anganwadis were in the main village. Tribal children in Tribal hamlets had no use of these anganwadis. We surveyed such 13 places and started Khelwadi (Play school) at 11 places in tribal hamlets. Children were given supplementary food. They were told stories giving information about fruits, birds etc. Now, there Khelwadis have been adopted by the government as anganwadi and we have been absorbed as anganwadi worker or helper. This was possible due to AUK"—Kamal Pawar, Karjat, District Raigad.

(4) "Earlier we were preparing check dam in the river with clay. They could not last long. The crabs used to break them. AUK gave us gunny bags. So, we could construct Vanrai check dams. This helped us a lot. Our agricultural production increased. These dams cannot be broken by crabs." Shivram Hunya Valvi, Dhadgaon, District Nandurbar.

(5) "I was selected by villagers for AUK. I was under pressure whether I would be able to do good work. But the objectives of AUK were very appealing. I was trained to understand issues about malnutrition and how to stop it, how to reduce child mortality. We got training about care of pregnant and lactating women, about taking weights of 0-3 children and plot the grade. I met anganwadi worker. She was happy since our work was complementary. We surveyed children 0-3 age group, pregnant and lactating women and prepared a record register. While taking weight, we told people about its

importance and relationship with malnutrition. I helped villagers to get *wadi* sanctioned from BAIF for 115 persons, 38 persons got fruit saplings from Agriculture Department, 7 persons got cooking gas from ITDP office. I also helped people to get their revenue card called 7/12 certificate. The *sattu* was greatly appreciated by children and they gained weight. Medicine box prevented people from travelling for medicine and losing wages. We helped on SHG of women to get a ration shop. AUK has been a good programme of development." Magan Damaji Valvi, Peer Supervisor.

Vaidu Training

Like other animals, human communities sought their food and medicine from the neighbourhood environment. The baseline survey under AUK all over Maharashtra tribal area brings out the range of marital ties ranging from 5 km. to 25 km. This means, the movement of women normally do not extend beyond this distance since all consanguineous and affinal kins are located within the radial distance. Due to extension of transport, migration for employment, visit to pilgrimage centres, the mobility has increased for men.

Tribal life is different from that of caste-peasantry socio-economic life, in the absence of division of labour which is inherent in caste groups, having traditional hereditary occupations, ranked on a hierarchical ladder. In tribal communities, everybody does all work without specialisation.

With reference to knowledge of medicinal herbs, all people have some basic knowledge of herbs to be used for common ailments. However, some persons have better knowledge of medicinal herbs and their uses, who are termed as *'Vaidus'*. There are different local terms in different tribal regions. In anthropological tribal monographs, the shamans or *Bhagats* who engage in magico-religious rituals for treatment of an ailment are discussed widely. There rites are claimed to have positive psychological effect which helps the process of cure.

Normally, the *Vaidus* give symptomatic and mono-therapy treatment. The herbs usually in the form of root, leaves, bark and fruits are used in raw form. It is not uncommon for a patient visiting a tribal herbalist (*Vaidu*) made to wait, until the herbalist goes to pick up fresh herbal material for treatment. There is very little processing of herbs.

Since *Vaidu* are the first defense available in the hamlet, village, or in a neighbourhood village, with knowledge of little traditions, (local health traditions), it was decided to upgrade the skills and knowledge of *Vaidus.* These local health traditions were generalised as textual great traditions, by the reflective scholars such as *Charak, Sushrut, Vagbhat. Vaidu* needed training in the processing of raw-herbal material into the drugs which could have better shelf life and accessibility. The Ayurvedic Pharma industry is preparing such drugs commercially, whereby the herbal material is mostly supplied by such *Vaidus* to contractors who supply them to industry. Some physicians who are producing such drugs in their house courtyards to dispense them to their own patients get the raw-material from *Vaidus* delivered directly to them.

The *Vaidus* were visited by AUK coordinators and volunteers to undertake a quick survey about their knowledge of herbs and the ailments for which they were used.

During March 2008 and February 2009, a four-day state-level *Vaidu* training was organised at Pune at which 53 *Vaidu* were trained to make the following drugs. A tribal Thakar *Vaidu* from one of the AUK centre in Karjat (District Raigad) who had undergone training in Kerala was the main resource person.

Training session was visited by a senior Ayurvedic physician from Pune, and CEO of Zhandu Pharmaceutical Works from Mumbai.

1. *Bala* oil
2. *Kudaghanvati*
3. *Nirgudi* oil
4. *Krimighna Vati*
5. *Rala* ointment
6. *Laghusut Shekhar*
7. *Shatavari Kalpa*
8. *Gandharva Haritki*
9. *Hingvashtak Churna* Powder.

Such training workshops were organised in other AUK

centres by the *Vaidus* from these centres who attended Pune workshops. The products made by these *Vaidus* were bought back by AUK to use in the Ayurvedic medical kits of the volunteers.

Initially, for Ayurvedic medical box, drugs were purchased at concessional rates from a local pharma manufacturing unit owned by a very senior Ayurvedic physician at Pune and from Zandu Pharma industry at Mumbai, under Corporate Social Responsibility Scheme.

Ailments treated by Tribal *Vaidus*

Sl. No.	*Name of Ailments*	*Maharashtra Herbs*
1.	Malaria	–
2.	Fever	6
3.	Jaundice	9
4.	Bone setting	1
5.	Piles	3
6.	Arthritis	5
7.	Cough and Cold	–
8.	Stomach pain	5
9.	Skin Disease	–
10.	Toothache	4
11.	Headache	1
12.	*Dhaat*	–
13.	T.B.	–
14.	Gynaec Problems	11
15.	Cancer	–
16.	Paralysis	1
17.	Filaria	–
18.	Snake/Scorpion Bite	10
19.	Diarrhoea	13
20.	Renal Calculi	10
21.	Worm Infestation	4
22.	Avoid Miscarriage	3
23.	For conception	5
24.	To increase weight	4
25.	Lactation + Recovery after delivery	7

Source: AUK Report submitted to Government of Maharashtra.

Response

Residential training workshop, for *Vaidu* were organised twice at

Dharni, where 33 *Vaidus* received training. The advantage of these workshops was communication and exchange of information and knowledge amongst the *Vaidus*. Otherwise there has been no formal or informal platform to bring the *Vaidus* together.

At a village Baru in Dharni, measles were reported with a potential risk of spreading it to villages in the neighbourhood. Gram Sabha were organised in these villages to inform the people and take special precautions about cleanliness, boiling drinking water and reporting fevers to volunteers. PHC was admitting patients with fever for investigation. In the villages, awareness marches were organised by Anganwadi worker, AUK volunteer, pada worker in collaboration with youth groups.

It was, however, found that children with measles were not being admitted to PHC since they were taking treatment from *Vaidu*. The said *Vaidu* who had attended AUK workshop was invited for a meeting with ANM, MPW and Anganwadi worker. The *Vaidu* agreed to tell people in the Gram Sabha to take treatment at PHC and use bleaching power in drinking water. With this intervention, measles was brought under control.

Other *Vaidus* from AUK centres revealed that they had a problem of storage of herbs for use all the year round while they were available in certain seasons of the year. Due to AUK training about processing of herbs, it became possible to store it in powder or oil form for future use. This resource of trained *Vaidu* need to be utilised in the formal health care system.

In Sindhudurg district adjoining Goa, at village Kochare in Vengurla taluka, *Vaidu* training workshops were organised twice, during May 2011 and February 2014. Unlike tribal *Vaidus*, trainees from this region were educated, majority of them having attended the school up to 10th standard. A batch of about 25 persons who were treating patients with herbs were selected for training. Couple of young persons, educated up to graduation wanted to start the vocation after the workshop. As at Pune, 9 types of drugs were selected for processing in a four-day workshop. Former Dean, Poddar Ayurved College, Mumbai and Director of Ayurved, Government of Maharashtra, gave lectures on the principles of Ayurveda.

Sindhudurg district has plants with bio-diversity. There is scope to further develop plantation of medicinal herbs in Sindhudurg and in the forests adjoining tribal areas.

Panchayat Raj Training

In accordance with Lincoln's definition of democracy, functioning democracy has to be operational through democratic decentralisation. Traditionally, Indian villages were governed by Panchayat, a body of village elders representing all caste groups, which adjudicated issues concerning village as a whole. For caste groups, there were separate inter-village caste panchayats.

With initiation of Community Development, statutory, elected bodies at the village, block and district level were established. There are District Development Boards and District Planning Committees which allocate funds to Panchayat Samiti and Gram Panchayat. With community development in 1952, a government functionary at the Gram Panchayat level, mainly for technical guidance in agriculture and to initiate and monitor schemes of rural development was a Gram Sevak, a Village Level Worker (VLW). Now, he is the Secretary of Gram Panchayat in charge of day-to-day development administration and accounts, while the elected Sarpanch is the Chairman of Gram Panchayat.

While discussing the issues of selection of villages for AUK project, we were advised by CEO of Nandurbar Zilla Parishad in July 2003 that we should take Gram Panchayat as the unit of action, since all development work of government functioned through Gram Panchayat. Unlike the traditional panchayats for each village, statutory panchayats have been group Gram Panchayats, i.e. one Gram Panchayat for a group of villages if population-wise, the villages are small. Members of panchayat are elected, now 50 per cent seats being reserved for women candidates including the positions of Sarpanch.

AUK realised that the newly elected Sarpanch, Up-Sarpanch and members had no knowledge of the powers, responsibilities of the Gram Panchayat. As they narrated, "The Gramsevak comes to Panchayat office, issues notice about the meeting under signature of Sarpanch or Up-Sarpanch, for other members. At the meeting, he announces that there are schemes from Panchayat Samiti and Agriculture Department, which we have to implement, our cooperation is necessary. The villagers should deposit house tax in Gram Panchayat to facilitate village development. The meeting ends after all members sign attendance register."

"Gram Sabha is convened twice or thrice in a year. Announcement by beating a drum is made about Gram Sabha. About 100-150 persons attend Gram Sabha. 15-20 women are persuaded to attend by ASHA, anganwadi worker and some SHG members.

Gram Sevak informs about schemes of development applicable to the village. If people express their concerns, Gramsevak informs them that he had noted them down. Gram Sabha ends."

We were further told that the proceedings were all in Marathi. "It is difficult for us to understand when we read the papers. The government employees take undue benefit of this weakness and do not allow us to understand our powers of execution."

A lady tribal Sarpanch said at the inaugural function of AUK at Karjat, District Raigad, that it took two years for her to understand that the Gramsevak was her employee and not the other way round. She was being treated by Gramsevak as his subordinate.

It was, therefore, decided to organise training of PRI for the Gram Panchayat members and office bearers under AUK jurisdiction, in the year 2007 and again in 2012 after the Panchayat elections.

Subjects Covered under Training

1. 73rd Constitutional Amendment which bestowed self-governance authority to tribals through PESA
2. Gram Sabha and monthly meeting
3. Powers of Sarpanch/Up-Sarpanch
4. Writing minutes and resolutions passed by Panchayat and Gram Sabha

5. Finance—income and expenditure
6. Budgeting
7. Selection of beneficiaries for government schemes
8. Education campaigns
9. Integrated child development schemes and services
10. Malnutrition causes and remedies
11. Women and children fund
12. Nirmal gram
13. Right to Information
14. Gramsevak's duties and responsibilities
15. Forest Rights Act etc.

A booklet on this subject prepared by AUK-MAAS was given to all trainees. The workshops were residential giving opportunity for all to interact freely.

Before AUK started, MAAS had organised such workshops exclusively for women members in Dhadgaon area. At the concluding session, BDO was present. It was a sight to see, women encircling the BDO after the function, asking him several questions about development issues in their respective villages.

Resource persons for AUK workshops have been State Project Coordinator, local MLA, Panchayat Samiti Sabhapati, social welfare chairman at district level, BDO etc. The Panchayat members also narrated their experiences. The PO of ITDP gave information about the schemes of development.

Response

"Such orientation of PRI members is very essential. As a Sarpanch, I had no knowledge of my powers. Now, I will select the needy beneficiaries for getting the benefits of the schemes." Sanjay Atram, Sarpanch, Shible, Zari-zamani, District Yavatmal.

Several of the AUK volunteers got elected as members, sarpanch/Up-Sarpanch of Gram Panchayats. In total, about 350 Gram Panchayat members from 9 centres attended training workshops.

Training at ARTI

Appropriate Rural Technology, India (ARTI) is a NGO

institution at Phaltan providing training in some skills to young persons. Plant nursery, Smokeless *Chulha* (hearth), Bio-gas, Bamboo products, vermin-composting, coal making etc. are some of the subjects in which training is provided. It has been a week-long residential training programme.

About 125 young persons from AUK centres including some volunteers were sponsored for training. A mould for making cement smokeless *chulha* was used for household production in Dharni centre. Material equivalent to two basketful of crushed stone and 2 kg. of cement was required to make a hearth (*chulha*). For exit of smoke, 10 feet long with 3 inch diameter pipe was required. All volunteers in Dharni installed these hearths in their houses. About 70 hearths were prepared. The problem of smoke pollution affecting women and children was solved.

Vermin-composting was another skill which was instantly adopted by people. This organic fertilizer was used for cotton and wheat crops. In four villages, about 250 farmers from the same and other villages visited vermin-composting sites. Wheat with the use of this organic fertilizer, produced 43 quintal quality wheat on about 2.5 acres of land against 18 quintal on other 2.5 acres without this fertilizer.

For plant nursery, training was given to make a slightly raised platform for growing plants to manage the required water. Excess water could drain off due to raised platform. This was a good livelihood alternative.

Bio-gas unit was installed at Bijudhavdi Ashram School, Dharni, to utilise the left-over food in the plates of students for making gas used for cooking.

Puppet Training

Puppetry in India is a common art form which is used for entertainment and for communicating new messages. Rajasthani puppets made of wooden materials are played by controlling or moving string tied around the fingers. Mr. Hemant Kanitkar with his wife established a NGO "The Puppet" basically to function as public education and awareness institution. Department of Science and Technology, Government of India, through its body established for science awareness gave a grant to "The Puppet" to develop their infrastructure and help other socially conscious NGOs to use puppets for public education.

AUK sent about 150 persons from their 8 centres in eight batches except from Etapalli, for residential training of making puppets and organising performances on issues for which AUK was functioning. There were basically finger puppets and shadow puppets. Head of a person has been the main part of the body of puppet. With colour of the face and expressions of eyes and clothes, the identity of age, gender could be communicated. The story and lyrics of the poem had to be composed in local dialect about different subjects.

Basically, the idea was to make people think about their ignorance, wrong ideas and solutions on various subjects. People said, we learnt the significant of issues such as:

1. Weighing of children and pregnant woman, by AUK volunteer and its registration.
2. Registration of birth, marriage, death with the Gram Panchayat.
3. Water borne diseases. Importance of treating drinking water with medicine given by Anganwadi worker or *pada* worker.
4. Doctor, ANM, Gramsevak give lot of information which we did not understand. But through puppetry, and in our own dialect, we understood the significance of messages.
5. Causes of malnutrition, how to identify and action to find the solutions.
6. We have understood the objectives and activities of AUK.

Among all the AUK centres, Dharni centre where Korku tribals speak Korku dialect, formed groups and gave performances of puppetry along with songs on various subjects. Chetna group presents a story of a person retrieving the date of birth of his son from AUK records and getting validated from Tehsildar. Jagriti group composed a story and a poem about superstition regarding health. A child with fever and diarrhoea is taken to a *Bhagat* by his alcoholic father and agrees to pay for sacrificial fowl or sheep. AUK volunteer takes the child to a doctor for proper treatment. Jatubaba group presents a story and poem about cleanliness through the medium of puppetry. A woman is polluting well water by cleaning the utensils and washing clothes at the well. Gram Panchayats imposes fine for this misbehaviour. Jai Durga group has presented puppet about malnutrition by preventing a marriage of a girl of 16 years instead of 18 years advocating that a baby born would be low birth weight baby.

AUK, Dharani organised an awareness campaign through rallies in 20 villages. 14 youth were selected and properly oriented for 3 days.

The team of 10 youth out of 14 trained for the purpose, presented small plays in 20 villages through stories regarding registration of birth, importance of education, nutrition and diet, superstitions, age at marriage, family planning, clean drinking water at the point of origin and in the house, urban youth interacting with tribal youth resulting in undesirable habits and behaviour etc. This team visited all the villages, sang songs and presented plays without any fee.

According to their records, about 7000 people in 20 villages were spectators from their progrmmes, about 4500 men and 2500 women.

Field Area: *Dais* & Volunteers, *Vaidu* (Herbalist), Puppet Training

Sr. No.	Area	Dai & Volunteers	Vaidu (Herbalist)	Puppet Trainees
1.	Akkalkuwa	163	33	20
2.	Dhadgaon	199	30	22
3.	Rajur	168	—	10
4.	Dharni	138	32	23
5.	Zarijamni	214	36	21
6.	Etapalli	211	23	—
7.	Karjat	209	30	20
8.	Jawhar	147	25	11
9.	Mokhada	187	34	22
	Total	**1636**	**243**	**149**

Source: AUK Report submitted to Government of Maharashtra.

Out of 1636 tribal women received *Dai* training, traditional *Dais* were about 500. Others included lady volunteers and village women.

Bamboo Handicraft Training

Bamboo is a natural product in the forests of tribal belts. By way of livelihood and skill development, training sessions for making artistic artifacts of bamboo were organised by AUK at four centres at Dhadgaon, Akkalkuwa, Dharni and Karjat which were attended by about 200 participants. Ten days training was provided at each centre by a professional trainer from Velhe in Pune district. Accordingly flower pots, model of house, wall hangings were made. Children in Biju Davdi Ashram School made about 1000 visiting cards made from bamboo which were purchased by ATC, Amravati ITDP. Winnowing fans used in every house for cleaning grains at household level were also made and were available for sale. Tribal artifacts are pieces of art work which could have good market, to be promoted by Cottage Industries Corporation and KVIC.

Some small works respecting the request of people about providing a drinking water tank for cattle by the side of bore well or a platform for washing clothes by women with a proper drainage, to avoid the slush of mud were carried out under AUK.

Similarly, the demand for soak pits by people where drainage could not carry water due to uneven levels of land in the village were also made under AUK programme in Zari-zamni area.

Adolescent Girls: Health Education

Discussion about child mortality and malnutrition in tribal areas bring out the issues of adolescent health, age at marriage of girls and birth parity. If adolescent girls and young mothers are anaemic or malnourished, low birth babies resulting in stunting, wasting etc. would be an obvious outcome. It is, therefore, necessary to address the issues of adolescent health. The girls in the ashram school are available for focused work, being educated, would be amenable to rational thinking and behaviour, and would occupy good positions in society afterwards. It was decided to address them on priority basis. Special orientation was arranged for them and pathological tests such as Hb estimation, weight, and height were recorded including, for out of school girls in the village.

Nutrition Grade of Girls: Ashram School

District	*Taluka*	*Ashram School*	*No. of Girls*	*BMI 12-16*	*BMI 17-18*	*BMI 19-20*	*BMI 20+*
Raigad	Karjat	Bhaliwadi	176	117	37	17	–
Thane	Jawhar	Sakur	172	62	34	44	32
Thane	Mokhada	Gonde, Chas, Pimpalpada	142	119	8	10	5
Gadchiroli	Etapalli	Hedri, Todsa	139	49	30	37	23
Amravati	Dharni	Bijudhawdi	75	32	14	19	10
		Total	**704**	**379**	**123**	**127**	**70**
		Average	**100**	**53.8**	**17.4**	**18**	**10.6**

Source: AUK Report submitted to Government of Maharashtra.

Hb Estimation of Girls: Ashram School

District	*Taluka*	*Ashram School*	*No. of Girls*	*10 gm+*	*9-10 gm*	*8-9 gm*	*7-8 gm*	*6-7 gm*
Raigad	Karjat	Bhaliwadi	27	13	11	3	–	–
Thane	Jawhar	Sakur	152	89	40	13	6	4
Thane	Mokhada	Gonde, Chas, Pimpalpada	134	91	27	11	5	–
Nandurbar	Dhadgaon	Chulwad, Asli, Sonkhurd	133	12	20	53	25	23
Gadchiroli	Etapali	Todsa, Burgi, Hedri	183	69	57	47	8	2
	Total		**629**	**274**	**155**	**127**	**44**	**29**
	Average		**100**	**43.5**	**24.6**	**20.1**	**7**	**4.6**

Source: AUK Report submitted to Government of Maharashtra.

It appears 70 per cent girls are chronically malnourished. The content of orientation sessions broadly covered:

1. Objectives
2. Stages of life and life cycle.
3. Physiological changes according to growing age.

4. Puberty, menstruation and hygiene. Pathological issues like stomach ache, white discharge etc.
5. *Food*: Concept of nutrition and balanced diet. Proteins, Vitamins, Micro-nutrients.
6. *Family*: Biological, Social, Psychological, Emotional needs.
7. *Marriage*: legal age and its importance, family planning.
8. Essentials of child rearing practices.

The adolescent girls were happy and demanded such orientation regularly.

Although a patriarchal society, in tribal communities, there is no positive discrimination against women. There is no dowry, but bride price. Maternal mortality is not economically affordable in tribal communities, supposedly due to custom of bride price. Amongst non-tribal castes and communities in India, with strong custom of dowry, in case of difficulty in labour, survival of new born baby may be preferred, in affinal family, to survival of mother. Among the non-tribals, termination of pregnancies with female foetus, identified through sonography, is not uncommon, due to dowry issues. Gender friendly sex-ratio is common in all tribal communities.

Information Centre: Reading Room

There was a demand from volunteers to have the useful books and other fiction in the villages. As a result, such reading centres were developed in each of the 9 AUK centres. Book like Marathi translation of "Where there is no doctor" or "Doctor for women" and some story books were kept in a room managed by a village committee of 5-7 members monitored by AUK volunteer. About 30-40 persons took benefit of this facility at each centre in a month. There has been a constant demand for more books.

At some reading rooms, application forms to take the benefit of government schemes were also kept and assistance provided to fill them for submission to appropriate authorities.

Check Dams

Tribal people in Dhadgaon and Akkalkuwa have been traditionally making check dams to hold the rain water flowing through small streams and canals. They were putting stone pieces in the stream and cover it with teak leaves and clay. However, at night, the crabs would make holes in the leaves and clay. So, everyday, people had to do the exercise and use the water till evening, by using diesel pump or through small drains.

AUK coordinators with the help of volunteers arranged village meetings to discuss the issues. Villagers agreed to do the work by contributing their labour provided the gunny bags were procured by AUK.

Estimates of empty bags in anganwadi after consumption of material supplied by government was made and BDO made the bags available. Simultaneously empty cement begs were purchased from the market. Subsequently, people procured the bags by themselves. As a result, production of wheat, gram, maize and vegetables increased without much expenditure.

In 9 villages in Akkalkuwa, under three Gram Panchayats, 25 hamlets were benefitted by constructing 28 check dams. About 45 tribal farmers could take the benefit of irrigation for increased production of cereal, pulses and vegetables including onion and garlic. Some of them planted water melons.

Chavdi (*Chaupal*)

Among the Kolam (PVTG), *Chavdi* is a cultural centre, meeting place, and a guest house of the Kolam tribal community, in Zari - zamni AUK centre, in Yavatmal District. *Chavdi* is a cultural identity of the Kolam. *Chavdi* is also a judicial place for the Kolam tribal Panchayat.

The lady AUK volunteer was giving information about supplementary nutritious food to a group of women with their children in the *chavdi*. In the meantime, it started raining heavily, and the women had to huddle up where the leaking roof of *Chavdi* could be avoided. After the meeting was over, as the rain stopped, one villager exclaimed, "You are talking about so many schemes. It would be better if you repair our *Chavdi,* so that we could organise the meetings peacefully, in a better way." As AUK agreed to this suggestion, another meeting with Kolams discussed about the requirement of material, such as tin-sheets, cement, sand, labour and transport. Villagers offered labour and transport as their contribution. Although there was a demand from 14 places out of 23, under AUK jurisdiction, AUK could repair only couple of *Chavdi,* since the basic objectives and the approved budget could not permit construction work of this type.

Couple of *Ghotuls*—youth dormitories among the Madia in Etapalli were also repaired on the same lines as Kolam *Chavdi.* These activities proved useful in winning the confidence of the people to facilitate meaningful dialogue with the community.

Holi at Kathi

Holi is the biggest festival among the Bhil and Pawra. In the Hindi speaking belt of north India, the lunar calendar ends with the full moon of Holi. Next day after Holi is the first day of the new year. Kathi Principality in the hills of Akrani in Nandurbar district had a Chieftain. Since his times, *Holi* has been celebrated as a very important festival with thousands of Bhil and Pawra dancing whole night. Early morning, at dawn, after the ritual worship, *Holi* sacred fire is lighted. A hill, the slopes of which form a natural stadium is full of people to watch the ritual. Within minutes after the fire is lighted, people after paying their respects to the fire, go back to their respective villages. Holi is celebrated in nearby villages for 2-3 days subsequently.

Among the Hindus, *Diwali* and *Holi* days are fixed as per Hindu almanac (*panchang*). Among the Bhils and Pawra of Akrani area, *Diwali* and *Holi* are celebrated, spread over a week or two, separately in various villages. The names of festivals are Hindu, not necessarily linked with Hindu mythological stories. These festivals are celebrated as occasions of gaiety, solidarity expressed through gatherings of tribal people in the area.

People from about 30-35 villages in the neighbourhood as also from Gujarat and Madhya Pradesh visit the place to participate and observe *Holi* dances of the people. There are no less than 20,000 people on the hills dancing and moving whole night. The dancers are bedecked with colourful dresses adorning peacock feathers, dancing bells, musical bottle gourds around their waists and on the ankles. There are small shops selling tea, snacks, trinkets and small oranges to quench the thirst for water. For water, people search for bore-well taps in the fields in the area.

AUK decided to provide drinking water to people by hiring a tanker with drinking water. About 10 taps were provided to avoid crowding. About 20-25 big glasses were also provided. 7-8 AUK volunteers from the villages/hamlets were monitoring the water supply which had to be replenished.

People were wondering as to why the government and elected representatives of the people could not provide drinking water at the time of *Holi*, which a voluntary organisation could organise. Such confidence building activities go a long way in eliciting people's participation in development governance.

Kolam Culture

At *'Dandar'* dance competition among the Kolams and Gonds of Zari-Zamni area, people have dancing programmes during *Dashahara* and *Diwali*, dedicated to the memory of their ancestors. People made a request to provide musical instruments to enhance the quality of traditional dance-drama events. AUK decided to sponsor the competitions, and musical instruments were supplied by way of prizes to the winners. People remarked that in order to preserve tribal culture, such events were necessary.

Lessons Learnt

Intervention activities were planned according to the conceptual framework of integrative aspect of culture, i.e. if change was desired in one aspect of culture, interventions in several other aspects had to be initiated. The components mainly focusing on health, education and livelihood were identified. The community had to manage these activities, monitored by volunteers, peer supervisors and local coordinators to attain sustainability. The capacity of the community had to be developed with knowledge and skills to undertake these activities. Variety of training programmes were designed towards this objective. Some services were offered which were urgent requirements, such as availability of medicines for common ailments. Besides making Ayurvedic medicines available, *Vaidus* with traditional knowledge of medicinal herbs were trained to process the herbs into medicines, increasing the shelf life and value addition in economic terms. Local innovations such as *Dai*-hut for institutional delivery would be useful to reduce neonatal mortality.

The important governance issue about planned change is to link macro- and micro-planning and implementation. The PRI have to be given financial, implementation and monitoring authority over the functioning of government schemes. Constant dialogue with the people is necessary, but possible, if the people have confidence with visible evidence, about the implementers, addressing their requirements and concerns.

In academic perspective, planning and implementing intervention activities, provides opportunities to test the concepts and hypotheses about sustainable socio-economic and cultural change. This experience would help in developing theories of change. In medical sciences, there is constant clamoring for research which should be translatable in action. Why should social science research be non-translatable? Do not have social sciences predictive value? There cannot be water-tight compartments between so-called basic research and applied research.

Intervention activities rooted in the academic conceptual framework has given good dividends to look back at the basic theories in social sciences in general, and anthropology in particular.

"Thus, my point is not just that research can help action, but also that involvement in action can enhance the quality or research. This statement is bound to raise some eyebrows. What about objectivity? Is personal commitment to a cause compatible with an objective reading of the facts? Is it not important to remove oneself from the situation in order to consider it in an objective light? To this I would respond, first of all, that inaction is not neutrality" (Jean Dreze, *Economic and Political Weekly*, March 2, 2002: 818).

"The case for action-based research appears to me to be particularly strong if the aim of research is to facilitate human advancement and social change. In the academic world, and particularly in development studies, there is often a presumption that this is the case. Most project proposals stress the importance of the proposed research for economic or social advancement, and academic papers routinely end with a section on "policy implications". In this perspective, however, the government is almost always perceived as the crucial agent of change, so that "better policies" become the focus of attention. Rarely is there much acknowledgement of the ability of people themselves to bring about change, and of the potential value of research in assisting the process. If the researcher addresses himself or herself to civil society rather than to the government, research grounded in public action (rather than in the world of policy advice) is likely to have special value" (Jean Dreze, *Economic and Political Weekly*, March 2, 2002: 817-819).

Working with the government system functioning through the vertical, hierarchical line departments was a limiting factor. The employees who are shirkers had an excuse for non-participation by saying that their department bosses had not given them any instructions to coordinate with NGO activities. Even the single window Tribal Development Department which had no cadre of their own at the village-hamlet level and had to function through the cadres of line departments faced these difficulties. The para-professional cadres like ASHA, anganwadi sevika, ANM etc. who had an organic link with the community, were co-operative in their individual capacities. The Revenue and Forest Department mindset inherited from the British Raj is not congenial to the development initiatives which necessitates community involvement and management. We were fortunate in having freedom of thought and action about planning and initiating people-centric activities validated through joint monitoring committees of government and us, at all levels, affirming the spirit of partnership.

C. GOVERNMENT-NGO PARTNERSHIP

Introduction

The Principal Secretary, Tribal Development Department, Government of Maharashtra had offered us to be the "partners in development". In the government order about sanctioning the project, mention has been made that "the project proposal was sought from the two organisations. The project was then considered and it was decided to sanction the project, as was submitted".

In response to the government's offer of partnership, in the proposal presented by us, we suggested joint committees of Government and AUK for coordination and monitoring the project, at all levels of functioning of the TDD.

1. Apex Committee at the Mantralaya level
   Chairman: Principal Secretary, TDD
   Secretary: State Coordinator, AUK
   Members: Project Director, AUK
   Tribal Commissioner, GoM
   The committee was to meet once in a six months.
2. State level Committee: At the Commissionarate level
   Chairman: Tribal Commissioner
   Secretary: State Co-ordinator, AUK
   Members: All ATC and PO (ITDP)
   Programme Directors: AUK
   Programme Coordinators, AUK as observers. The committee was supposed to meet every quarter.
3. Regional level/Field level Committee: at the level of Additional Tribal Commissioners
   The jurisdiction of each regional committee was limited to the geographical jurisdiction of the additional Tribal Commissioner as the head of all ITDP in that region.
   Chairman: Additional Tribal Commissioner
   Secretary: Taluka Project Co-ordinator AUK
   Members: PO ITDP, BDO, Panchayat Samiti Sabhapati
   State Project Coordinator, AUK; Assistant Taluka Project Coordinator.

This Committee was scheduled to meet every two months.

The draft minutes of all these meetings were prepared by the Secretary of the Committee and finalised after the approval of the Chairman.

The partnership principle was translated in creating a structure, with Government functionary as Chairman and AUK paid functionary as the Secretary of all committees. We understand that the government had to report to the Hon. High Court periodically.

Altogether Apex Committee met formally 6 times during 2005-2012; State-level committee met 10 times during the period and field level regional committees met 7 times under the Chairmanship of ATC or in his absence with PO ITDP in chair. Besides the formal, minuted meetings, there were several informal meetings of the Project Directors with the Secretary, Commissioner, ATC and PO of ITDP. Likewise, at the field level, taluka coordinators used to report to the PO, ITDP periodically and accompanied him on his tour in the field area.

Report of activities every six months were sent to all concerned which were scrutinised at the Commissionarate and Mantralaya-level and the doubts if any were cleared by the State coordinator visiting Commissioners office at Nasik and by the Taluka coordinators in ITDP office. Usually, all meetings lasted for about an hour.

Meetings began with submission of reports and PP presentation of the work done after the previous meeting. During discussion, suggestions were offered by the Chairman and other government functionaries. The limiting factors were the transfers of government functionaries at all levels, which necessitated fresh briefing to the new incumbent.

Some of the suggestions made at Mantralaya and Commissionarate-level are as under:

1. To ensure registration of all births and deaths of 0-5 age group with Gramsevak, Anganwadi and ANM.
2. To reconfirm child deaths in Mokhada, Akole and Akkalkuwa since they appeared less than average expected deaths.

3. Awareness campaigns about personal hygiene, alcoholism, age at marriage and birthing parity.
4. To enhance coordination with government department such as ITDP, Panchayat Samiti, ICDS and PHC.
5. Constitute a Taluka-level coordination committee between PHC, Anganwadi and ITDP.
6. Submit activity chart with expected budget outlay for a year for financial planning and performance audit.
7. Performance note for Bombay High Court.
8. Present proposals for starting anganwadi (Khelwadi) in uncovered hamlets.
9. Grades 3 and 4 malnourished children to be admitted to hospital and monitor their health status.
10. Statistics from Anganwadi, AUK and other NGOs is different. Better coordination with ICDS.
11. AUK village-level statistics of malnutrition and child mortality to be scrutinised at Taluka-level AUK, before sending it to Pune office. Data need to be analysed before sending as Post office.
12. Monitor closely Pregnancy, Maternity and growth of infant up to 1 year.
13. Continue with supplementary nutritious *sattu*, medicines, *Dai* training and *Dai*-hut, health education and health check-up of adolescent girls.
14. Ensure accessibility of government health care to people. Health camps, Medicine box, institutional delivery, 100 per cent immunisation, anganwadi children to be weighed and examined regularly, registration of pregnant and lactating mothers to be focused.
15. Statistical documentation of programmes being implemented, comparing with baseline survey of 2005. Documentation in the context of human development index.
16. Separate report for Dharani centre of AUK, in view of Melghat constantly in media.
17. Provide Family Health Card to all families under AUK.
18. Prevalence of Anaemia and institutional delivery data to be collected.

19. Boards of AUK be prominently displayed on the main roads in road junctions leading to AUK villages.
20. Prepare village-wise development projects and send to PO/ATC.
21. Kitchen gardens in Ashram School with the help of teachers and students.
22. Information of malnourished children to PO office and Rajmata Jijau Mission.
23. Field report of AUK every month to PO/ATC.
24. Impact of AUK on child mortality and malnourishment to be statistically, analysed.
25. Comparative analysis of children's weights between those supplied with and not supplied with *Sattu*.
26. You should publicise your work through documentation, photographs, CDs etc.
27. Submit proposal for adding more tribal areas in AUK including Nasik tribal area.
28. Submit proposal with budget for mini-Anganwadis as Khelwadi in your area.
29. TDD have no workers at village-level like the revenue/ forest development. AUK volunteers have to reach TDD scheme to people. Suggest scheme for this.
30. Suggest beneficiaries for livelihood schemes focusing on families with Grade 3 and 4 children.
31. Follow up of Matrutva Anudan Yojana.
32. Prepare schemes other than TDD schemes in consultation with PO.
33. Health education to adolescent girls in ashram school.
34. Present cash flow every month to release the grants.
35. Lady volunteers be given ASHA training.
36. Undertake disability survey.
37. Suggest about requirements of road, school, hand-pump, sub-centre, check dams etc. in Katkariwadi hamlets.
38. As NGO to analyse the real causes of child mortality despite implementation of schemes.
39. Ashramshala need to be developed as development centre.

40. Organic farming and vermin-composting to be taught to tribal farmers, for profits.
41. Monthly field report of AUK to be given to Panchayat Samiti, Tehsil office, Sabhapati, MLA and other people's representatives for better coordination.
42. Volunteers to be given identity cards for better coordination with government offices.
43. Joint meetings of Sarpanch, Garmsevak, *Talathi* (*Patwari*), Anganwadi, ASHA periodically.
44. To form farmers saving group like SHG to get benefits of Panchayat Samiti schemes.

These suggestions emerging out of discussions in the joint meetings were followed up and the action taken report was sent to respective authorities as also presented in the subsequent meetings. Due to this arrangement of joint committees, there was no confrontation between the Government officials and AUK coordinators.

AUK thus could emerge as a model of government-NGO partnership. The respective Ministers of Tribal Development were also accessible and helped in regard to recommending funds for release to Finance Ministry.

During initial stage of AUK, the Principal Secretary, TDD had suggested MAAS-CRHP to accept the responsibility as mother-NGO for tribal development to organise networking of NGOs and Government. However, we suggested to take up this additional responsibility only after getting some experience of AUK, doing focused work. Otherwise there could be risk of frittering away our focus and energy in administrative work.

AUK: Convocation Ceremony and Valedictory Function Nasik: 22 November, 2012

As per government order dated 27 February, 2004, AUK was sanctioned jointly to two organisations, namely CRHP, Jamkhed and MAAS, Pune for a period of 5 years. However, due to Parliamentary elections around the same time, the first instalment of grant was delivered in August 2004, i.e. in the financial year 2004-05. The project was to end by March 2009 as per G.R., but AUK kept on getting yearly no-cost extension until March 2013, when officially the bank accounts were closed.

Major activities had to be tapered down after March 2012. During all these years, periodic reports were presented at the joint meetings between the government and AUK functionaries held at the Mantralaya level, Commissionarate-level and at each ITDP centre as statutorily agreed in the G.R.

Before the final report was drafted and submitted to the Government, it was decided to have a state-level confluence of all the AUK workers at one place to provide them opportunities to interact with each other and to make presentations publicly in front of the Ministers, Government functionaries and media.

The place was to be chosen to find residential accommodation for about 500 persons and a place for meeting which could be covered in case of unseasonal rain. The implementing office of Tribal Development Department in Maharashtra, by way of Commissionarate is located at Nasik. Nasik being a pilgrimage centre hosting *Sinhastha* or *Ardha-Kumbha Mela* occasionally, by the side of sacred Godawari river which originates at Nasik, such place was available which is normally used by the *sadhus* during these events.

The dignitaries present for the inaugural function included Sri Padmakar Valvi, Minister for Youth Welfare and Sport who was earlier Minister of State for Tribal Development, Tribal Commissioner and Additional Tribal Commissioner. Hon. Minister for Tribal Development, Sri Babanrao Pachpute and former Minister for Tribal Development who sanctioned AUK project, Sri Madhukar Pichad, then President of Nationalist Congress Party (NCP) could not be present due to some urgent government and Party meeting at Mumbai. In the afternoon session, Sri Vinayakdada Patil, former Minister of Forests, Government of Maharashtra addressed the gathering. Certificates of work were given to all tribal volunteers, peer supervisors, assistant coordinators and coordinators.

Three lady and four men volunteers from five AUK centres addressed the gathering, and expressed their gratitude for getting an opportunity to work for their people which helped develop their own capabilities.

"There was lot of malnutrition in our area with several Grade 3 and 4 children. By taking the weights of children regularly, we could improve the situation by giving supplementary nutritious *Sattu*. Meal to pregnant women helped to improve birth weight of babies. By making *Sattu* in the village through SHG, we could get livelihood at the doorstep. We could get exposure to mainstream society through our training at different places."

"After joining AUK, we were given training every month. We were giving medicine for ailments. We got seeds for kitchen garden. We were organising meetings of women, of pregnant women. We told them what to eat, what medicine to take. Girls in the schools, ashram schools had no privacy of bathing. We provided those facilities. Our new born babies had no proper clothes to cover. By giving cotton wrappings and clothes, babies got the warmth as in the uterus."

"We provided solar lamps in the school which helped students to study without electrcity bills. In the ashram school, we used waste water for kitchen garden and herbal plants. We examined Hb of adolescent girls and gave them medicine."

"Government anganwadis were in the main village. We tribals did not get their benefit. AUK started 13 Khelwadis which now have been taken over by the government as anganwadis."

"We in Akkalkuwa used to make check dams of clay. AUK gave us cement gunny bags to make the check dams. This irrigation has resulted in increased agricultural production."

The Tribal Commissioner, himself a tribal, while addressing the audience remarked that "this partnership programme between the government and voluntary organisation has been very successful. We in the government implement several schemes spending crores of rupees. But this programme has proved that without community involvement nothing can succeed. He appealed to 500 tribal workers in the *pandal* to develop partnership with the government. People should evaluate government programmes".

"Even if 552 Government ashram schools receive vegetables from you, you will stand to gain economically. There is a need of land development and skill development. Our economy is a survival economy not a development economy. It is necessary to remove our ignorance. AUK has shown the way. You 500 workers have to prepare your peers to undertake the work of AUK."

Advocate Padmakar Valvi, himself a Bhil and Minister of youth affairs and sports, earlier Minister of State, Tribal Development while addressing the gathering complimented AUK for organising this confluence of tribal workers from different parts of Maharashtra. The Minister shared the bitter fact about tribal belts continuing to remain backward despite large sums of money spent on these areas. He said, "the schemes were very good but implementation was very poor. You have shown that with little honorarium, you could achieve good results, in addressing malnutrition."

"Today we need good tribal workers, not the leaders, you have to protect your own land from alienation. You have to be alert and protect your interests. We need good teachers and good doctors. Skill development of tribal people is very important for their development."

In the afternoon, Shri Vinayakdada Patil who was a Senior Minister earlier addressed the gathering. He said, "The tribal issues should not be taken for granted. We have to understand their issues from their perspectives. Malnutrition is a general problem. Money alone would not solve it. It is necessary to have knowledge about solving the issues in terms of tradition and science. Development among all groups is not similar. The gap has to be addressed. NGOs can help in this process. You should not feel shy of your language. You should put up your views in your language."

The programme also provided opportunities to tribals to present their music and dance performances whole night before they started departing to their own places in chartered buses next day morning. It was very important, particularly for tribal women, that those who had not gone beyond 20 km of their marriage distance travelled long distances from Gadchiroli, Yavatmal, Dharni and Nandurbar hilly areas.

Among the tribal workers, 52 per cent were men and 48 per cent were women. About 40 per cent of them were in the age group of 30-40 years. 51 per cent of them were educated up to 10th standard and 14 per cent were illiterate. 97 per cent of the volunteers had a combination of agriculture and agricultural labour as their occupation. 25 per cent of them had exclusively landless labour as their occupation.

At Nasik confluence, about 600 persons from different tribal areas attended the ceremony which besides volunteers and other workers included Sarpanch, Police Patil and some tribal villagers.

Among the 287 volunteers who filled AUK forms about their background, 35 wrote some comments on the form. Mainly, they wanted such AUK programme to continue, since besides tribals getting benefits, they personally benefited by way of their personality and knowledge development, enhancing their self-confidence and self-esteem. Many of them could become ASHA, Gram Panchayat membership and leadership positions due to work experience in AUK.

Outcome: Government–NGO Partnership

Development in the social sector, of the marginalised people, is not possible without community involvement and community management. Government systems emerged in human history as regulatory authorities to ensure law and order, to regulate the production and markets, for peaceful living of the citizens. There has been a difference between village as a part of a larger unit for economic, social and defense requirements and the geographically isolated tribal communities, living in symbiotic relationship with the nature, for their day-today requirements of food and shelter. However, when these simple people become a part of a large nation-state, they get a right of equality of opportunity to enjoy the quality of life, commensurate with other citizens.

The centralised planning and implementation by those who have no familiarity with the concerns of these communities cannot look at issues from the perspective of the people. Government rules are not region or village or group specific. They lack flexibility. It is, therefore, considered desirable that people's groups or representatives should have a constant dialogue with the government system.

People who lived by collection of food from nature cannot adjust with the regulations of having been denied their basic resources by declaring them as national resources. It is, therefore, desirable to function with the people in partnership for development. AUK project has been a sincere and successful effort in functioning partnership with the government.

Annexure I
Impact of Meals to Pregnant Women

—Anjali Radkar

Setting

This data is a subset of the data that has been collected for the large scale intervention project under—Adivasi Utthan Programme (AUP). The project is run in the entire tribal area of Maharashtra covering 9 Tehsils from 7 Districts.

The study looks at malnutrition of the tribal children at large. Main thrust of the project is the intervention in the tribal areas of Maharashtra where large scale malnutrition has been documented.

Intervention

1. Weighing of all the children under three years. It also includes the birth weights of the children born in the study period. All the children under 3 years of age are weighed every month to monitor the malnutrition closely and thus to reduce the severity of malnutrition in tribal areas of the State.
2. Provide nutrition supplements for pregnant and lactating women and children below 3 years of age. Lactating mothers are provided with supplementary food in the form of fortified *Sattu*. Children less than 3 years of age also are provided with *Sattu*.
3. Provide one full meal to pregnant women registered for antenatal care.

All the pregnant women who are registered for ANC under government health facility means the women with confirmed pregnancy are provided with one full meal. This is with the understanding that the women are so poor that even the pregnant woman cannot have one full meal and that affects the maternal health and hence the child health.

Data

To get the real picture and also to find out whether the intervention works, the data is recorded in the form of the cohort.

These are 2 cohorts: Cohort for children and cohort for women.

1. Cohort of children born in the months of August 2008 to March 2009. Using this data birth cohort for every month can be prepared.
2. Cohort of pregnant women who are registered for antenatal care (ANC) in the government health facility.

Information on the weights of children born during August 2008 to March 2009 are recorded for every month to look at their malnutrition status.

Pregnant women in the project area were provided a meal under this programme. The programme started in September 2008 and continued till March 2009. As stated before, these are the women who have confirmed their pregnancy and have antenatal card with them.

Locale of the Study

Study is carried out in 9 tribal tehsils from 7 districts and in Maharashtra. They are as follows:

Table 1: Tehsils and districts under study

Sl. No.	*Districts*	*Tehsils*
1.	Ahmednagar	Akole
2.	Thane	Jawhar, Mokhada
3.	Yavatmal	Zari-Zamni
4.	Amravati	Dharni
5.	Gadchiroli	Etapalli
6.	Nandurbar	Dhadgaon, Akkalkuwa
7.	Raigad	Karjat

Importance of this Study

This study is focused on the tribal population where the data is available by tribe. In many cases the data is available at aggregate level as Scheduled Tribes, which does not reflect the variation between the tribes. Using the available data comparisons between the tribes are not possible.

Another advantage is that in the village no sampling is done. All the children or pregnant women in the village are included in the study for the intervention.

It is difficult to get the dedicated educated workers to work at village-level to record the information. For this study a local person who can measure the weights of children and women has been appointed and provided with the ledgers to record every pregnancy and every child born. There is a possibility that the workers at the village. In spite of the training and follow-up by the supervisors at the tehsil, some errors in recording and reporting the weights have been observed. Considering the uniformity in errors of reporting across the study area, the data has been analysed. It might not give the accurate values of the weights, but they do show the trends in the weights of children and pregnant women to infer about the intervention.

Major Findings of the Study

The findings would be reported for each tehsil separately. The numbers for each tehsil are small but each one has it peculiarity depending on the tribe which is found in majority in that area.

One most important finding of this study, which is common everywhere is awareness about the health of the children among tribal women. When the health worker visits the house every month for recording the weight, there is some short talk of the worker with the mother. This talk itself is important as mothers start observing their children. In case when the child is sick mother discusses it with the worker and if the worker sees some problem, he/she advise the woman to take the child to health centre. This visit in itself is a major intervention in this project. Child health has been improved because of this visit, though it is difficult to quantify its importance.

For calculating the grades of malnutrition, growth charts prepared by volunteers are used.

The report would be presented in order:

1. Dharni
2. Mokhada
3. Dhadgaon
4. Zari-zamni
5. Karjat
6. Etapalli
7. Jawhar
8. Akole
9. Akkalkuwa

Analysis of the data for each tehsil has been presented initially for children and then for women.

Entire Sample

Children Cohort—Entire sample

Total number of children born in the study area during the study period is 2548.

Table 2: Distribution of children born in study area during the study period by place of residence

Characteristics of women	*Number*	*Per cent*
Dharni	342	13.4
Mokhada	355	13.9
Dhadgaon	397	15.6
Zari-zamni	154	6.0
Karjat	132	5.2
Etapalli	212	8.3
Jawhar	353	13.9
Akole	206	8.1
Akkalkuwa	397	15.6
Total	**2548**	**100.0**

Highest number of children is born in Dhadgaon (15.6%) and Akkalkuwa (15.6%) during the study period, followed by

Mokhada and Jawhar, 13.9 per cent each whereas the least number is in Karjat.

Around 300 children are born in every month from August 2008 to February 2009. Children born in July are also weighed like August born children, so their information is included in the analysis.

Sex-ratio at birth is 1015, favourable for females. Fifteen more females are born per 1000 males. This is unlike other sections of the population. In tribals, status of women is comparatively higher.

The prominent tribe here is Bhil (27.8%), followed by Mahadev Koli and Korku (10.9% each), followed by Thakar (9.3%). Other prominent tribes include Madia, Kokna, Warli, Dhor Koli and Pawra.

Among 2548 children born 23 deaths are reported—16 males and 7 females. It is also reflected here that male is a weaker sex compared to female. Extent of deaths is 0.9 per cent. Sixteen of these children are weighed at the time of birth. The distribution of them shows that 6 were in the normal category, 4 in grade I of malnutrition, 2 in grade II, grade III and grade IV each. At the time of the birth if the children are in grade II, grade III and grade IV of malnutrition meaning they are high risk children.

Table 3: Distribution of children born during July 2008-March 2009 by their background characteristics

Characteristics of Children	*Number*	*Per cent*
Month of Birth		
July	21	0.8
August	329	12.9
September	284	11.2
October	339	13.3
November	301	11.8
December	362	14.2
January	372	14.6
February	299	11.7
March	240	9.4
No information	1	—

Characteristics of Children	Number	Per cent
Sex		
Male	1260	49.6
Female	1279	50.4
No information	9	—
Tribes		
Bhil	708	27.8
Mahadev Koli	277	10.9
Korku	277	10.9
Thakar	236	9.3
Madia	182	7.1
Kokana	177	6.9
Warli	144	5.6
Katkari	103	4.0
Dhor Koli	98	3.8
Pawra	79	3.1
Other	267	10.6
Total	**2548**	**100.0**

As far as malnutrition is concerned birth weight of the children is an important determinant. It also is an indicator of health of the mother. In the study area mean birth weight of the children is recorded as 2745.10 grams.

Most of the newborns lose up to 10 per cent weight initially and regain birth weight by 10 days and thereafter the weight gain is around 200 gms per week in the first 3 months, 150 gms per week in the next 3 months and 100 gms per week in the next 6 months (Elizabeth, 2005).

Weight of the children is steadily increasing from birth to 4 months. The increase in first month is 488.21 grams, in second 467.90 grams, in third 453.12 grams, in fourth 536.91 and then fifth month there is a dip to 399.53 grams, which again goes up. The average weight gain seems to be less among these children. It can be the effect of malnutrition of mother also. If there is no enough breast milk for the infant, how it would gain weight. We do not have the concept of weaning food as such in India. Tribal population cannot be the exception.

Table 4: Average birth weight and weight gain of children by age

Weight	*Birth*	*1 Month*	*2 Months*	*3 Months*	*4 Months*	*5 Months*	*6 Months*	*7 Months*
In grams	2745.10	3252.02	3724.00	4174.48	4712.08	5091.14	5524.26	5931.11
No. of children	2265	2060	1700	1338	944	643	340	176
Difference in average weight		488.21	467.90	453.12	536.91	399.53	422.89	415.77
No. of children		1844	1668	1329	936	642	332	168

Table 5: Weights of the children at different ages by grade of malnutrition

Time Period	*Number*	*Per cent*
Birth		
Normal	1101	48.8
Grade I	954	42.1
Grade II	163	7.2
Grade III	22	1.0
Grade IV	25	1.1
Missing	283	—
Month 1		
Normal	776	37.7
Grade I	985	47.8
Grade II	254	12.3
Grade III	30	1.5
Grade IV	15	0.7
Missing	488	—
Month 2		
Normal	662	38.9
Grade I	534	31.4
Grade II	448	26.4
Grade III	41	2.4
Grade IV	15	0.9
Missing	848	—
Month 3		
Normal	480	35.9
Grade I	497	37.1
Grade II	203	15.2
Grade III	141	10.5
Grade IV	17	1.3
Missing	1210	—
Month 4		
Normal	376	39.8
Grade I	310	32.8
Grade II	204	21.6
Grade III	42	4.4
Grade IV	12	1.3
Missing	1604	—
Month 5		
Normal	248	38.6
Grade I	213	33.1
Grade II	147	22.9
Grade III	25	3.9
Grade IV	10	1.6
Missing	1905	—
Month 6		
Normal	132	38.8
Grade I	109	32.1
Grade II	73	21.5

(Contd.)

Time Period	*Number*	*Per cent*
Grade III	20	5.9
Grade IV	6	1.8
Missing	2208	—
Month 7		
Normal	63	35.8
Grade I	68	38.8
Grade II	28	15.9
Grade III	14	8.0
Grade IV	3	1.7
Missing	2372	—
Total	**2548**	**100.0**

Source: AUK Report submitted to Government of Maharashtra.

At the time of birth 49 per cent children are in the normal category, which fluctuate between 35 per cent and 39 per cent in next 7 months. Similarly, the share of children in the different grades of malnutrition is increasing. Meaning malnutrition among the children is increasing. It can be because of two reasons. One reason is the errors are recording the weight of the children, as it is difficult to weight small children and especially when they are not well. And the other reason is the malnutrition of mothers. If mothers themselves are underweight and children are not spaced then how can they provide enough for the new born. For maternal and child health lactating mothers should be provided supplementation at least in the poor tribal areas.

Table 6: Distribution of children in grades of malnutrition at birth and at 7 months

Grade at birth	*Grade–7 Month*					*Total*
	Normal	*Grade I*	*Grade II*	*Grade III*	*Grade IV*	
Normal	16	15	5	2	–	38
Grade I	18	31	11	4	–	64
Grade II	2	3	4	8	–	17
Grade III	–	–	–	–	3	3
Total	**36**	**49**	**20**	**14**	**3**	**122**

Source: AUK Report submitted to Government of Maharashtra.

This analysis pertains to the same child, meaning what is the nutrition status of each child at the end of 7th month. This is also a time when the child is not fully on breast milk. The weaning has begun at this stage. Then how the child copes up is tried to capture here. This information is available only 122 children for who birth weight and weight in seventh month is available. It shows that among 38 children who were normal at the time of birth, 18 have slipped in grade I and II in grade II malnutrition. Those who were in grade I malnutrition, 18 are normal in 7th month, 31 are in grade I, 11 in grade II and 4 went to grade III. Similarly, among 17 who were in grade II, 5 improved, 4 remained in the same grade and 8 deteriorated in the grade. All 3 at grade III at the time of birth slipped into grade IV. There is a very little improvement in spite of the intervention. In fact available data shows that there is a need for a strong intervention for mothers because at the time of the birth only 3 children were high risk (grade III) which have become 17 in 7 months (Grades III and IV).

Table 7: Difference in malnutrition grades of children

Difference in grades	*Number of children*	*Grade gone down*	*No change in the grade*	*Grade improved*
Birth and 1 month	1844	576 (31.2)	1027 (55.7)	241 (13.1)
1 month and 2 months	1668	445 (26.7)	1041 (62.4)	182 (10.9)
2 months and 3 months	1329	277 (20.8)	901 (67.8)	151 (11.4)
3 months and 4 months	936	141 (15.1)	628 (67.2)	167 (17.7)
4 months and 5 months	642	90 (14.0)	459 (71.5)	93 (14.5)
5 months and 6 months	332	44 (13.3)	259 (78.0)	29 (8.7)
6 months and 7 months	168	16 (9.5)	136 (81.0)	16 (9.5)

Note: Values given in parentheses denotes the percentage.

Source: AUK Report submitted to Government of Maharashtra.

This is the overall analysis of all the children at each age. Difference in the malnutrition grades shows that share of children going down in malnutrition grade is decreasing. Similarly, the share of those maintaining their grade is increasing. However, improvement in the grades does not show any trend.

Women Cohort—Entire Sample

In this study 3217 women are provided one meal.

Table 8: Distribution of enroled pregnant women by place of residence

Characteristics of Women	*Number*	*Per cent*
Dharni	282	8.8
Mokhada	354	11.0
Dhadgaon	835	26.0
Zari-zamni	150	4.7
Karjat	260	8.1
Etapalli	255	7.9
Jawhar	520	16.2
Akole	187	5.8
Akkalkuwa	374	11.6
Total	**3217**	**100.0**

Source: AUK Report submitted to Government of Maharashtra.

Women are not equally distributed by place of residence. Maximum number women come from Dhadgaon (26.0%) and the least from Zari-zamni (4.7%).

Table 9: Characteristics of the enroled pregnant women

Characteristics of Women	*Number*	*Per cent*
Tribe		
Bhil	1057	32.9
Thakar	313	9.7
Mahadev Koli	237	7.4
Kokna	235	7.3
Korku	230	7.2
Madia	206	6.4
Warli	183	5.7
Katkari	182	5.6
Dhor Koli	146	4.5

(Contd.)

Characteristics of Women	*Number*	*Per cent*
Pawra	145	4.5
Other	283	8.8
Month enrolled for programme	1403	47.3
September	344	11.6
October	327	11.0
November	308	10.4
December	277	9.3
January	174	5.4
February	131	4.4
March	253	—
Total	**3217**	**100.0**

Source: AUK Report submitted to Government of Maharashtra.

Share of Bhils in this sample is about one-third, followed by Thakar (9.7%), Mahadev Koli (7.4%), Kokna (7.3%) and Korku (7.2%). Other listed tribes have their share just about 5 per cent each. Thus, Bhils dominate this sample.

This programme has started in September 2008 so over 47 per cent have enrolled in September. These are the women at various stages of pregnancy. As expected, the share of women getting enrolled for this programme gradually goes down.

Health of pregnant women and success of the pregnancy outcome apart from its other determinants depend on the biological characteristics of the women. Among the most important are age and birth order. In this study it is important to note the gestation period also considering that they are getting one full meal in the programme.

Table 10: Biological Characteristics of the Women

Biological characteristics of women	*Number*	*Per cent*
Age		
15–19	272	9.5
20–24	1497	52.3
25–29	780	27.2
30–34	227	7.9
35–39	68	2.4

(Contd.)

Biological characteristics of women	Number	Per cent
40–44	15	0.5
45–49	7	0.2
No information	351	—
Order of pregnancy		
1	959	31.8
2	881	29.3
3	579	19.2
4	281	9.3
5	143	4.7
6	67	2.2
7	46	1.5
8	35	1.2
9	11	0.4
10	6	0.2
11	1	0.0
12	2	0.1
No information	206	—
Month of pregnancy		
1	16	0.7
2	14	0.6
3	86	3.6
4	1306	54.1
5	416	17.2
6	219	9.1
7	148	6.1
8	104	4.3
9	105	4.3
No information	803	—
Total	**3217**	**100.0**

Source: AUK Report submitted to Government of Maharashtra.

Being the tribal women their childbearing starts early. Around 10 per cent women are in the ages 15–19 and in all 89 per cent of them are below 30 years. Over 80 per cent births are up to birth order 3 and just about 20 per cent births are the higher order births. Actually, these 20 per cent pregnancies are high-risk from maternal health as also malnutrition point of view.

It is seen here that over 54 per cent women have started

taking meal in 4th month of the pregnancy followed by 17 per cent in 5th and 9 per cent in 6th month. Just about 4 to 6 per cent each have registered in the programme in 7th, 8th and 9th month. About 5 per cent of the women have started taking meal before completion of 4 months of pregnancy.

Table 11: Average duration of pregnancy by month of enrollment in the programme

Month of enrollment	*Mean duration of pregnancy at enrollment*	*Number of women*
September	5.61	909
October	4.44	314
November	4.32	291
December	4.28	287
January	4.28	276
February	4.39	110
March	4.89	70
Total	**4.87**	**2257**

Source: AUK Report submitted to Government of Maharashtra.

This programme has started in September 2008 so all those who were pregnant at that time have registered for the meal irrespective of their duration of pregnancy. It is reflected in the higher mean duration in September. Once the women know about the programme almost all of them joined in immediately after they got their pregnancy confirmed in the hospital in 4th month.

Range for the number of meals taken by pregnant women in this programme is 2 to 162, with mean as 45 meals. On an average, pregnant women got the food for about one and a half month. This also would benefit the women. Mean difference in the eight gain of the women is presented in Table 12.

Weight of the pregnant mothers is recorded for every month since they are enrolled. Between September and November weight gain is just about 1 kg, which goes up in the next month t 1.12 kg and drops down again to about 1.01 kg the next month. It is difficult to attribute this weight gain to the meal programme.

Table 12: Mean difference in the weights in different months of enrolled pregnant women

Months	*Number of women*	*Mean difference in weights*
October weight – September weight	500	0.92
November weight – October weight	570	0.98
December weight – November weight	586	1.12
January weight – December weight	615	1.01

Source: AUK Report submitted to Government of Maharashtra.

Outcome

The whole idea of providing the meal to pregnant women is that they should give birth to the healthy baby to help reduce malnutrition.

Data on the birth weight of the children to the mothers enrolled in meal programme is very deficient. The data is available only for 1079 births which forms just one-third. Of course, there are few women here, who did not give the birth in the study period.

Thus, an attempt has been made here to analyse the available data on birth weight.

Among the births to the women who were taking a meal in the programme, data on the birth weight is available for 1057. Among these 1057 women—

284 women gave birth to children ≤ 2.500 kg It is 26.9%
773 women gave birth to children > 2.500 kg It is 73.1%

That means LBW children are just 26.9 per cent which are about 30 per cent in the population. Means giving one full meal to pregnant women helps. Only in 14 cases birth weight is less than 2 kg.

Mean weight of the children to mothers who have received meals is 2.76 kg. That means average baby to women who received the meals is normal weight baby.

Reference

Elizabeth K.E., 2005, *Nutrition and Child Development*, III Edition, Paras Medical Publisher, Hyderabad, India, p. 31.

Annexure II

Initiation of Major Activities

Sl. No.	Activities	Starting Month
1.	Coordinators' Workshop	September-2004
2.	Volunteers' Training	January-2005
3.	Distribution of Weighing Scales	June-2005
4.	Distribution of Medicine Kit to volunteers	June-2005
5.	Seeds for Kitchen Garden	June-July-2005
6.	Cloth wrappings to new born	August-2005
7.	*Dai* Training	September-2005
8.	Health Camp	September-2005
9.	Base Line Survey	December-2005
10.	Ready-to-eat Nutrition Supplement	July-2006
11.	Ayurvedic Kit	August-2006
12.	Tailoring Training	2006
13.	Panchayat Raj Training	September-2006
14.	Health Education and Check Up	January-2007
15.	*Dai*-hut	January-2007
16.	Khelwadi (Mini Anganwadi)	January-2007
17.	Ideal Ashram School	January-2007
18.	Library in Village	January-2007
19.	Puppetry Training	April-2007
20.	Appropriate Technology Training	May-2007
21.	Indoor Residential Food for Acute Malnourished	September-2007
22.	*Vaidu* Training	October-2007
23.	Nurseries	2007-2008
24.	Bamboo Handicraft Training	2007-2008
25.	Check Dam	2007-2008
26.	Food to pregnant women	August-2008
27.	Ideal Anganwadi	July-2011
28.	Volunteers Certificate Award Ceremony, Nasik	22 November, 2012
29.	Submission of Dharani Report	7 December, 2012
30.	Submission of Final Report	October 2013

Beneficiaries of Major AUK Programmes

1. Activity: Orientation and Training

Sl. No.	Activity	No. of Beneficiary
1.	*Dai* Training: Birthing and Neonatal Care	500 *Dai*
2.	*Vaidu* (Herbalist): Processing of herbs to make drugs	349 *Vaidu*
3.	Panchayat Raj about powers and responsibilities	344 GP members
4.	ARTI institution about appropriate technology	145 persons
5.	PUPPET institution about puppetry	150 persons

(Contd.)

Sl. No.	Activity	No. of Beneficiary
6.	Tailoring	295 women
7.	Bamboo artifacts	184 persons
8.	AUK Tribal volunteers about AUK activities	500 volunteers
9.	AUK Peer supervisors (*Margadarshak*)	80 persons
	Total trained	**2547 Tribal persons**

2. *Activity: Health Care*

Sl. No.	Activity	No. of Beneficiary
1.	Utilization of medicinal kit with volunteers	70,380 persons per year
2.	Benefit of Health Camps	7,928 persons
3.	Weighing of children by volunteers	11,500 children per month
4.	Cotton wrappings to new born babies	10,334 infants
5.	Deliveries conducted at *Dai*-hut (10)	80
6.	Health check-up of adolescent school girls	1740 girls

3. *Activity: Food and Nutrition Supplements*

Sl. No.	Activity	Average per Month
1.	Ready-to-eat *Sattu* to children – 6 months – 3 years age (July-2006 – August-2008)	11500
2.	*Sattu* – 6 months – 15 months children: (September-2008 – Nov. 2009)	2026
3.	Lactating women: *Sattu* 3 Kg per month: (June-2007 to August-2008)	2400
4.	Lactating women: Fortified *Sattu* with Ayurvedic drugs *Shatavari, Ashwagandha, Pimpli, Jyesthamadh* – 25 gm each to 1 Kg *Sattu*	2400
5.	Pregnant women: *Sattu* 3 Kg per month: (June-2007 to August-2008)	2000
6.	Pregnant women: One full meal per day (September-2008 to March-2009)	2031
7.	Kitchen Garden Seeds of vegetables (2005–2010)	34202

4. Activity: Education Programmes

Sl. No.	Activity	No. of Beneficiary
1.	Khelwadi (Mini Anganwadi)	382 children
2.	Development of Ideal Anganwadi	12
3.	Health Education: Adolescent girls	3346
4.	Reading and discussing booklets on pregnancy and child care with pregnant women (during meal programme)	3000 pregnant women
5.	Health related books to Ashram Schools	37 Ashram Schools
6.	Computer training in Ashram Schools	240 Teachers
7.	Ideal Ashram School	Biju Dhavdi, Tal. Dharni, District Amraoti.
8.	Special Coaching about English and Mathematics	290 Students
9.	Library and Information Centres (92)	3943 Registered Members

Activity: Other Development Programmes

Sl. No.	Activity	No. of Beneficiary
1.	Repair and Construction of Bathrooms-Toilets for girls	7 Ashram Schools
2.	Repairing of Ghotul and Kolam *Chavdi*	7 Villages
3.	Vanrai Check dams (Dhadgaon & Akkalkuwa)	65 places
4.	Herbal medicine nursery	14 Ashram Schools
5.	Fish Nursaries	15 SHG and 239 Families
6.	Soak Pits	200 places

Nutrition Supplement

	Beneficiaries during May 2008			Beneficiaries during December 2008		Clothes & Covering for new born
	Pregnant women	Lactating women	Children (6 months to 3 Years)	Full square meal for pregnant women	Fortified Nutrition supplement for lactating women	June 2005 to December 2008
Akole	316	294	2078	186	187	786
Akkalkuwa	254	193	1330	247	325	1151
Dhadgoan	316	294	2400	395	503	2162
Dharani	212	152	1093	189	270	1123
Etapalli	127	95	708	97	163	734
Jawhar	215	204	1250	298	277	1012
Karjat	144	117	729	170	153	344
Mokhada	273	248	1301	317	387	1173
Zarijamani	111	118	702	132	148	585
Total	**1968**	**1715**	**11591**	**2031**	**2413**	**8970**

Annexure III

Report of the Tour of Dhadgaon and Akkalkuwa

Dates: 20-22 July, 2003
Members: Dr. R.S. Arole, Prof. R.K. Mutatkar and Sri P.S. Agashe
Meeting with Janardan Walvi, Rampur, Tal. Shahada on 20th evening and 21st morning. His analysis and suggestions about tribal education:

1. Idea of Ashram School with 11 acres of land was to be an instrument of area development.
2. Ashram Schools up to 5th standard in difficult areas, beyond 5th a central school with emphasis on agriculture, and farm based industry.
3. No book in local language such as Bhilori but teachers undergoing D.Ed. be trained in the dialect for better communication with the primary level students.

4. Co-education up to 5th standard, beyond 5th standard separate Ashram Schools for girls.
5. Ashram schools have made students dependent on the system. On earlier occasions, every Sunday, students had to cook and manage the Ashram school without the employees.
6. Educated students of higher class do not participate in traditional production activities, but prefer to spend time on recreation provided by mass media, listening film music and cricket commentaries.
7. More vocational courses are needed even up to 10th standard.

Twenty first morning we visited Kakarda Ashram School and Mandavi Ashram School for girls on way to Dhadgaon. At both places, the prayers were on. Prayer session was used for giving national news and some general knowledge such as capitals of States. Kakarda School had a hall which could be used for training purposes. The Head Mistress of girls ashram school reported that several girls were sick everyday. She also reported that the girls were given information about menstrual issues and welcomed further training in such matters. This was the only *ashram* for girls in the taluka. More hostels than ashram schools were recommended for adolescent girls. About 30 girls appear for SSC each year with 70 per cent passout rate. Some of them also go for higher education at Shahada and Dhadgaon.

After brief interaction with teachers at institution of Janardan Maharaj, Rural Hospital was visited. There was a tribal doctor couple, with MBBS degree, and BMO with BAMS degree and 7 years of working at Dhadgaon, and his BAMS wife. In this 30-beded hospital, there were adult cases of diarrhoea. There was a lady patient with eclampsia with IV. Dr. Arole recommended food intake through mouth. RH had a jeep and new ambulance. There was adequate budget for taking patients to Dhule, nor could patients afford to pay for diesel for the jeep. Also there were no facilities for emergency surgery except tubectomy. There was no anaesthetist in the district and no blood bank in public sector. There was an anesthetist at Shahada and a private blood bank at Nandurbar. The BMO gave following information about grassroots level health manpower infrastructure in the taluka. There were 120 anganwadi workers with equal number of helpers, 120 mini-anganwadi workers, and 225 trained *dais* who were paid Rs. 40 on the day of training once in three months. 544 *Pada* workers appointed for 6 months, functioning mainly as *Sandeshvahak*, (communicating information to referrals) most of them males. Payments to *Pada* workers were very irregular. Due to poor institutional delivery at PHC level, *dais* could not be shown live demonstration of delivery. They were only trained with the help of models. He said *Pada* workers were found very useful, particularly, during monsoon since it was not possible for the health workers to reach the places due to difficult terrain and altitudes of *padas*.

The BMO thought that replacement of male *Pada* workers by females may create an agitational problem.

We met the BDO who made the following points:

1. There were only 25 Gram Panchayats for 163 revenue villages and 260 official *padas* in Dhadgaon Tehsil. Scattered settlements with few huts were more than 1000.
2. *Pada* should be taken as unit for EGS, like approach road and sanitation, digging well.
3. He recommended EGS on one's own field like land levelling and bunding, to prevent migration.
4. Recommended Narmada belt on priority basis for health activities under proposed *pada* scheme.
5. The postings in these areas should not be considered as punishment posts since it ultimately became punishment to people by having incompetent staff.
6. Looking at the difficult terrain, staff beyond the age of 50 should not be appointed since they would not have physical energy to cope up with the terrain.
7. Staff should be rewarded with one increment for three years service in this area and they should be allowed to go to the plains after one year of service even if no reliever reports in time.

8. *Pada* worker should work through Panchayat system with linkage to ICDS.
9. Change from male to female *Pada* worker should have clearcut administrative instructions. She should not be burdened with too many and too much records like 14 registers with ICDS workers. Illiteracy is not a problem if the records are kept by somebody, not necessarily by the worker.
10. A *dai* or a herbalist (*Bhagat*) could be considered for *Pada* worker.
11. Training clusters will have to be identified in various places in the Taluka/Block.

After visiting PHC at Kathi where the ANM was present, who could give all the information with confidence, we moved to see Molgi PHC. There was a tribal doctor, MBBS, who thought that BAMS was not useful for emergency, otherwise there was no difference between MBBS and BAMS. He agreed that *Pada* worker be a women to concentrate on IMR and MMR.

On 22nd July there were discussions with PO of ITDP, Mr. Bhalerao, with the Collector, and with the CEO of Zilla Parishad. Collector accepted the suggestion about incorporating the blood bank in the special action plan for Dhadgaon and Akkalkuwa.

The RH at Taloda and civil hospital at Nandurbar were also visited. RH Taloda had good functioning infrastructure, and competent ANM, who took us around the hospital. The lady gynaecologist had gone to civil hospital, Nandurbar, as per her schedule of 2 days a week. Water shortage was serious problem which was brought to the notice of the Collector, and he said that decision to solve the problem was taken. RH was clean despite water shortage.

At the civil hospital, the wards were fully occupied. The paediatrician was officiating as the civil surgeon. He reported that surgery was a problem due to non-availability of blood and an anaesthetist. However, there was a private blood bank in the town and anaesthetist from Shahada offered his voluntary services as charity. A new 100 beded hospital was under construction, at Nandurbar.

Sickle Cell as a tribal health problem was discussed, for which some counselling centres at few places were proposed. There were cases of adult diarrhoea in the wards. It was reported that the male adults consumed water in the fields in rainy season and got infection. The children in the house did not get diarrhoea in this season. The scheme whereby school children were trained to put chlorine drops in the household supply had been showing good results. It was discussed that the post-graduate residents be posted to RH and civil hospital to provide their speciality at these places.

There was overwhelming movement of private jeeps which were overflowing with passengers, about 30-40, including on the roof, were strikingly visible on the roads in Akrani and Akkalkuwa. The transport is available, but is it usable for the patients?

How are the health facilities accessible to tribal people in difficult terrain?

Annexure IV

Epidemiological case study about Tribal Malnutrition, an intervention research project

Statement of the Problem

1. Media reports about mal-nutrition deaths in Tribal areas of Maharashtra.
2. PILs on this issue in various courts.
3. *Suo Motu* Action by Bombay High Court against Government of Maharashtra.
4. Government offered the project to two NGOs jointly—MAAS and CRHP.

Project Design

1. Conceptual issue of treating mal-nutrition in isolation or as one programme of health, health itself being an aspect of culture which is an integrated whole.
2. Comprehensive and Sustainable Human Development

of the Tribal People of Maharashtra—Briefly called as Adivasi ttthan Karyakram.

3. Health as an entry point of development. (*Alama Ata*—Primary health care approach—inter-sect oral development—non-health sector making an impact on health sector.

Strategy of Implementation

1. Confidence Building Activities, medicine box in every hamlet.
2. Capacity Building activities.
3. Activities having a direct bearing on mal nutrition, such as supplementary ready-to-eat nutritious food for babies, lactating women and pregnant women.
4. Indirect activities addressing issues of mal-nutrition, such as kitchen garden, irrigation bunds, fish nurseries'.
5. Training in appropriate technology such as bio-gas, smokeless *chulha*, bamboo work, drug processing, soak-pits, *dai*-huts.
6. Model Anganwadi and Ashram School.

Human Resources

1. About 250 male and 250 female community volunteers selected by the community to cover about 250 villages and hamlets with a tribal population of about 1,50,000.

Expected Outcomes

1. Reduction of mal-nutrition as per Anganwadi gradation.
2. Capacity building of community volunteers.
3. Government NGO Partnership.

Documentation

1. Weights of new born baby.
2. Monthly weights of children up to two years of age.
3. Weight gain of pregnant women.
4. Monthly report of activities by Co-ordinators.

Analysis

1. Cohort analysis of new born baby's up to two years of age.
2. Babies born to pregnant women under feeding programme.
3. Qualitative analysis of monthly reports.

Chapter 6

Epilogue

"What has been the impact of government policies on tribal livelihoods? Where should Central and State Governments focus to improve the situation? To answer these questions we quote in detail from a Planning Commission (2000) document":

> "As tribal people in India perilously, sometimes hopelessly, grapple with these tragic consequences, the small clutch of bureaucratic programmes have done little to assist the precipitous pauperization, exploitation and disintegration of tribal communities. Tribal people respond occasionally with anger and assertion, but often also in anomie and despair, because the following persistent problems have by and large remained unattended to: land alienation, indebtedness, relation with forests, and government monopoly over MFPs, and non-implementation of the Forest Rights Act, 2006; ineffective implementation of Panchayats (Extension to the Scheduled Areas) Act of 1996 (PESA, 1996) for Schedule V Areas; involuntary displacement due to development projects and lack of proper rehabilitation; shifting cultivation, such as *podu*; poor utilization of government funds; and poor delivery of government programmes" (N.C. Saxena, former Secretary, Planning Commission, GoI, in *'Seminar'* – *'The Malnourished Tribal'* Journal No. 661, September 2014, 16-17) (*Children of a Lesser God* by N.C. Saxena).

The Constitution of India has advocated the Principle of Equity, Equality of opportunity in emphasising that all citizens of India should be a part of "We, the People of India". Towards that purpose every adult is given a single vote belonging to all castes, religious groups, gender etc. to choose or reject their elected representatives.

In order to quicken the process of effective functioning as one Nation-State, the concept of "Backward" has also been introduced in the Constitution so that some groups of people who for historical or geographical hardships may lay behind in getting the benefits of equal opportunity, may jump the time by following affirmative policy and action, for some duration of time. For the purpose of the Constitution, some groups would be deemed to be Scheduled Castes and Scheduled Tribes *vide* Articles 341 and 342 respectively. Further provisions have been made in the Constitution for representation in the governance by introducing such concepts as Scheduled Area for Scheduled Tribes. The Governors have been bestowed with special Constitutional powers to directly intervene in favour of safeguarding and promoting the interests of tribal communities lest the State Governments dominated by non-tribal representatives in the legislatures and as Executive, forget or ignore the spirit of the Constitution in elevating the marginalised communities to be equal partners as citizens of one Nation-State. Respecting the traditions of self-governance and tribal people protecting the forest resources and other natural resources for centuries, PESA and Forest Rights Act have been enacted. Distinct Tribal Development Departments, Tribal Sub-Plan, Tribal Research and Training Institutes have been created. Some tribal states, districts and blocks/talukas have been formed to promote self-governance and development paradigms, in tune with their culture. Now, even some tribal universities have been established which are expected to focus on research, training and interventions about tribal regions and communities. However, what is lacking is a National Tribal Policy which continues to be in a draft stage, awaiting the formal approval of the Parliament and the President.

All these positive steps initiated in the process of freedom struggle, by such leaders as Mahatma Gandhi, Jawaharlal Nehru, Dr. B.R. Ambedkar and many others culminated in the Constituent Assembly to provide statutory status to the marginalised groups. The infrastructure of administration and finance to implement these provisions have been created. Despite all these, malnutrition and child mortality, level of illiteracy and poverty are distinctly visible and measurable in comparison to other social, ethnic groups who form the bulk of Indian peasantry.

What was the position of tribal communities before Independence, on 15 August, 1947?

Traditionally, tribal communities are identified or branded as examples of ancient human communities who provide insights in the evolution of organisation of Man-Man, Man-Environment and Man-Supernatural relationships. It is from the studies of "queer customs" of such communities by voyagers, turned anthropologists, that the theories of culture and concept of psychic unity of mankind developed. The conquests of their territories for natural resources impoverished their lives into subjugation and exploitation. In countries like India, references to tribal people are found in the mythologies of *Ramayana* and *Mahabharata*. The tribal people are believed to have retracted to inaccessible hills and deep forests for their safety and security, and remained into relative time freeze, due to geographical isolation and encapsulation.

The development of roads and transport to commercially exploit the natural forest resources and the establishment of regulatory forest department with police uniforms, gradually led to denial or restriction to tribal communities, their traditional access to forest, their home, for collection of food and slash and burn agricultural practices.

The British Regime was not for the development of the people or the country. The visible development by way of transport and communication, selective education, was a tool and technique for rule of the majority by small number of the British. Otherwise a small nation with limited population could not have ruled several nations in different continents. There was a principle of indirect rule, governing through kings, chieftains, *jagirdars* and *zamindars*. Tribal areas were governed by chieftains.

After Independence, the lofty ideal of rural reconstruction extended to tribal areas by way of community development blocks. As a natural process, tribal people could not use the opportunities since they were not educationally equipped to do so, thus remaining backward and shy. In the process, with a view to exploit natural and forest resources, as national wealth, land alienation and restrictions on the collection of forest food continued resulting into malnutrition.

Across the country, even among the higher castes in urban centres, infant and neo-natal mortality could not be controlled, Up to 1931 Census, the population in India appeared to be stabilised in terms of fertility and mortality balancing each other. The hang over of the experiences of infant and child mortality in rural and urban areas, as destiny, has been the stumbling block against population control.

Despite best efforts in trying to develop the tribal areas through area development approach, and tribal people through education and reservation in employment, the tribal talukas, districts and states are ranked low according to human development index and remain so through decades.

Issues as to what is special about tribal problems of poverty and malnourishment that require special attention and different strategy have been debated. The solution offered has been administrative, in terms of having more public facilities in health care by way of reduced population ratio, as compared to mainstream society, or earmarking special budgets for development. Although, it is theoretically recognised that nothing in tribal development could give good results without the involvement of people, which led to PESA and FRA, and which established single window Tribal Development Department for inter-sectoral coordination, on the ground, the policies do not get translated into effective action. These are also areas of operational and epidemiological research in tribal public administration and in tribal public health.

Moreover, ST is not a uniform category of living. It is an administrative category to facilitate administration and measure the outcome to compare with other such categories like SC, OBC and others. People live in their ethnic groups such as Warli,

Thakar, Katkari, Mahadeo Koli, Gonds, Kolam etc. and they are not equal on the socio-economic scale. No doubt, this reality is recognised by way of branding some of them as PVTG.

The tribal people have been living together and governing themselves at the village and hamlet level for centuries. We have created administrative category of group Gram Panchayat as per our numerical, administrative and budgetary formula, which becomes a non-functional development entity in the tribal belt with scattered habitat in difficult terrain. The revenue pattern of one *patwari/talathi* for a number of villages also gets applied to development sector whereby one Gram Sevak (Secretary of Gram Panchayat) may look after more than one such group Gram Panchayat. As a result, the concept of Gram Sabha and their expected frequent meetings are more in the registers of records, than on the ground. The visual anecdotes about a Gram Panchayat meeting not lasting for more than few minutes after signing the attendance meeting, by the Secretary of Gram Panchayat, are no fiction, but facts.

In the AUK and BAIF projects, funded by the government, those with B.Sc. (Ag.) degree were preferred and appointed as project assistants in the field, with an idea to promote agricultural activities. Male village volunteers were also chosen in equal proportion to female volunteers in AUK, with the same purpose in view. Coincidentally, the government decided to fill the vacant posts of *Gram Sevaks*, on contractual basis, and selected those with Bachelor's degree in agriculture. Although, the contractual emoluments were exactly half of what we had offered them, all B.Sc. (Ag.) left the jobs in both AUK and BAIF, to join the contractual positions in the government. *Gram Sevak* as Secretary of Gram Panchayat has financial authority, jointly with the Sarpanch.

One of the basic questions in planned change is, can the social change be brought about successfully by the paid employees of the government or even of the NGOs? What is the function and commitment of the employees, to whom? The pattern of administration boils down to regulatory issues of rules to be followed uniformly across the State or Country. People do not lead their lives according to government rules. They live as per patterns and norms of their cultural and social groups. They have to live in their kin groups, in the neighbourhood groups and in their respective peer groups at the places of their interaction with others, whether in the families, at the school, on the field or at some other work place.

The knowledge and goods generated by science and technology whether in production or in the kitchen with food, diet and nutrition, or with disease control and cure, at individual or at the level of public, need to be accessible to all tribal people. How to do it?

Should the strategies adopted at the macro-level regions of states and nation, for development, be the same in tribal belt? Even Symington in 1938 while studying the issues of poverty, indebtedness and exploitation in West Khandesh (Nandurbar since 1998) in Dhule district, opined that for the tribal people, different strategies were needed. He wanted the tribals to be treated like a child holding his hand, to support him while walking.

The Constitutional and universally acceptable human rights accept right to life and right of health as fundamental rights which are open to judicial review. The food security issues about poor people in general and tribals in particular have been discussed in the High Courts and Supreme Court several times. The vote bank pressures prevail upon the governments to take temporary measures for controlling malnutrition not leading to mortality. The Tribal Development department thus get reduced to survival schemes rather than sustainable development schemes. Failure of one scheme leads to floating a parallel scheme with changed nomenclature.

This book on Tribal Health and Malnutrition has presented the flexible, people-centric approach and activities perused jointly by two voluntary organisations. One of them CRHP, essentially known as a health NGO who pioneered and developed Jamkhed model by involving the illiterate, marginalised village women in community health by developing their capabilities, has evolved from the curative to promotive-preventive strategies into comprehensive development of the people. Another voluntary institution, the Maharashtra

Association of Anthropological Sciences, with an academic base of university level in teaching and research in Anthropology, which is the only academic discipline dealing with the study of Mankind in totality, through pre-historical and historical times to the contemporary issues, after decolonisation in the world. So, the two organisations with different origins have merged with a common objective of comprehensive and sustainable human development. Although, Anthropology is not a study of tribal people alone, since no other academic discipline ventures to interact with the tribal people in their natural habitat, tribal studies continue to be the exclusive preserve of Anthropology. The pioneering studies of isolated communities have led to development of basic theories of culture, integration, cultural relativism, and culture and personality etc. validated subsequently by the primary health care approach advocating inter-sectoral coordination and slogans such as, "think globally, act locally."

Cause of Public Concern

There is widespread media coverage about deaths of tribal children supposedly due to mal-nutrition/under-nutrition during monsoon as has been reported every year for the last twenty years. It is also reported that the Hon'able Ministers of Health visit the hospitals or primary health centres and enquire about the lapses on the part of the staff on duty. It is quite interesting that the Minister for Tribal Development is not primarily accountable for malnutrition deaths. The department only doles out the money to health department.

"There is a clear case for coordinated action between concerned Ministries, given that chronic undernutrition in *adivasi* children is influenced by multiple factors: poverty, household food insecurity, maternal undernutrition before and during pregnancy, frequent infections or disease, poor care and feeding practices especially in the first two years of life, inadequate health services and unsafe water and sanitation. At least six Ministries directly play a role in Tribal Affairs, Health and Family Welfare, Women and Child Development, Consumer

Affairs, Food and Public Distribution, Rural Development and Drinking Water and Sanitation. Have these Ministries and their respective State departments made a special effort to reach out to *adivasis*?" (*Journal 'Seminar' – 'The Malnourished Tribal'* Journal No. 661, September 2014, p. 43; *'Mind the Gap'* by Biraj Swain and Vani Sethi).

There have also been PILs about tribal child malnutrition leading to mortality. The interesting techno-managerial responses in the judicial courts to these deaths amount to defending with an argument that the deaths were due to diarrhoea and pneumonia, and not due to malnutrition. Actually in the year 2004, MAAS and CRHP-Jamkhed were jointly offered a project by the Ministry of Tribal Development, Government of Maharashtra as a result of *suo motu* injunction by the Bombay High Court. The sanctioned Adivasi Utthan Karyakram for five years got extended to eight years ending 31st March, 2013, as a result of perfunctory (irregular) release of funds.

The concerns have been : (1) Although, the deaths of tribal children in Grade III and IV admitted to an institution like PHC or rural hospital could be prevented by emergency crisis management, can it address the issue of under-nutrition? (2) After the discharge of children from the institution, what is the safeguard that these children would not relapse into Grade III and IV, which would necessitate re-entry in the institution?

AUK tried to develop a sustainable model which could be replicable in the government system of tribal development by addressing the issue of under-nutrition in a comprehensive manner.

Outcome and Recommendations

What has been attained over a period of eight years which is measurable in quantitative and qualitative terms and is sustainable and replicable? What has been the process of transformation? Who have been the actors or catalysts of change? How does AUK represent the State, as a sampling frame, in terms of geographical coverage and tribal groups?

The Government of Maharashtra reposed complete confidence in the joint functioning of two NGOs in innovating several programmes to effectively address the issues of malnutrition, by interventions in all aspects of life, maintaining the balance of priorities of different components of life. The programme has been administered by following two basic strategies of confidence building of the people in the programme and about the organisations, followed by capacity building of the people to initiate and monitor the implementation of various components of the programme. This process has developed their capabilities, their self-confidence and self-esteem. The intervention goods like supplementary ready-to-eat food or new born baby clothes or weighing machines were supplied first time. Later the same were managed by SHGs and trained tribal volunteers. The issues of livelihood, food security or migration for living, are linked with policies about land ownership, forest use and vocational education etc. which requires inter-sectoral programmes, to be monitored with supervisory authority by the TDD.

Outcome

1. Spot feeding of pregnant women with one time full meal immediately after the pregnancy is registered with the ANM has shown increase in birth weight of new born babies. Spot feeding was done in the house of a tribal volunteer of AUK to all pregnant women of the village/ hamlet. Purchasing of raw-material was done by the volunteer from local or weekly market, without vouchers. Volunteers and his/her young children were permitted free meal by way of labour charges. Pregnant woman was allowed to have her young child for a free meal with her. AUK employees were not permitted to make purchases for this programme.
2. *Supplementary food*: pre-cooked ready-to-eat powder (*sattu*) of baked wheat and *chana dal* (Bengal gram) was given initially to children of 6 months to 3 years age and later reduced to 2 years due to financial crunch.
3. To address the issue of under-nourished lactating women, this supplementary food was fortified with

Ayurvedic tonics like *Shatavari, Pimpli, Jyeshthamadh* and *Ashwagandha* to improve lactation. The production of supplementary food was done by women's self-help groups. This resulted in drastic reduction of Grades III and IV children and increase in normal grade as per Anganwadi parameters.

4. To provide vitamins and micro-nutrients, seeds of plant vegetables for the kitchen garden were supplied free to the families with under-nourished children and pregnant women. Later, the tribal volunteers were provided free seeds.
5. Cotton new born baby clothes including a cap were supplied free to new born babies to protect from respiratory infections. This was linked with recording of birth weight of the baby and registration of birth.
6. In the house of every volunteer, a box of medical kit for common ailments was provided for free distribution to the patients; later on Ayurvedic drugs were also added to this medicinal kit.
7. Seeds of fish were provided in selected areas for fish nursery and production, for free consumption.
8. Plant nurseries were promoted, specifically in ashram schools.
9. A separate *Dai*-hut was constructed in a village of the *Dai* who was in great demand, for institutional delivery in a sanitary condition.
10. In view of the tribal volunteers weighing the children in their respective homes every month, people understood the relationship of weight and mal-nutrition. This developed the mindset to take action in case of loss of weight.
11. Volunteers developed capacity to weigh and plot the gradation chart of weights as per Anganwadi pattern.
12. The training of Volunteers, Gram Panchayat members, herbalists (*Vaidu*), *Dai* etc. about making bamboo artifacts, making and playing puppets, production of smokeless hearth, tailoring etc. developed their self-confidence and self-esteem. Many volunteers improved

their social status by way of becoming Anganwadi worker, ASHA, Gram Panchayat member, Sarpanch etc.

13. In some talukas like Karjat in Raigad, Zari-Zamani in Yeotmal, Jawhar in Thane and Etapalli in Gadchiroli, the Anganwadis located in the main village could not cater to the needs of tribal children from hamlets. There was also a social distance between the caste peasants in the main village and the tribals in the hamlets. AUK started the Anganwadis in the hamlets with the title "Khelwadi" as recommended by the then Tribal Commissioner. Several of these Khelwadis have been taken over by the government as Mini-Anganwadi.
14. The model of partnership through joint monitoring committees of the government and AUK as a voluntary agency, to undertake constructive programmes have given positive results.

In short, the main outcome of AUK activities, besides reducing mal-nutrition of tribal children has been the human resource development of tribal volunteers to develop their capacities to undertake tribal development work in their respective villages. This also helped better utilization of government schemes. This trained manpower can undertake benchmark surveys in the tribal area and administer community management.

Recommendations

1. The activities carried out by AUK are replicable in terms of logistics and financial viability. The ITDP, therefore, can undertake these activities as a government programme. In fact, some of the programmes have already been implemented in some ITDP project areas.
2. The government under the initiative of AUK had formed a coordination committee at the taluka-level of ITDP PO, PHC Medical Officer and AUK Coordinator to meet every month to monitor the mal-nutrition issues. In the absence of AUK, committee can be re-organized to include Tehsildar, BDO and Anganwadi Supervisor. ITDP PO would be the convener of the committee.

Health

1. Anganwadi as an institution has a very important role to play in areas of health and education. It has to develop as a nodal agency for health of women and children, and for non-formal education. There has to be a closer link between ICDS and ITDP with control by the community.
2. Orientation programme about health and development issues for Mahila Mandals, women members of Gram Panchayat and SHGs should be organized by the ITDP every quarter in every village.
3. Health camps focusing on woman and child health be organized every quarter at the PHC, Anganwadi, Ashram Schools or Garm Panchayat Bhavan.
4. Medical examination of children from Ashram School and other schools be undertaken every quarter with participation of the school teachers.

Education

1. Ashram Schools need to be developed as information centre about government schemes.
2. The curriculum of Ashram School need to be development oriented as was originally recommended by the Vandrekar Committee about starting of Ashram Schools. The Board of Secondary Education need to re-organize their curriculum and certification to incorporate the special needs of tribal development.
3. The vocational education need to start from the V Std. since many tribal students drop out before reaching the X Std., required for ITI entrance.
4. The girls' ashram schools need to cater to training in nutrition, women's health, child rearing and nursing.
5. NDA Khadakwasla, Pune, has a special curriculum for trainee officers to meet with defence requirements. However, they are awarded the graduation degree by JNU, Delhi for this curriculum. Similar arrangement can be made for secondary education in tribal schools.

6. Computer training on a large scale has to be undertaken for the teachers and students. Alternative energy requirement is necessary for functioning of computers, due to meager electricity supply by state electricity board.
7. Among the PVTG, Katkari are the most migrant, and treated with contempt by other tribal groups. It is necessary to have separate ashram schools for their children at least up to IV Std. to get them oriented to education and muster enough confidence to interact with children and teachers of other tribal groups, later in other ashram schools.

Government Sector Recommendations

1. Since the Tribal Development Department has no authority to monitor the activities of line departments, which receive TSP funds, it is necessary to at least have senior officers of respective line departments with the Tribal Development Commissioner on deputation to monitor the expenditure and outcomes.
2. ITDP PO need to have the status and powers equivalent to District Collector and CEO of ZP for better coordination.
3. Group Gram Panchayat in tribal area turns the PRI into a passive entity. The principle of one village—one Gram Panchayat—one Gram Sevak, and Gram Sabha for each hamlet, need to be followed to pursue the spirit of PESA.
4. Gram Panchayat Members need to receive development orientation every two years. All legislation about tribal issues including the issues of pseudo tribalism need to be introduced in its orientation.
5. There need to be separate orientation to women members of Gram Panchayat focusing on health.
6. The staff of Tribal Development Department including the ITDP staff need to be frequently oriented about development issues, preferably at the Tribal Research and Training Institute (TRTI). The curriculum can be designed by experts with experience.
7. Every hamlet need to have a Mini Anganwadi, or Anganwadi. Anganwadi workers need refresher training in nutrition and home health care, including AYUSH.

8. The tribal manpower of about 550 persons who have been trained under AUK can be utilized for undertaking benchmark survey of entire tribal population of Maharashtra, under the guidance of MAAS with technical support from TRTI, if necessary.
9. *Research:*

   High level committee under the chairmanship of Prof. Xaxa (pronounced as *khakha*) has recommended, from the public health point of view, certain aspects of tribal health research. These are:

   (a) Epidemiology, disease patterns and mortality rates in Scheduled Areas.

   (b) Traditional belief systems and practices, and effective communication methods.

   (c) Tribal healing systems.

   (d) Methods of health care delivery in Scheduled Areas.

   The AYUSH (Ayurveda, Yoga, Unani, Siddha, and Homoeopathy) Department and the Indian Council of Medical Research should incorporate these into their scope of working (p. 249).

   (*Ref.: Report of the High Level Committee on Socio-Economic, Health and Educational Status of Tribal Communities of India,* Ministry of Tribal Affairs, Government of India, May 2014.)

Some of the programmes developed by AUK have been adopted by the government as their regular programmes, thus extending the benefits to all tribal people, and making it sustainable at the government level. To make it sustainable at the people's level, will require further in-puts in skill development and capacity building of the people to become a part of the cultural life style.

When development has to be achieved in a given direction, no doubt, respecting the spirit of the Constitution, time bound planning process becomes a centralised agenda. There is a feeling that experienced bureaucracy can hasten the implementation of programmes. However, the experience is that the bureaucracy is used to mindset of revenue overriding development issues. Although, democratic decentralisation on paper is up to the Gram

Panchayat level, it cannot function effectively at least in tribal areas. In Maharashtra, a high level committee to look into the regional imbalances, treating all tribal areas as one separate region, under the chairmanship of a senior, retired bureaucrat, Shri Vijay Kelkar, has submitted its report. The government has yet to take a decision on the report.

Democratic set up of governance has to give primacy to the people's sector. We find, the primacy is given to the government sector. Government system functioning through line depart-ments with independent cadres of each department functioning up to taluka, Gram Panchayat or even village-level is unmindful of the people's sector. They create their own structures like district, taluka, block, group Gram Panchayat etc. Single window departments like the TDD without their own cadres have to function through the unwilling cadres of line departments.

Kelkar Committee has pointed out these administrative anomalies.

Administrative Fragmentation of Tribal Areas

"Following the Presidential Order of 1985, the Scheduled Areas and TSP areas were supposedly made coterminus in Maharashtra. However, considerable anomalies still exist. About 49 per cent of the tribal population lives within the Scheduled Areas where as remaining 51 per cent lives outside. Some of them are covered by what is termed as "Outside Tribal Sub-Plan (OTSP)" programmes, but they do not enjoy the Constitutional safeguards meant for Scheduled Areas. In several places, an Integrated Tribal Development Project (ITDP) area is spread over different talukas, but not covering the entire district. The administration therein is divided between Revenue, Rural Development, Forest and the Tribal Development Departments. However, except for the TDD, the officers from other departments such as the Collector, CEO Zilla Parishad, BDO, Tahsildar, have to look after programes in the Scheduled Areas as well as the Non-Scheduled Areas. Hence, the governance in the districts is not tribal centric."

Governance Issues: PESA

"One of the major difficulties in Maharashtra PESA has been the inappropriate definition of a village and the village assembly (*Gram Sabha*). Instead of making the *Gram Sabha* of an individual hamlet (*wadi, pada, tola, pod, mohalla* or village) as the seat of decision making, the *Gramsabha* of a *Grampanchayat* (as per the Maharashtra Gram Panchayat Act, 1958) has been authorized. As it is known, the *Gram Panchayats* encompass several villages and hamlets and hence cannot become the true locale of self-governance."

Limitations of Tribal Sub-Plan and the Development Programmes

"Moreover, the TSP budget provision is, in principle, an additional provision to bring tribal people to the level of the rest of the population. Hence, other services or expenses which should be uniformly spread over the entire state should not be spent from the TSP. The TSP budget is often used as substitution and not as additionality to the general budget" (pp. 219-220).

Anthropology as a an academic discipline is people-centric. The basic agenda of anthropology has been to understand people and their lives through their perspectives, their eyes, specs, lens, as expressed with different terms having the same meaning. This is achieved by living with the people, ideally for one year, since an year is the unit of life, which repeats itself, what is referred to as "going native". If anthropologists have to study the totality, the whole, of contemporary processes of change, one would have to understand the government sector also and the ground level reality of interaction between the people' sector and the government sector. .

This book has documented the processes going beyond the academic agenda of study at the micro-level and understanding of emic perspectives. We have planned and implemented the interventions to address the issues of malnutrition. We have learnt that this new role would help to develop the knowledge discipline to evolve into a professional discipline.

The academic issue of research and objectivity in Anthropology pertains to the role of Anthropologists in planning and implementing the interventions. This debate probably is a hang-over of colonial times. So-called value neutrality tacitly becomes pro-establishment. If the establishment is anti-people, or lack the capacity and sensitivity to address the concerns of the people, which are guaranteed by the Constitution, and accepted internationally as human rights, anthropologists have to face the danger of being branded as colonial anthropologists and get marginalised by economists in national reconstruction. Anthropology as a discipline studying Mankind and Man as an inseparable part of nature, with other living beings, has to do advocacy in support of basic values of Man.

In terms of developing knowledge for its own sake, the experience gained by "going native" by living with the people to understand the emic perspectives, has to be fortified with experience of initiating the process of change. The Western anthropologists were called upon to advise the respective imperial powers during Second World War. Whose interest were they serving?

These are areas of academic debates. This book primarily documents the processes and outcomes of interventions to develop a sustainable model of human development.

The then Hon. President of India, Sri Pranab Mukherjee while inaugurating the golden jubilee celebrations of the Tribal Research and Training Institute, Pune on 28.12.2013 has referred to the objective of integration of tribal communities in India as under:

> "I would like to say that there is much to learn and appreciate from the tribal societies. At a time when the entire country is gripped by concerns about women's safety and security as well as by moral challenges, a peek into gender behaviour and relations in tribal communities hold significant lessons for the society at large. As much as we ought to learn from tribal people, we have a duty to empower plural tribal streams and contribute to that guiding spirit of our Constitution: "We, The People of India"."

References

Adiseshiah, Malcolm, 1973, Review Committee of the Indian Council of Social Science Research, ICSSR, New Delhi.

Bhanage, N.P., 1993, *Tribal Commissions and Committees in India*, Himalaya Publishing House, Bombay.

Biraj Swain and Sethi, Vani, 2014, *Mind the Gap*, in *Seminar—The Malnourished Tribal*, No. 661, New Delhi.

Dubos, Rene, 1965, *Man Adapting*, Yale University Press, New Haven.

Dreze, Jean, 2002, *On Research and Action* in *Economic and Political Weekly*, Mumbai, pp. 817-819.

Gopalan, C., 1989, *Nutritive Value of Indian Foods*, National Institute of Nutrition (ICMR).

Government of India, Ministry of Tribal Affairs, 2014, *Report of the High Level Committee on Socio-Economic, Health and Educational Status of Tribal Communities of India*, New Delhi.

Government of Maharashtra, 2002, *Maharashtra Human Development Report*, Mumbai.

Government of Maharashtra, 2012, *Maharashtra Human Development Report*, Sage Publications, New Delhi.

Government of Maharashtra, Planning Department, 2013, *High Level Committee on Balanced Regional Development Issues in Maharashtra (Kelkar Committee)*, Mumbai.

Herskovits, Melville, 1948, *Man and His Works*, Alfred A. Knopf, New York.

ICSSR, 1972, *A Survey of Research in Sociology and Social Anthropology*, Vol. III, New Delhi.

ICSSR, 1973, *A Report on Social Sciences in India : Retrospective and Prospective*, Vol. II, New Delhi.

Kluckhohn, Clyde, 1985, *Mirror for Man*, University of Arizona Press.

Kulkarni, Sumati, 1990, "Demographic Aspects of Poverty", in Tarlok Singh (ed.), *Social Science Research and Problem of Poverty*, Concept Publishing Co., New Delhi.

McElroy, Ann and Townsend, Patricia K., 1985, *Medical Anthropology in Ecological Perspective*, Westview Press.

Mander, Harsh, 2014, *Unequal destinies*, in *Seminar – The Malnourished Tribal*, No. 661, New Delhi.

Montagu, Ashley, 1985, Foreword to *Mirror for Man* by Kluckhohn, Clyde, University of Arizona Press.

Mead, Margaret (ed.), 1955, *Cultural Patterns and Technical Change*, UNESCO, The New American Library, New York.

Mukhopadhyay, Kanchan, 2011, "Anthropology of Food in India: The Scope and the Prospect", in *Journal of the Indian Anthropological Society*, Volume 46-2,3, Kolkata.

Mutatkar, R.K., 1981, *Social and Economic Aspects of Leprosy*, WHO, Geneva.

Mutatkar, R.K., 2004, *Nandurbar Report on Health and Education*, IGIDR, Mumbai.

Mutatkar, R.K., 2016, *AYUSH in Public Health*, Vols. I and II, Concept Publishing Co. Pvt. Ltd., New Delhi.

Mutatkar, Kalpana, 2013, Practicing Medical Anthropology: Addressing Malnutrition among Tribal Children, in Bhat, *et al.* (ed.) *Explorations in Indian Medical Anthropology*, Vol. II, Concept Publishing Co. Pvt. Ltd., New Delhi.

Mutatkar, Rohit, 2012, *Background Paper for MHDR 2012*, Sage Publications, New Delhi.

Pangariya, Arvind, 2012, *The Myth of Child Malnutrition in India*, IIPS, Mumbai.

Pandit, C.G., 1982, *My World of Preventive Medicine*, ICMR, New Delhi.

Roy Burman, B.K., 1990, "Development and Poverty among the Tribals", in Tarlok Singh (ed.), *Social Science Research and Problem of Poverty*, Concept Publishing Co., New Delhi.

Saxena, N.C., 2014, *Children of a lesser god*, in *Seminar – The Malnourished Tribal*, No. 661, New Delhi.

Sethi, Vani, 2014, *The Problem* in, Seminar – *The Malnourished Tribal*, No. 661, New Delhi,.

Sukhatme, P.V., 1982, *Newer Concepts in Nutrition and their Implications for Policy*, Maharashtra Association for the Cultivation of Science, (MACS), Pune.

Sukhatme, P.V., 1990, "Relationship between Poverty and Malnutrition" in Tarlok Singh (ed.), *Social Science Research and Problem of Poverty*, Concept Publishing Co., New Delhi.

Tata Institute of Social Sciences, 2015, *Tribal Sub-plan in Maharashtra: A Diagnostic Study*, Mumbai.

Tata Institute of Social Sciences, 2015, *A Tribal Atlas for Maharashtra*, Mumbai.

Tarlok Singh (ed.), 1990, *Social Science Research and Problem of Poverty*, Concept Publishing Co., New Delhi.

Uma Datta Roy Choudhury, *et al.*, 1990, "Central Statistical Organization: Poverty Concept and Measurement" in Tarlok Singh (ed.), *Social Science Research and Problem of Poverty*, Concept Publishing Co, New Delhi.

Valiathan, M.S., 2003, *The Legacy of Caraka* (Charak), Orient Longmans, Chennai.

Vogel, Virgil J., 1970, *American Indian Medicine*, University of Oklahoma Press.

Index